Textbook of
PSYCHIATRY

Textbook of
PSYCHIATRY

As per the Competency-based Medical Education Curriculum (NMC)

Praveen Tripathi MBBS MD
Consultant Psychiatrist
Renowa Care
Noida, Uttar Pradesh, India
and
New Delhi, India

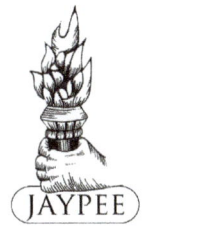

JAYPEE BROTHERS MEDICAL PUBLISHERS
The Health Sciences Publisher
New Delhi | London

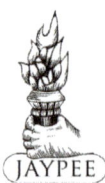 **Jaypee Brothers Medical Publishers (P) Ltd**

Headquarters
EMCA House
23/23-B, Ansari Road, Daryaganj
New Delhi 110 002, India
Landline: +91-11-23272143, +91-11-23272703
+91-11-23282021, +91-11-23245672
E-mail: jaypee@jaypeebrothers.com

Corporate Office
Jaypee Brothers Medical Publishers (P) Ltd.
4838/24, Ansari Road, Daryaganj
New Delhi 110 002, India
Phone: +91-11-43574357
Fax: +91-11-43574314
E-mail: jaypee@jaypeebrothers.com

Overseas Office
JP Medical Ltd.
83, Victoria Street, London
SW1H 0HW (UK)
Phone: +44-20 3170 8910
Fax: +44(0)20 3008 6180
E-mail: info@jpmedpub.com

Website: www.jaypeebrothers.com
Website: www.jaypeedigital.com

© 2023, Jaypee Brothers Medical Publishers

The views and opinions expressed in this book are solely those of the original contributor(s)/author(s) and do not necessarily represent those of editor(s) or publisher of the book.

All rights reserved. No part of this publication may be reproduced, stored or transmitted in any form or by any means, electronic, mechanical, photocopying, recording or otherwise, without the prior permission in writing of the publishers.

All brand names and product names used in this book are trade names, service marks, trademarks or registered trademarks of their respective owners. The publisher is not associated with any product or vendor mentioned in this book.

Medical knowledge and practice change constantly. This book is designed to provide accurate, authoritative information about the subject matter in question. However, readers are advised to check the most current information available on procedures included and check information from the manufacturer of each product to be administered, to verify the recommended dose, formula, method and duration of administration, adverse effects and contraindications. It is the responsibility of the practitioner to take all appropriate safety precautions. Neither the publisher nor the author(s)/editor(s) assume any liability for any injury and/or damage to persons or property arising from or related to use of material in this book.

This book is sold on the understanding that the publisher is not engaged in providing professional medical services. If such advice or services are required, the services of a competent medical professional should be sought.

Every effort has been made where necessary to contact holders of copyright to obtain permission to reproduce copyright material. If any have been inadvertently overlooked, the publisher will be pleased to make the necessary arrangements at the first opportunity.

Inquiries for bulk sales may be solicited at: jaypee@jaypeebrothers.com

*Textbook of Psychiatry / **Praveen Tripathi***

First Edition: **2023**

ISBN: 978-93-5696-169-2

Dedicated to

My Parents

CONTRIBUTORS

Anweshan Ghosh
Senior Resident
Institute of Psychiatry
Kolkata, West Bengal, India

Hiral Kotadia
Associate Professor
Department of Psychiatry
Sri Aurobindo Medical College and Post Graduate Institute
Indore, Madhya Pradesh, India

Meha Jain
Child Psychologist
Department of Paediatrics
All India Institute of Medical Sciences
Patna, Bihar, India

Padma Angmo
Consultant
Department of Psychiatry
Sonam Norboo Memorial Hospital
Leh, Ladakh, India

Priyanka Goyal
Consultant Psychiatrist
Renowa Care
Noida, Uttar Pradesh, India

Snehanky Chattopadhyay
Consultant, Clinical Psychology
Renowa Care
Noida, Uttar Pradesh, India

Sujita Kumar Kar
Additional Professor
Department of Psychiatry
King George's Medical University
Lucknow, Uttar Pradesh, India

Swayam Prava Baral
Assistant Professor
Department of Psychiatry
Sri Jagannath Medical College and Hospital
Puri, Odisha, India

Vijay Niranjan
Assistant Professor
Department of Psychiatry
Mahatma Gandhi Memorial Medical College
Indore, Madhya Pradesh, India

Vivek Attri
Junior Resident
All India Institute of Medical Sciences
Kalyani, West Bengal, India

PREFACE

Psychiatry is one of the most exciting subjects in medical sciences. The human brain, its structure, it's functioning, its disorders, everything about it is fascinating.

Despite this, unfortunately, many students fail to develop a connection with the subject of psychiatry. I believe there are two reasons for the same:

1. Our psychiatry books are difficult to understand for an undergraduate as they are full of terms alien to an average student.
2. Clinical exposure in psychiatry is limited, as most students don't go to psychiatry postings.

This issue could be solved if a textbook is written, keeping an undergraduate student in mind, with the use of simpler language and lots of clinical examples to explain the concepts. And this book has been written keeping exactly these goals in mind. My experience of writing 'Review of Psychiatry' book and the feedback that the book got also came in handy while deciding the content of this textbook. Having taught lakhs of students for PG medical entrance preparation has kept me aware of the changing pattern of questions in these exams. While writing content, I have tried to balance conceptual learning and the relevance for various entrance examinations.

Writing this textbook was perhaps one of the toughest things that I have accomplished in my life. In today's world, where instant gratification has become a rule, and most of us are more comfortable recording a video and seeing the response to it immediately, writing a textbook, reading and revising the content and putting years of work into it was not easy.

It took more than 3 years to finish the first draft and then 6 months more to write the final draft of this book. In the last 6 months, during which the book's content was finalised, my life revolved around this textbook, and it was pretty stressful, but today, when I am writing this preface, all those efforts appear to be so worth it. I feel immense satisfaction as this book has turned out to be exactly how I had envisioned.

I have included the recent advances in psychiatry, especially in biological psychiatry, in the content; at the same time, I have included certain topics such as psychoanalysis which may not be so relevant in today's clinical practice but have a remarkable historical significance.

In the end, I want to say that a lot of honest efforts has gone into the writing of this book. Not only I but all the co-authors have tried their best to provide a textbook that meets the requirements of the students, and we are very hopeful that students will get massively benefitted from this book.

January, 2023

Dr Praveen Tripathi MBBS MD
Instagram: @drpraveentripathiacad
Twitter: @drpraveenpsy

ACKNOWLEDGEMENTS

There is an old saying, 'It takes a village to raise a child'; this saying is apt for a book too. Many individuals have contributed to the completion of this book. Perhaps, the most important being my patients. For any doctor, patients are the most important teacher. Listening to their experiences enriches our clinical knowledge, and that clinical knowledge is what we pen down when we write a book on a clinical subject. I am eternally grateful to my patients for sharing their lives with me, and I hope that I could provide them with some support in their struggles.

I am always thankful to my parents, who have steadfastly supported me in all I do. I am grateful to my wife, Dr Priyanka Goyal, who takes care of our clinical work and often has to put in double the effort as I get occupied with academic work. This, I feel, is a blessing in disguise for our patients, as she is a better psychiatrist than me. Without her stepping up, finishing the book would have been impossible.

It goes without saying that the co-authors of the chapters were instrumental in completing this book. Not only they did a great job, but they also tolerated my repeated requests to make changes to the manuscript. A big thanks to all of them, Dr Sujita Kumar Kar, Dr Hiral Kotadia, Dr Priyanka Goyal, Dr Vijay Niranjan, Dr Anweshan Ghosh, Dr Swayam Prava Baral, Dr Padma Angmo, Ms Meha Jain and Ms Snehanky Chattopadhyay.

A special note of thanks to Dr Vivek Attri, who helped with the proofreading and editing of the content. He pointed out some crucial mistakes and made important additions to the content. His dedication towards psychiatry is inspirational for everyone around him, including me. Thanks, Dr Vivek, for being there.

I also want to thank Dr Abhishek Pratap Singh, my senior from IHBAS (Institute of Human Behaviour and Allied Sciences), New Delhi, India and one of the best psychiatrists I have ever met, for what he has taught me. Even today, whenever I need a suggestion regarding a difficult case, I reach out to him, and somehow, he always has an answer. Thank you, Sir!

I am thankful to the entire production and publishing teams at Jaypee Brothers Medical Publishers (P) Ltd, New Delhi, India for their continuous support. I would like to express my debts of gratitude to Shri Jitender P Vij (Group Chairman), Mr Ankit Vij (Managing Director), Mr MS Mani (Group President), and a special thank to Ms Chetna Malhotra (Senior Director – Professional Publishing, Marketing and Business Development) for always being there to listen the issues and solve them. Dr Madhu Choudhary (Director – Educational Publishing) and Dr Aditya Tayal (Team Lead – UG Publishing) have been crucial for the completion of the work, and I thank them for staying patient even during times when my work became irregular.

And in the end, I want to thank my beloved students. I feel indebted towards them; they have always been there, accepting my work, recognising my work and staying open to my teaching and writing style. A teacher is nothing without his students, and I always keep that in mind.

Dr Praveen Tripathi
January, 2023

CONTENTS

CHAPTER 1: **Basics of Psychiatry** 1
Praveen Tripathi, Priyanka Goyal

CHAPTER 2: **Schizophrenia and Other Primary Psychotic Disorders** 11
Praveen Tripathi, Priyanka Goyal

CHAPTER 3: **Mood Disorders (Depressive Disorders)** 28
Praveen Tripathi, Priyanka Goyal

CHAPTER 4: **Mood Disorders (Bipolar and Related Disorders)** 40
Praveen Tripathi, Priyanka Goyal

CHAPTER 5: **Anxiety or Fear-related Disorders** 50
Praveen Tripathi, Priyanka Goyal

CHAPTER 6: **Obsessive-compulsive and Related Disorders** 58
Praveen Tripathi, Priyanka Goyal

CHAPTER 7: **Impulse Control Disorders** 64
Praveen Tripathi, Priyanka Goyal

CHAPTER 8: **Disorders Specifically Associated with Stress** 66
Sujita Kumar Kar, Praveen Tripathi

CHAPTER 9: **Somatic Symptoms and Related Disorders** 72
Vijay Niranjan, Swayam Prava Baral, Praveen Tripathi

CHAPTER 10: **Dissociative Disorders** 80
Vijay Niranjan, Swayam Prava Baral, Praveen Tripathi

CHAPTER 11: **Substance Related and Addictive Disorders** 83
Praveen Tripathi, Anweshan Ghosh

CHAPTER 12: **Neurocognitive Disorders** 97
Sujita Kumar Kar, Praveen Tripathi

CHAPTER 13: **Personality Disorders** 109
Padma Angmo, Praveen Tripathi

CHAPTER 14: Eating Disorders — 117
Praveen Tripathi, Priyanka Goyal

CHAPTER 15: Sleep Disorders — 122
Praveen Tripathi, Vijay Niranjan

CHAPTER 16: Sexual Disorders — 130
Sujita Kumar Kar, Praveen Tripathi

CHAPTER 17: Child Psychiatry — 139
Hiral Kotadia, Praveen Tripathi

CHAPTER 18: Psychoanalysis — 150
Praveen Tripathi, Priyanka Goyal

CHAPTER 19: Other Somatic Therapies — 156
Praveen Tripathi, Priyanka Goyal

CHAPTER 20: Psychological Theories and Interventions — 160
Meha Jain, Snehanky Chattopadhyay, Sujita Kumar Kar, Praveen Tripathi

CHAPTER 21: Forensic Psychiatry — 167
Vijay Niranjan, Praveen Tripathi

CHAPTER 22: Community Psychiatry — 172
Sujita Kumar Kar

Index — 175

COMPETENCY TABLE

Number	COMPETENCY The student should be able to	Core (Y/N)	Chapter number	Page numbers
PS1.1	Establish rapport and empathy with patients	Y	1	1–10
PS1.2	Describe the components of communication	Y		
PS3.3	Elicit, present and document a history in patients presenting with a mental disorder	Y		
PS3.4	Describe the importance of establishing rapport with patients	Y		
PS3.5	Perform, demonstrate and document a mini-mental examination	Y		
PS3.6	Describe and discuss biological, psychological and social factors and their interactions in the causation of mental disorders	Y		
PS3.12	Describe, discuss and distinguish psychotic and non-psychotic (mood, anxiety, stress related) disorders	Y		
PS4.1	Describe the magnitude and aetiology of alcohol and substance use disorders	Y	11	83–96
PS4.2	Elicit, describe and document clinical features of alcohol and substance use disorders	Y		
PS4.3	Enumerate and describe the indications and interpret laboratory and other tests used in alcohol and substance abuse disorders	Y		
PS4.4	Describe the treatment of alcohol and substance abuse disorders including behavioural and pharmacologic therapy	Y		
PS4.5	Demonstrate family education in a patient with alcohol and substance abuse in a simulated environment	Y		
PS4.6	Enumerate and describe the pharmacologic basis and side effects of drugs used in alcohol and substance abuse	Y		
PS4.7	Enumerate the appropriate conditions for specialist referral in patients with alcohol and substance abuse disorders	Y		
PS5.1	Classify and describe the magnitude and aetiology of schizophrenia and other psychotic disorders	Y	2	11–27
PS5.2	Enumerate, elicit, describe and document clinical features, positives	Y		
PS5.3	Describe the treatment of schizophrenia including behavioural and pharmacologic therapy	Y		
PS5.4	Demonstrate family education in a patient with schizophrenia in a simulated environment	Y		
PS5.5	Enumerate and describe the pharmacologic basis and side effects of drugs used in schizophrenia	Y		
PS5.6	Enumerate the appropriate conditions for specialist referral in patients with psychotic disorders	Y		

Competency Table

Number	COMPETENCY The student should be able to	Core (Y/N)	Chapter number	Page numbers
PS6.1	Classify and describe the magnitude and aetiology of depression	Y	3	28–39
PS6.2	Enumerate, elicit, describe and document clinical features in patients with depression	Y		
PS6.3	Enumerate and describe the indications and interpret laboratory and other tests used in depression	Y		
PS6.4	Describe the treatment of depression including behavioural and pharmacologic therapy	Y		
PS6.5	Demonstrate family education in a patient with depression in a simulated environment	Y		
PS6.6	Enumerate and describe the pharmacologic basis and side effects of drugs used in depression	Y		
PS6.7	Enumerate the appropriate conditions for specialist referral in patients with depression	Y		
PS7.1	Classify and describe the magnitude and aetiology of bipolar disorders	Y	4	40–49
PS7.2	Enumerate, elicit, describe and document clinical features in patients with bipolar disorders	Y		
PS7.3	Enumerate and describe the indications and interpret laboratory and other tests used in bipolar disorders	Y		
PS7.4	Describe the treatment of bipolar disorders including behavioural and pharmacologic therapy	Y		
PS7.5	Demonstrate family education in a patient with bipolar disorders in a simulated environment	Y		
PS7.6	Enumerate and describe the pharmacologic basis and side effects of drugs used in bipolar disorders	Y		
PS7.7	Enumerate the appropriate conditions for specialist referral in patients with bipolar disorders	Y		
PS8.1	Enumerate and describe the magnitude and aetiology of anxiety disorders	Y	5	50–57
PS8.2	Enumerate, elicit, describe and document clinical features in patients with anxiety disorders	Y		
PS8.3	Enumerate and describe the indications and interpret laboratory and other tests used in anxiety disorders	Y		
PS8.4	Describe the treatment of anxiety disorders including behavioural and pharmacologic therapy	Y		
PS8.5	Demonstrate family education in a patient with anxiety disorders in a simulated environment	Y		
PS8.6	Enumerate and describe the pharmacologic basis and side effects of drugs used in anxiety disorders	Y		
PS8.7	Enumerate the appropriate conditions for specialist referral in anxiety disorders	Y		

Number	COMPETENCY The student should be able to	Core (Y/N)	Chapter number	Page numbers
PS9.1	Enumerate and describe the magnitude and aetiology of stress related disorders	Y	8	66–71
PS9.2	Enumerate, elicit, describe and document clinical features in patients with stress related disorders	Y		
PS9.3	Enumerate and describe the indications and interpret laboratory and other tests used in stress related disorders	Y		
PS9.4	Describe the treatment of stress related disorders including behavioural and psychosocial therapy	Y		
PS9.5	Demonstrate family education in a patient with stress related disorders in a simulated environment	Y		
PS9.6	Enumerate and describe the pharmacologic basis and side effects of drugs used in stress related disorders	Y		
PS9.7	Enumerate the appropriate conditions for specialist referral in stress disorders	Y		
PS10.1	Enumerate and describe the magnitude and aetiology of somatoform, dissociative and conversion disorders	Y	9 10	72–79 80–82
PS10.2	Enumerate, elicit, describe and document clinical features in patients with somatoform, dissociative and conversion disorders	Y		
PS10.3	Enumerate and describe the indications and interpret laboratory and other tests used in somatoform, dissociative and conversion disorders	Y		
PS10.4	Describe the treatment of somatoform disorders including behavioural, psychosocial and pharmacologic therapy	Y		
PS10.5	Demonstrate family education in a patient with somatoform, dissociative and conversion disorders in a simulated environment	Y		
PS10.6	Enumerate and describe the pharmacologic basis and side effects of drugs used in somatoform, dissociative and conversion disorders	Y		
PS10.7	Enumerate the appropriate conditions for specialist referral in patients with somatoform dissociative and conversion disorders	Y		
PS11.1	Enumerate and describe the magnitude and aetiology of personality disorders	Y	13	109–116
PS11.2	Enumerate, elicit, describe and document clinical features in patients with personality disorders	Y		
PS11.3	Enumerate and describe the indications and interpret laboratory and other tests used in personality disorders	Y		
PS11.4	Describe the treatment of personality disorders including behavioural, psychosocial and pharmacologic therapy	Y		
PS11.5	Demonstrate family education in a patient with personality disorders in a simulated environment	Y		
PS11.6	Enumerate and describe the pharmacologic basis and side effects of drugs used in personality disorders	Y		
PS11.7	Enumerate the appropriate conditions for specialist referral	Y		

Competency Table

Number	COMPETENCY – The student should be able to	Core (Y/N)	Chapter number	Page numbers
PS13.1	Enumerate and describe the magnitude and aetiology of psychosexual and gender identity disorders	Y	16	130–138
PS13.2	Enumerate, elicit, describe and document clinical features in patients with magnitude and aetiology of psychosexual and gender identity disorders	Y		
PS13.3	Enumerate and describe the indications and interpret laboratory and other tests used in psychosexual and gender identity disorders	Y		
PS13.4	Describe the treatment of psychosexual and gender identity disorders including behavioural, psychosocial and pharmacologic therapy	Y		
PS13.5	Demonstrate family education in a patient with psychosexual and gender identity disorders in a simulated environment	Y		
PS13.6	Enumerate and describe the pharmacologic basis and side effects of drugs used in psychosexual and gender identity disorders	Y		
PS13.7	Enumerate the appropriate conditions for specialist referral	Y		
PS14.1	Enumerate and describe the magnitude and aetiology of psychiatric disorders occurring in childhood and adolescence	Y	17	139–149
PS14.2	Enumerate, elicit, describe and document clinical features in patients with psychiatric disorders occurring in childhood and adolescence	Y		
PS14.3	Describe the treatment of stress related disorders including behavioural, psychosocial and pharmacologic therapy	Y		
PS14.4	Demonstrate family education in a patient with psychiatric disorders occurring in childhood and adolescence in a simulated environment	Y		
PS14.5	Enumerate and describe the pharmacologic basis and side effects of drugs used in psychiatric disorders occurring in childhood and adolescence	Y		
PS14.6	Enumerate the appropriate conditions for specialist referral in children and adolescents with psychiatric disorders	Y		
PS18.2	Enumerate the indications for modified electroconvulsive therapy	Y	19	156–159
PS18.3	Enumerate and describe the principles and role of psychosocial interventions in psychiatric illness including psychotherapy, behavioral therapy and rehabilitation	Y		
PS19.1	Describe the relevance, role and status of community psychiatry	Y	22	172–174
PS19.2	Describe the objectives strategies and contents of the National Mental Health Programme	Y		
PS19.3	Describe and discuss the basic legal and ethical issues in psychiatry	Y		

1. Basics of Psychiatry

Praveen Tripathi, Priyanka Goyal

PS1.1	Establish rapport and empathy with patients
PS1.2	Describe the components of communication
PS3.3	Elicit, present and document a history in patients presenting with a mental disorder
PS3.4	Describe the importance of establishing rapport with patients
PS3.5	Perform, demonstrate and document a mini-mental examination
PS3.6	Describe and discuss biological, psychological and social factors and their interactions in the causation of mental disorders
PS3.12	Describe, discuss and distinguish psychotic and non-psychotic (mood, anxiety, stress related) disorders

INTRODUCTION

The branch of medicine that deals with the morbid psychological processes is called **Psychiatry**. The term 'Psychiatry' was coined by a German physician, Johann Christian Reil.

Psychiatry is quite similar to the other branches of medicine and follows the same scientific principles for diagnosis and treatment. As of now, in Psychiatry, detailed history taking and clinical examination are the backbone of the diagnostic process, and investigations play a limited role. However, as knowledge about the development of psychiatric disorders improves and structural and functional neuroimaging techniques become more refined, it can be envisaged that such neuroimaging techniques will be used as diagnostic tools in the future.

A good clinical interview is a prerequisite for detailed history taking. Let's understand the process of interviewing a patient with a psychiatric illness.

PSYCHIATRIC INTERVIEW

A comprehensive interview with the patient is the most important tool available to the doctor. A good psychiatric interview serves two purposes:
1. It helps collect information, which in turn helps reach the diagnosis according to specific standard criteria.
2. It helps establish a sound **patient–doctor relationship** that in itself has a therapeutic effect (i.e., it helps in the treatment).

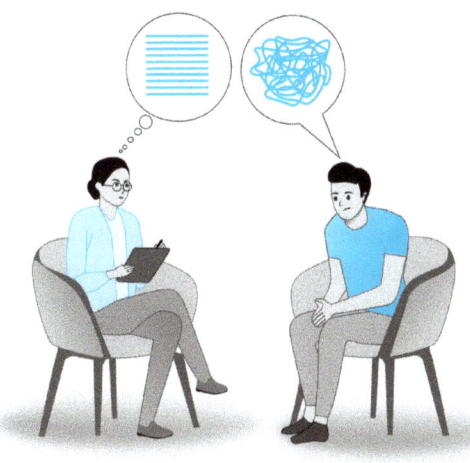

Fig. 1.1: A psychiatric interview.

The following principles are followed while conducting a psychiatric interview:
- **Introduction and consent:** At the onset, the psychiatrist should introduce himself and explain the purpose of the interview. If the patient has not taken the appointment himself and has been referred by some agency (e.g., court), that should be clearly conveyed. The psychiatrist should start the interview only after taking consent from the patient.
- **Privacy and confidentiality:** The importance of privacy and confidentiality while interviewing a patient with a psychiatric disorder cannot be overemphasised.

The interview should be held in a comfortable place where patients' privacy is ensured. Often, patients are hesitant to discuss personal issues, and assurance about confidentiality can be beneficial. A psychiatrist should not disclose any information obtained during the interview without permission from the patient. Any exceptions to this rule (e.g., in case of a court seeking information) should be clearly informed to the patient.

- **Empathy:** Empathy is a valuable tool that must be used while conducting a psychiatric interview. Empathy involves understanding the thinking and behaviour of the patient by putting oneself in the patient's shoes. It involves the psychiatrist asking himself, 'If I were in the place of this patient, what would I experience' and using the answer to understand the patient's experiences. Empathy is different from '**sympathy**'; sympathy is keeping a considerate view of another person's hardship.
- **Patient–doctor relationship:** The relationship between patient and doctor plays a vital role in the treatment process. The term used earlier, "doctor-patient relationship", has now been replaced with "patient-doctor relationship" to emphasize that it is the patient towards whom treatment is centred (patient-centred). While interacting with the patient, a doctor must make him feel safe and comfortable. Patients' problems must be understood carefully. The patient should feel that the doctor is genuinely interested in him and cares for him. Throughout the interview, the doctor should maintain a nonjudgmental attitude, reflected in his verbal and non-verbal responses. All these measures help develop rapport between the patient and the doctor. **Rapport** is defined as a 'close and harmonious relationship between the patient and the doctor.'
- **Safety and comfort:** The patient should feel safe and comfortable during the interview. It is advised that both patient and doctor be seated in chairs of similar heights so that no one towers over the other and the patient feels a sense of friendliness and comfort. A distance of around 4-6 feet between patient and psychiatrist is recommended. Patients, especially those with psychosis and those who may be feeling threatened, must be reassured that they are safe and sufficient staff is available to ensure the same. Similarly, the doctor's safety must also be ensured. The doctor should terminate the interview immediately if he feels that the patient is becoming aggressive. An exit door for the doctor should be available to leave the interview room without passing across the patient.
- **Open-ended and closed-ended questions:** At the beginning of the interview, it is preferable to ask open-ended questions such as "what problems are you facing?". Later on, 'closed-ended questions' such as "do you feel more depressed in the morning or evening?" can be asked to find out the specific details.

HISTORY TAKING IN PSYCHIATRY

Following the principles mentioned above, a comprehensive interview should be done, and the information received should be organised under the following heads.

Identifying Data

The basic information about the patient that includes name, age, sex, residence, education, occupation, marital status, religion, socioeconomic status, type of family, and domicile (rural/urban) should be noted. If any medicolegal case is ongoing, that too should be noted.

Informants

The individuals providing information about the patient and the illness are called 'informants'. Details of informants should be duly noted. The patient should always be one of the informants unless entirely uncooperative or unable to provide the information. A comment on the **reliability** of informants should be made.

An informant is considered reliable if the following five parameters (5 C's) are fulfilled:

1. **Consistency:** If the informant provides the same information across the interviews, he is considered to be consistent. A consistent informant will provide the same history, whether the consultant or a medical student is taking the interview.
2. **Coherence:** Coherence is assessed depending on whether the different pieces of information provided by the informant are logically connected or not.
3. **Chronological information:** The informant should be able to provide the information in a chronological sequence. For example, if the patient has been symptomatic for a year, the informant should be able to answer questions like 'How did the illness start?', 'What were the initial symptoms?' 'How each symptom progressed over time', etc.
4. **Closeness with the patient:** It should be assessed whether the informant is close enough to the patient to have an accurate account of information. For example, if the informant lives in a different city and communicates with the patient once a month, irrespective of the relationship with the patient, he cannot be considered a 'close' informant.
5. **Concern with the patient:** It should be assessed whether the informant is genuinely concerned with the patient and if there is a possibility of '**malafide intention**' (dishonest intention). For example, if the informant is in a legal dispute with the patient, the informant's intentions should be evaluated carefully before accepting the information provided.

Along with assessing the reliability of the informant, an assessment of the '**adequacy**' of information provided should also be done. If the information provided is enough to reach a diagnosis, it is considered 'adequate'.

Presenting Complaints/Chief Complaints

Presenting complaints are the complaints for which the patient/informant has sought help. The patient's version (e.g., my family member wants to kill me) and the informant's version (e.g., the patient is suspicious of the family members) may be different. Both must be recorded in patient's/informant's own words. All the complaints should be recorded in chronological order.

The term '**chief complaints**' is sometimes used as a synonym for "presenting complaints"; however, strictly speaking, chief complaints are the complaints that the physician finds to be most important for the case formulation after hearing the narratives of the patient and the informants.

Additional points must be noted after describing the chief complaints.

These include:
1. **Onset of illness:** The onset of illness is defined based on the time duration in which the patient went from having 'no symptoms' to a state with a 'clear presence' of symptoms. The following are the types of onset:
   - **Abrupt onset** (in <2 days)
   - **Acute onset** (in <2 weeks)
   - **Subacute onset** (between 2 weeks to 3 months)
   - **Insidious onset** (>3 months)
2. **Duration:** The duration of each symptom should be mentioned separately
3. **Course of illness:** The 'course' describes whether the symptoms have been improving/deteriorating/are stable with time.
4. **Predisposing factors:** Any factor (e.g., family history) that makes it more likely for an individual to develop a psychiatric disorder should be mentioned.
5. **Precipitating factor:** Any factor (e.g., divorce resulting in the onset of a depressive episode) that resulted in the onset of illness should be mentioned.
6. **Perpetuating factor:** Any factor (e.g., poor relationship between the patient and the spouse) resulting in the continuation of symptoms should be mentioned.

History of Present Illness

This section provides a detailed description of the presenting/chief complaints chronologically. The evolution of symptoms throughout illness is described, and details about biological functions (sleep, appetite, and sexual functioning) are mentioned.

Past Psychiatric and Medical History

In this section, details about any past psychiatric disorders are recorded. Relevant information about past treatments, such as the use of psychotropics/admission to psychiatric facilities/use of alternative forms of medicine, is also recorded. History of any significant medical or surgical illness is also noted.

Treatment History

Details of treatment received (including medications, psychotherapy and other treatment modalities like electroconvulsive therapy) during the current illness/past illness are recorded. Along with the details of the types and dosages of medications used, other relevant points such as the side effects, treatment compliance (whether the treatment was taken as prescribed or not), and drug allergies are also noted.

Family History

Details about both '**family of origin**' (patients' parents, grandparents, and siblings) and '**family of procreation**' (patient's spouse, children, and grandchildren, as applicable) should be recorded. A '**family tree**' is usually drawn with details about three generations (patients' generation, patient's parent's generation, and patient's children's generation) and relevant information is added.

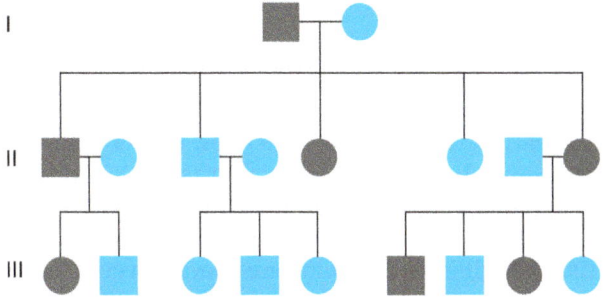

Following should be recorded in the family history:
- Type of family (nuclear, extended nuclear or joint)
- Details (name, age, relationship with patient) of the family members
- History of any psychiatric illness/relevant medical illness and, if available, treatment details
- History of substance abuse, suicides, missing persons in the family

Current social situation like socioeconomic status, per capita income, head of the family, and attitudes/beliefs of the family towards the patient's psychiatric illness should also be noted.

Personal History/Developmental History

Different parts of personal/developmental history will be relevant for different patients, and personal history must be individualised according to the case. It is important to take consent from the patient before exploring personal history as some topics, such as sexual history, may make the patient uncomfortable. Usually, it is recorded under the following headings.

Perinatal History

Records any relevant events in the prenatal, natal or postnatal period such as prenatal infections/drug use during pregnancy/complications during delivery, perinatal complications like jaundice, etc.

Childhood History

The history of developmental milestones is essential. In individual cases, relevant history, such as regarding breastfeeding and weaning, any history of maternal deprivation, toilet training, etc., may be important.

Educational History

Academic qualifications, performance during school and college, relationship with teachers and peers, any learning difficulties, etc., should be recorded.

Occupational History

Age at which work was started, number and types of jobs held, reasons for leaving the job, performance at the job and any difficulties with peers and officials should be recorded. Current job status and any stressors on the occupational front should be noted.

Sexual and Marital History

History about masturbation, sexual desire, sexual orientation, etc., may be relevant in individual cases. History about current sexual partners, safe sexual practices, and contraceptive methods may be required in certain cases. Marital history includes details about the age at marriage, arranged versus love marriage, overall relationship with spouse, and any marital difficulties. Not all points are relevant in every patient; the interviewer should use his judgement while taking sexual and marital history.

Menstrual History

In females, details like age at menarche, regularity and duration of menses, last menstrual period, any menstrual disturbances should be recorded.

Medicolegal History

In case of medicolegal issues, relevant details should be recorded.

Psychoactive Substance Abuse History

Details should be recorded about all the psychoactive substances that the patient has ever used. Details like age at initiation, amount used, route of intake, any history of craving/withdrawal symptoms/tolerance and social, occupational and personal impairment because of substance use must be duly noted.

Premorbid Personality

Here, the important personality traits of the patient before the onset of illness are noted. Certain kinds of personality traits are seen for years before the onset of psychiatric disorders. For example, a significant proportion of persons who develop schizophrenia have been quiet, introverted individuals with limited ability to express and feel emotions.

During the assessment of premorbid personality, information from guardians is taken about social relationships, predominant mood state, intellectual activities, interests, hobbies, interpersonal relationships, attitude towards work and responsibility, religious activities and fantasy life.

EXAMINATION

General Physical Examination and Systemic Examination

A detailed general physical and systemic examination should be carried out on all the patients. The format for the same can be referred to from any standard textbook of medicine.

Mental Status Examination

The clinical examination in psychiatry, wherein the clinician records the psychiatric signs and symptoms, is known as mental status examination (MSE). It can be considered the psychiatric equivalent of physical examination in medicine.

Following are the components of MSE.

General Appearance and Behaviour

The patient's appearance is described along with any gross abnormalities. In some cases, the general appearance may provide clues about the diagnosis. For example, a patient who enters the doctor's room wearing yellow pants, a pink shirt, blue glasses and starts dancing impromptu might be having symptoms of mania. Obviously, to make the diagnosis, the required criteria must be met. Still, the general appearance and behaviour may provide a clue. Hygiene and grooming of the patient are also noted. The patient's approach towards the interview is also described (i.e., cooperative/uncooperative/unconcerned).

Motor Activity

Motor activity during the interview may be described as normal, decreased (e.g., patients with depression may move slowly, called **decreased psychomotor activity**) or increased (e.g., patient in a manic state may keep on roaming around the room throughout the interview, called **increased psychomotor activity**). Any abnormal motor movements such as tremors should also be noted.

Speech

Various aspects of speech such as **rate** (the speed of speech), **tone**, **volume** (the number of words spoken), and the **spontaneity** of speech (whether the patient speaks on his own or not) are noted. Speech may give important clues about the diagnosis too. For example, a manic patient often has an increased rate and volume of speech.

Mood and Affect

Both the terms "affect" and "mood" are used to describe the emotions or emotional state.

'Mood' is the sustained (long-term) and internal emotional state that influences the way the world is perceived. For example, a person who has been feeling low internally for a long time and finds everything in his surroundings dull and boring would be described as having a 'depressed mood.'

'Affect' is the short-lived and external expression of internal emotions, that can be observed. For example, the person mentioned above during the interview avoided looking into the eyes of the examiner and started crying. His facial expression and crying would be interpreted as depressed 'affect'. It is the external expression of an underlying depressed mood.

The terms' affect and mood are at times used interchangeably.

Affect and mood are further described under the following three heads:

- **Quality:** It refers to the predominant emotional state. The quality of affect may vary from happiness, sadness to anger and anxiety. A few common abnormalities of the quality of affect/mood include:
  - *Euphoric mood (elevation of mood):* Euphoria refers to a state of excessive happiness without any apparent reason. It is usually seen in patients with mania or hypomania.
  - *Depressed mood:* Excessive sadness, usually seen in patients with depression.
- **Fluctuations:** It refers to changes in mood/affect. Usually, affect fluctuates in response to internal and external stimuli; however, abnormal fluctuations can be present in certain pathological states. The common disturbances or fluctuations include:
  - **Labile mood (emotional lability):** It is defined as excessive variations in the mood without any apparent reason. For example, a man suddenly started crying and the next moment started laughing without any apparent reason. The labile mood is usually seen in mania.
  - **Affective flattening:** In affective flattening, the emotional state does not change, irrespective of the situation. The patient does not experience any emotions in this condition, and his affect remains the same. For example, a patient with schizophrenia would not look happy during the festivals and did not appear sad when his mother died. His affect remained the same irrespective of the situation.
- **Appropriateness and congruency:** Appropriateness of affect is described in relation to the **social situation**. For example, at a funeral, the expected emotional state is sadness. Hence, being sad at a funeral is an 'appropriate affect'. If a man starts laughing and looks happy at a funeral, it would be diagnosed as 'inappropriate affect'.

Congruency of affect is described in relation to the **thought content**. Congruency describes whether the person's emotional state is in sync with his thought/speech. For example, if a man is thinking about or talking about the events which led to his mother's death, he is expected to be sad. Hence, appearing sad while talking about the mother's death is a congruent affect. If a person looks happy and smiles while describing his mother's death, it would be considered incongruent affect.

It must be stressed that while 'appropriateness' of affect is described after comparing the current affect with the expected affect in a given social situation, the 'congruence' is described after comparing the current affect with the expected affect in the context of the patient's thoughts.

Few other important disturbances of emotions include:
- **Alexithymia:** It is the inability to understand the emotions of others and the inability to express emotions of self. Although alexithymia is closely related to affective flattening, alexithymia is defined as a lack of words to describe emotions' rather than the absence of emotions.
- **Anhedonia:** It is an inability to experience pleasure in usually pleasurable activities. The patient may not enjoy activities like listening to music or playing a game, which was pleasurable in the past. Anhedonia can be present in patients with depression and schizophrenia.

NEUROANATOMICAL SUBSTRATE OF EMOTIONS

Limbic system (which includes the hippocampus, amygdala, hypothalamus, cingulate gyrus and related thalamic and cortical areas) is the neural substrate for the emotional experiences. The regulation of emotions is a function of the frontal lobe.

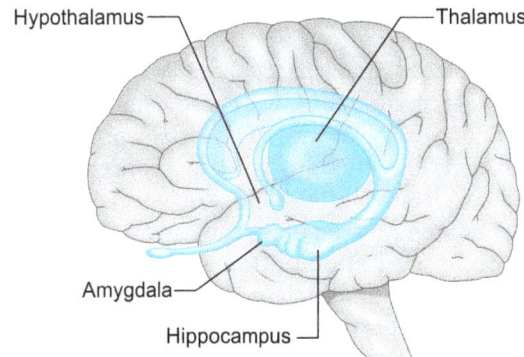

Fig. 1.2: The limbic system.

Perception

Perception is the process of recognition and interpretation of sensory information. The five basic perceptions include auditory, visual, tactile, olfactory, and gustatory. Perceptual disturbances are common in psychiatric disorders, and the two important disturbances of perception are:

Illusions: Illusion is defined as a 'false perception of a real object'. For example, a man mistakes a rope for a snake and gets frightened.

Hallucinations: Hallucination is defined as 'false perception in the absence of any object or stimulus'. For example, a patient with delirium reported seeing snakes on the ground of his room when there was nothing there in reality. Hallucinations have the following properties, and all these properties must be present to diagnose a perception as a hallucination:

- Hallucinations occur in the absence of any sensory or perceptual stimulus.
- Hallucinations are as vivid (clear or detailed) as true perceptions. This means that the person who experiences hallucinations can give a detailed description of what he is perceiving.
- Hallucinations are experienced in the outer objective space. This means that the patient experiences the source

of hallucinations to be in the outer world. For example, a patient with auditory hallucinations will report that the voices are coming from outside, such as from the wall or outside the house.

> **Pseudohallucinations** are experienced in the inner subjective space or originating from, within the mind. For example, a patient with auditory pseudohallucinations reported that the voices are originating from within his mind and not from outside.

- Hallucinations are not under the wilful control of the patient. This means that the patient can neither start the hallucinations nor can he stop them.

Hallucinations can occur in any modality. The **most common** type of hallucinations in psychiatric disorders are **auditory hallucinations**. The most common hallucinations in organic psychiatric disorders (such as delirium) are visual hallucinations. In patients with temporal lobe epilepsy, all kinds of hallucinations can be present, including olfactory and tactile hallucinations. Tactile hallucinations are a typical feature of cocaine intoxication.

Few specific hallucinations:
- **Hypnagogic hallucinations:** These hallucinations occur while falling asleep or while going to sleep. Since the term 'hypnagogic' has the word 'go' in it, it is easy to remember that they occur while "going" to sleep. Hypnagogic hallucinations are seen in narcolepsy.
- **Hypnopompic hallucinations:** These hallucinations occur while getting up from sleep. They are also often present in patients with narcolepsy.
- **Reflex hallucinations (synesthesia):** In reflex hallucinations, stimulus in one sensory modality results in hallucinations in another sensory modality. For example, a patient reported that whenever he sees a white bulb (i.e., stimulus in visual modality), he starts hearing voices of god (hallucinations in auditory modality). Reflex hallucinations are a feature of cannabis and lysergic acid diethylamide (and other hallucinogens) intoxication.
- **Functional hallucinations:** In functional hallucinations, stimulus in one sensory modality produces hallucinations in the same sensory modality. For example, a patient reported that whenever he heard the sound of a ticking clock (stimulus in auditory modality), he would also start hearing voices of god (hallucinations in auditory modality).

Thought (Cognition)

The terms "thought" and "cognition" are at times used interchangeably; however, in a stricter sense, cognition is the mental process of acquiring knowledge which includes thoughts but also experiences and sensations. The thought disturbances are primary in many psychiatric disorders such as schizophrenia.

Thought and its disturbances can be described under the following headings:

Disorders of the Stream of thought (or flow of thought): These can be further subdivided into—

Disorders of thought tempo: Thought tempo basically refers to the speed with which thoughts appear in mind. The disturbances of thought tempo include—
- **Flight of ideas:** Here, the thoughts follow each other rapidly, and the connection between successive thoughts appears to be due to chance factors such as rhyming. It is usually seen in patients with **mania**. For example, on being asked about his hometown, a patient with mania responded, "I live in Delhi…my cat has a big belly…I like to eat Jelly…Lilly Lilly Lilly".
- **Inhibition or slowing of thinking:** Here, thoughts come to mind very slowly, and the thought progression is slow. This is usually seen in patients with **depression**.
- **Circumstantiality:** In circumstantiality, the thinking progresses slowly with the inclusion of unnecessary details and goes round and round before **reaching the final goal**. For example, a medical student was asked about his preferred branch in postgraduation, and he replied, "Sir, in the first year, I was very interested in physiology; however, in the second year, I started liking pathology. In the third year, ophthalmology was my favourite subject. However, in the final year, I realised that I have a lot of passion for orthopaedics, and I like putting casts and working with POP. I also think that after MBBS, one should get married as soon as possible and that no one should have more than two kids…Well, you see, I like pediatrics as a subject and want to do my postgraduation in pediatrics". In this example, the thought process progressed with the inclusion of lots of irrelevant details; however, in the end, the goal was reached as the student said that he wanted to become a paediatrician.

Many influential authors, such as Nancy C Andreasen, consider circumstantiality a formal thought disorder.

Disorders of continuity of thinking: These include—
- **Perseveration:** It is the repetition of the same response beyond the point of relevance. For example, a patient was asked the following questions.
  Q. 1: What is your name?
  Ans. Mahesh Kumar
  Q. 2: Where do you live?
  Ans: Mahesh Kumar
  Q. 3: How many children do you have?
  Ans: Mahesh Kumar.

  It must be noted that the perseveration is in response to a question and is not spontaneous.
- **Thought block:** In this disturbance, the stream of thought suddenly stops, leaving a 'blank'. And then, a completely new thought begins. Thought block is seen in patients with schizophrenia, and it might also be seen in patients with severe anxiety.

Disorders of form of thought: Form refers to the "organisation" of thinking. When thoughts are well organised, there is a connection between various components of the single thought and also between successive thoughts. In disorders of the form of thought or '**formal thought**

disorders', there is a disturbance in the organisation of the thinking. The disorganisation of thought is manifested as 'disorganised speech', as thoughts usually get expressed in speech only.

The important formal thought disorders include:

- **Derailment:** In derailment, the association between the successive thoughts is disturbed. For example, a patient said, "Jawahar Lal Nehru was India's first prime minister, and he was a leader of the congress party. Sachin Tendulkar scored 100 international hundreds".

  In this example, there is no link between the first thought about Nehru and the second thought about Tendulkar.

- **Loosening of association:** Here, the connection is lost between the components of a single thought. For example, a patient said, "I thought it would rain today and Amitabh Bachchan is a famous actor". In this example, the phrase before the 'and' is disconnected from the phrase after the 'and' and hence exemplifies the loosening of association.

- **Incoherence:** Incoherence is characterised by a complete lack of organisation that makes the thought incomprehensible and impossible to understand. For example, a patient with incoherence said, "India me Churchgate pulses cricket computer". This thought does not convey any meaningful information.

- **Tangentiality:** In tangentiality, the answer is related to the question in some distant way, but the goal of the thought is never reached. For example, a patient was asked about his favourite Bollywood actor. He replied, "Well, you see, the Hindi movies are still male-centric and usually deal with relationship issues, whereas the Hollywood movies have lots of action and science fiction. I think the Hindi Film Industry is growing rapidly, and it's a good medium for the entertainment of masses".

  In this example, the patient's answer was distantly related to the question. However, the exact answer was never given, or in other words, the 'goal' of the thought was never reached. In contrast, in circumstantiality, despite the inclusion of many unnecessary details, the thought's goal is finally reached.

- **Neologism:** Neologism is the coining of a new word whose derivation cannot be understood. For example, a patient used the word "tintintapa" for the pen. Here the patient has devised a new word for pen, and the reason for the same is beyond understanding. The presence of neologism is highly suggestive of schizophrenia.

- **Word approximations (metonyms):** Metonyms are old words used in a new or unconventional manner. The meaning is readily evident, though the word in itself might appear strange. For example, a patient used the word "time vessel" for watch and "hand shoes" for gloves. Now using the term 'time vessel' for a watch is understandable to some extent, but still, it is an unconventional use.

- **Clanging (clang associations):** Here, the words are associated with each other as they sound similar, and there is a lack of any meaningful connection between the words. For example, a patient said, 'I make sense out of nonsense, and nonsense is the essence of the turbulence of life'. In 'flight of ideas', clanging is frequently observed.

Disorders of content of thought: 'Content' of thought refers to what a person is actually thinking about. The most important disorder of content of thought is 'delusion'.

Delusion: Defined as a false, unshakeable belief that is out of keeping with the person's social and cultural background.' There are three aspects to the definition of delusion:

1. **False belief:** It means that the belief is factually incorrect.
2. **Unshakeable belief:** It means that the patient continues to hold the belief despite the presence of evidence to the contrary.
3. **Out of keeping with the person's social and cultural background:** It means that the person's background can't explain the belief. For example: Say, a patient from a particular tribal area where superstitions are widespread, develops a belief that black magic is causing him health issues. When this patient's background is taken into account, it becomes understandable why the patient is holding this belief. Hence, the patient would not be diagnosed with a delusion.

The following are the common types of delusions:

- **Delusion of persecution:** It is the **most common** type of delusion. The patient with this delusion believes that he is being harmed. For example, a patient claimed that Indian police and CBI were hatching a conspiracy to kill him.

- **Delusion of reference:** The patient believes that neutral events happening around him are somehow related to him. For example, a patient claimed that the tube light of his apartment was flickering as there was a camera fitted inside through which his movements were being recorded.

- **Delusion of grandeur or grandiosity:** The patient believes he has an exceptional identity or power. For example, a patient claimed that he is the reincarnation of Lord Hanuman and can carry the mountains on his shoulders.

- **Delusion of love (erotomania, fantasy lover syndrome):** Patients develop a false belief that someone is in love with them. It is also known as **de Clerambault syndrome**. For example, a rickshaw puller claimed that Katrina Kaif was in love with him. He admitted that he had never met her or communicated with her; nonetheless, he insisted that Katrina Kaif secretly loved him.

- **Nihilistic delusion (delusion of negation, Cotard's syndrome):** Here, the patients may deny the existence of their body, their mind, or the world in general. They may claim that everybody is dead, the world has stopped, etc. The basic theme of this delusion is the "end of existence".

- **Delusion of enormity:** Sometimes nihilistic delusions are associated with 'delusions of enormity', in which the patient may believe that some of their actions may cause a catastrophe. For example, a patient reported that he tries to hold on to urine for as long as possible, as he believes that his urine may cause floods in the entire country.

- **Delusion of infidelity (delusion of jealousy):** The patient has a false belief that his partner/spouse is having an affair. It is also called **morbid jealousy** (pathological jealousy) or **Othello syndrome** (named after the famous Shakespeare play)

- **Delusion of guilt:** Here, the patient develops guilt at a delusional level. The patient may claim that he is an evil person and has committed unpardonable sins. This delusion is usually seen in patients with severe depression.

> **BIZARRE VERSUS NON-BIZARRE DELUSIONS**
>
> ❖ **Bizarre delusions:** The term 'bizarre' is used for those delusions which are **scientifically impossible** and **culturally implausible** (understandable). For example, a patient had a delusion that aliens stole his heart and lungs, and now he is living without those organs.
> ❖ **Non-bizarre delusions:** These delusions are possible in the sense that the content of the delusion can actually happen in the real world. For example, a patient developed a delusion that his family members wanted to take away his property.
>
> In the previous diagnostic systems (DSM-IV), the presence of bizarre delusion was given special importance in the criteria of schizophrenia, but the same was removed in DSM-5.

Disorders of possession of thought: Usually, people experience that their thoughts belong to themselves and no one else can influence their thinking process. There is also a sense of control over one's thinking. Or in other words, usually, people experience that they are in possession of their thoughts.

In the disturbances of possession of thought, the patient either experiences that others are tampering with his thoughts or that he has lost control over the thoughts.

The disorders of possession include the following:

A. **Obsessions:** Here, a thought comes repeatedly into the patient's mind against his will. The patient recognises the thought as his own, is distressed by the repetitive and intrusive nature of the thought and tries to stop it. The patient feels that he has lost control over his thoughts. The patient also understands that the thoughts coming to his mind are senseless and irrational. Obsessions are **'ego dystonic'** (i.e., unwanted and unacceptable). Some authors consider 'obsessions' as disorders of the content of thought.

B. **Thought alienation:** Here, the patient experiences that his thoughts are under the control of an external agency or that others are interfering with his thought process. Thought alienation phenomenon can be of the following types:
- **Thought insertion:** The patient feels that some external agency is inserting thoughts into his mind. For example, a patient said, 'doctor yesterday, I was sitting silently on my balcony and was thinking about the weather when I had a thought 'you must make an omelette for breakfast tomorrow', doctor, my neighbour used some weird technology and implanted that thought in my mind, I felt really upset'.
- **Thought withdrawal:** Patient experiences that his thoughts are being withdrawn/stolen from his mind by an external agency. For example, a patient said, 'doctor, yesterday, I was sitting silently on my balcony and was thinking about the weather when suddenly my mind went blank; I could not think of anything for a while; my neighbour used some weird technology and stole all my thoughts, I felt really upset'.
- **Thought broadcast:** Patient experiences that thoughts are escaping his mind and others can access them. For example, a patient said, "doctor, yesterday, I was sitting silently on my balcony and thought that I should go into the kitchen and make an omelette, and the next thing I saw was that my neighbour was standing on his balcony with eggs in his hands. Doctor, my thoughts about making omelette floated to him, and he knew what I was thinking about; I felt really upset".

Higher Mental Functions

In this component of MSE, various higher mental functions are assessed. These include:

Attention

Attention is the ability to attend to a specific stimulus without getting distracted. In clinical practice, attention is tested using **Digit Repetition Test (Digit Span Test)**. The test involves the examiner saying some numbers and the patient repeating them. The examiner starts with a single digit and gradually proceeds to a two-digit sequence, three-digit sequence, and so on until the patient fails to repeat.

For example: 2, 2-5, 3-8-7, 4-9-8-0, 1-3-2-5-8-7

An inability to repeat at least **five digits** indicates defective attention.

Concentration

Concentration is the ability to sustain attention for a longer duration. It is usually tested by **Serial Seven Subtraction Test**, in which the patient is asked to serially subtract 7s from 100 (100, 93, 86, 79....)

Memory

Memory is evaluated under the following three heads:

1. **Immediate memory:** It is the ability to recall information after an interval of a few seconds. The term "**working memory**" is sometimes used as a synonym for immediate memory, though there are finer differences between the two. Immediate memory is tested by Digit Repetition Test or Serial Seven Subtraction Tests.
2. **Recent memory:** It is the ability to recall information after minutes, hours or days. A commonly used test to evaluate recent memory is "24-hour recall," The patient is asked simple questions about events in the last 24 hours, such as 'What did he have in the meal the last night?', 'How did he reach the hospital?', etc. Orientation to the time, place and person also tests recent memory.
3. **Remote memory:** It is the ability to recall the information after years. It includes recall of both personal events and historical events. The examples of questions asked are 'Where did you go to school?', 'When was your first child born?', 'Name four past prime ministers of India?'.

Intelligence

It is usually tested by asking questions about general information and assessing calculation skills.

Abstract Thinking

Abstract thinking is the ability to form concepts and make generalisations.

It can be assessed by:
- **Proverb testing:** Here, the patient is asked to explain the meaning of proverbs. For example, patient was asked to explain the meaning of the proverb 'A stitch in time saves nine' or some other proverb that is commonly used in the region. And the explanation is assessed for the degree of abstraction. If the patient's explanation is 'A small effort at the right time may save a huge effort later', it demonstrates abstract thinking. On the other hand, if the patient's explanation is 'One stitch in the cloth at the right time can prevent nine stitches', it suggests 'concrete thinking'.
- **Similarities testing:** Here, the patient is asked to explain the similarities between two objects, e.g., 'What is the similarity is between a chair and a table?" If the patient answers that 'both are pieces of furniture', it would suggest that patient has abstract thinking and can conceptualise at a higher level. On the other hand, if the patient answers that 'both are kept on the floor', it would suggest an absence of a higher level of thinking (known as concrete thinking).

Judgment

It is the ability to respond appropriately in a particular situation. There are three types of judgments, and all are tested separately:

1. **Test judgment:** Here, a test situation is given, and the patient is asked to tell the appropriate response in that situation. The commonly asked question is what would the patient do if he sees a "house on fire" or "an addressed envelope lying on the ground." If the patient responds that he will "call the fire brigade" or "drop it in the letterbox", respectively, it suggests intact judgment.
2. **Personal judgment:** Here, the patient is asked about the plans for his future life, and the response is assessed.
3. **Social judgment:** Here, the patient's ability to interact appropriately in social situations is assessed.

Insight

Insight is defined as the 'awareness and understanding of the illness'. Insight can be rated on a five-point scale as described below:

- **Grade 1:** Complete denial of insight (absent insight) (e.g., I don't have any problem)
- **Grade 2:** Some awareness of being sick but denying it at the same time (e.g., At times, I hear some voices, but there is no illness)
- **Grade 3:** Awareness of being sick but attributing the symptoms to external or physical factors (e.g., Yes, I hear voices, and it is because my neighbours have installed a hidden speaker to trouble me)
- **Grade 4:** Awareness of illness without any accompanying changes in behaviour (intellectual insight) (e.g., I know I have schizophrenia, but I don't want to take any medicines or treatment)
- **Grade 5:** Awareness of illness along with the accompanying changes in the behaviour (emotional insight, the highest level of insight) (e.g., I have schizophrenia, and I want to take regular medications to prevent any relapses)

Classification

At present, there are two major classificatory systems in psychiatry.
1. **ICD-11 (International classification of diseases, 11th edition):** ICD is a diagnostic system published by WHO. Its latest edition is ICD-11 which was presented at the world health assembly in May, 2019 for adoption by member states and came into effect in February, 2022.
2. **DSM-5 (Diagnostic and statistical manual of mental disorders):** DSM is published by American Psychiatric Association. The fifth edition of DSM (DSM-5) was published in 2013. The revised version, **DSM-5-TR**, was published in March, 2022.

In DSM-IV, a multiaxial system was used for making a comprehensive clinical diagnosis, according to which a diagnosis was given on the following axes:

- **Axis I:** Clinical psychiatry diagnosis (the psychiatry diagnosis is coded)
- **Axis II:** Personality disorders and mental retardation (any personality disorder or mental retardation is coded)
- **Axis III:** Medical conditions (any accompanying medical illness is coded)
- **Axis IV:** Psychosocial problems (any psychosocial issues such as poor relationship with spouse, etc., is coded)
- **Axis V:** Global assessment of functioning (it is a measure of patients functioning in the last year)

In DSM-5, the concept of multiaxial diagnoses was removed. In DSM-5, axis I, II, and III of DSM-IV were combined, and axis IV and V are to be described separately.

Other Classifications

Psychiatric disorders have been classified in multiple ways. One of the classifications divides psychiatric disorders into organic versus functional psychiatric disorders, and another classification divides them into psychoses versus neuroses.
- **Organic versus functional (nonorganic) mental disorders:** This was the first major classification of psychiatric/mental disorders.
  - **Organic mental disorders:** The disorders caused by demonstrable brain disturbances were classified as organic mental disorders (primary brain disturbances or systemic disturbances known to affect brain parenchyma). For example: Delirium, dementia, etc.
  - **Functional (nonorganic) mental disorders:** The disorders in which no demonstrable disturbance of brain parenchyma could be found were called functional mental disorders. For example: Schizophrenia, mania, etc.

This classification tried to differentiate the disorders of the brain (i.e., organic mental disorders) from those of the mind (i.e., functional mental disorders). However, this classification is considered arbitrary since it's possible to demonstrate brain parenchyma disturbances even in the so-called "functional" mental disorders with the advancement of science. The terms 'organic' and 'functional' are still used widely, more so by non-psychiatric doctors.

- **Psychoses versus neuroses:** The functional disorders were further classified into psychotic disorders (psychoses) and neurotic disorders (neuroses).
  - **Psychoses:** The main characteristic of psychotic disorder includes lack of awareness of illness (or lack of insight) and impaired reality testing (i.e., the patients loses contact with reality and starts living in a fantasy world created by their ill minds). Schizophrenia and bipolar disorder are examples of psychotic disorders. Delusions and hallucinations are the prototype psychotic symptoms.
  - **Neuroses:** Neurotic disorders are characterised by awareness of the illness (insight is present), and reality contact is also intact. For example: Anxiety disorders and depression.

Again, this classification is arbitrary as many patients with psychotic disorders such as schizophrenia have insight into their illness and patients with neurotic disorders may lack insight.

Research Domain Criterion

One of the major critiques of current classification systems (i.e., ICD-11 and DSM-5) is that they are syndrome based classifications. The term 'syndrome' is used for a group of symptoms that occur together and are unique as a group. So, a diagnosis of "schizophrenia" is given if a patient has a particular group of symptoms (i.e., delusion, hallucinations, and disorganisation).

Though helpful in clinical practice, the syndrome-based classification is still considered problematic as any definitive classification should be based on aetiology. In fact, studies have suggested that the current psychiatric disorders such as 'schizophrenia' may actually represent many different 'diseases', all of which have a similar presentation but are different as far as underlying cause and pathology is concerned.

To address this lacuna, the NIMH (national institute of mental health, USA) has funded a research framework called **RDoC (research domain criterion)**. RDoC aims to create new approaches for the investigation of mental disorders.

An RDoC matrix has been developed, which describes major 'domains' of human functioning.

These 'domains' include:
- **Negative valence systems:** These systems are responsible for responding to negative (or aversive) situations or contexts, such as anxiety or fear.
- **Positive valence systems:** These systems are responsible for responding to positive situations or contexts, such as reward seeking.
- **Cognitive systems:** These are responsible for cognitive functions such as attention, memory, etc.
- **Systems for social processes:** These systems are responsible for social responses such as interpersonal relations.
- **Arousal/Regulatory systems:** These systems are responsible for functions such as arousal, sleep-wakefulness, circadian rhythms, etc.
- **Sensorimotor systems:** These systems are primarily responsible for the control of motor behaviours.

These domains have been further divided into "constructs", which describe different aspects of overall functions. For example, negative valence system has constructs like fear, anxiety, loss, etc., which define particular negative contexts.

Further, these domains and constructs are measured using different methods called "units of analysis". Units of analysis include neurocircuitry, molecular, genetic and behavioural assessment. For example, a particular cognitive function, say attention, is regulated by a specific circuit in the brain. Now, abnormal functioning of this circuit may result in poor attention, which may further present clinically as a child with attention deficits while attending class and resulting in poor scholastic performance. This child will get a diagnosis of attention deficit hyperactivity disorder (according to ICD-11 or DSM-5). Once RDoC is fully developed, it is expected that a more precise diagnosis in terms of specific neurocircuit abnormality, genetic or molecular factors involved, would be given. And this precision diagnosis would guide the treatment better too. RDoC is a work in progress.

CASE BASED MCQ

A 25-year-old male presented to the psychiatry emergency along with his family members. During the interview, the patient appeared cheerful and cooperative. The patient claimed that he has special powers and can change the route of rivers and oceans; when asked how he does that, his response was, "I am the chosen one; I will save this world from destruction." Which of the following is likely present in the patient?
a. Delusion of persecution
b. Delusion of grandiosity
c. Delusion of reference
d. Delusion of infidelity

Ans. b. Delusion of grandiosity

SUGGESTED READINGS

1. Boland R, Verduin M, Ruiz P, Shah A, Sadock B. Kaplan & Sadock's synopsis of psychiatry. 12th ed. Philadelphia: Wolters Kluwer; 2020.
2. Casey P, Kelly B, Fish F. Fish's clinical psychopathology: signs and symptoms in psychiatry. 4th ed. New York: Cambridge University Press; 2019.
3. Oyebode F. Sims' Symptoms in the Mind: Textbook of Descriptive Psychopathology. 6th ed. Elsevier; 2018.
4. Andreasen NC. Scale for the assessment of thought, language, and communication (TLC). Schizophrenia bulletin. 1986;12(3):473.
5. Strub R, Black F, Geschwind N, Strub A. The mental status examination in neurology. 4th ed. Philadelphia: F.A. Davis Company; 2000.
6. Research Domain Criteria (RDoC) [Internet]. National Institute of Mental Health (NIMH). 2021 [cited 9 December 2021]. Available from: https://www.nimh.nih.gov/research/research-funded-by-nimh/rdoc

2. Schizophrenia and Other Primary Psychotic Disorders

Praveen Tripathi, Priyanka Goyal

PS5.1	Classify and describe the magnitude and aetiology of schizophrenia and other psychotic disorders
PS5.2	Enumerate, elicit, describe and document clinical features, positives
PS5.3	Describe the treatment of schizophrenia including behavioural and pharmacologic therapy
PS5.4	Demonstrate family education in a patient with schizophrenia in a simulated environment
PS5.5	Enumerate and describe the pharmacologic basis and side effects of drugs used in schizophrenia
PS5.6	Enumerate the appropriate conditions for specialist referral in patients with psychotic disorders

Schizophrenia is the prototype of psychotic disorders. It is one of the "**serious mental disorders**" and possibly evokes more curiosity and interest in the general public than any other psychiatric disorder. It causes immense health, social, and economic burdens that affect the patients, caregivers, and society at large.

HISTORY

The understanding of schizophrenia has evolved over time, with the contribution of many eminent personalities.

Emil Kraepelin

Based on the symptoms and course of illness, Emil Kraepelin classified psychiatric disorders into the following two major categories:

1. **Dementia praecox:** It was characterised by symptoms of delusions and hallucinations, a **long-term deteriorating course** and gradual **cognitive decline** (i.e., gradual decline of cognitive functions such as memory, attention and goal-directed behaviour). Kraepelin believed that this disorder was caused by a neurodegenerative process and emphasised on cognitive decline (hence the term dementia) and early age at onset (hence the term praecox). Later, Eugen Bleuler, a Swiss psychiatrist, renamed "dementia praecox" as "schizophrenia", which is the current name of this disorder.
2. **Manic-depressive psychosis:** It was characterised by distinct manic and depressive episodes. The patient would have **episodic illness** alternating with periods of normal functioning, unlike dementia praecox, which was a continuous and progressively deteriorating illness.

Table 2.1: Dementia praecox and manic depressive psychosis.

	Dementia praecox	Manic depressive psychosis
Clinical features	Delusions and hallucinations	Distinct manic and depressive episodes
Course	Continuous and deteriorating	Episodic
Cognitive decline	Present	Absent

Further, unlike dementia praecox, there was **no cognitive decline** in manic depressive psychosis. Later "manic depressive psychosis" was renamed "bipolar disorder" (**Table 2.1**).

Eugen Bleuler

Bleuler coined the term "**schizophrenia**". The term "schizophrenia" is derived from the Greek words schizein (which means splitting) and phrene (which refers to mind). The term 'schizophrenia' literally means 'splitting of mental functions', which refers to the loss of coherent mental functioning seen in schizophrenia. Schizophrenia is not the same as "split personality". The "split personality" or "multiple personality disorder" is a personality disorder and should not be confused with schizophrenia.

Bleuler observed that the illness was not always associated with a cognitive decline and did not always have an early onset, as suggested by the Kraepelin. Bleuler described four fundamental (primary) symptoms, which he believed were diagnostic of schizophrenia. These are often referred to as 4 A's of Bleuler (**Table 2.2**).

Kurt Schneider

Schneider described a list of eleven symptoms that were seen frequently in patients with schizophrenia and could be used for making the diagnosis. However, Schneider had stressed that these symptoms, referred to as **First Rank Symptoms**, could be seen in other psychiatric disorders too and are not specific to schizophrenia **(Table 2.3)**. These include:

PRIMARY AND SECONDARY DELUSIONS

- **Primary delusions:** These delusions arise as a direct result of a morbid psychological process caused by the underlying disorder
- **Secondary delusions:** These develop secondarily to some other psychopathology. For example, a patient who had auditory hallucinations and heard a voice that repeatedly said, "you will be killed", started believing that "somebody wants to kill him". This "delusion of persecution" that developed is a secondary delusion as it developed secondarily to the auditory hallucinations.

Table 2.2: Four A's of Bleuler.

Autism	The term "autism" refers to the withdrawn behaviour wherein the patient is preoccupied with his thoughts and appears uninterested in external events. Bleuler's "autism" should not be confused with the childhood disorder of "autism", which is a distinct clinical entity
Ambivalence	Ambivalence refers to the inability to take decisions. Patients with ambivalence face difficulty in deciding for or against. For example, while walking, a patient with schizophrenia suddenly appeared confused as he could not decide whether to put his foot forward or backwards
Affect disturbances	It refers to emotional disturbances such as inappropriate affect
Association disturbances	It refers to disturbances in the organisation of thought, such as loosening of associations

Note: Apart from the fundamental symptoms, Bleuler also described the accessory (secondary) symptoms of schizophrenia, such as delusions and hallucinations.

Table 2.3: Schneiderian first-rank symptoms (SFRS).

The 11 SFRS can be further clubbed into subgroups:	
Three thought alienation phenomena (passivity of thought)	In the thought alienation phenomenon, the patient experiences that his internal thought processes can be influenced or tampered with by others. Three types of thought alienation have been described as first-rank symptoms. These include: 1. **Thought insertion:** In thought insertion, the patient experiences thoughts being inserted into his mind by an external force 2. **Thought withdrawal:** In thought withdrawal, the patient experiences that thoughts are being taken away from his mind by an external force 3. **Thought broadcast:** In thought broadcast, the patient experiences that thoughts are "escaping" his mind and others can access them
Three "made" phenomenon	Here, the patient experiences that his actions, emotions or drives are being controlled by external forces. Three types of made phenomenon are included in SFRS: 1. **Made volition (passivity of volition):** Here, the patient experiences that an external agency is controlling his actions. For example, a patient with schizophrenia would repeatedly attempt to touch the blades of a running fan. When asked for the reason, he replied, 'I don't want to touch the fan, but I am being made to. An alien control my hands and makes me do all these dangerous activities. I am helpless" 2. **Made affect (passivity of emotion):** Here, the patient experiences that an external force is controlling his emotions. For example, a patient said, "at times I start laughing loudly, and at times I cry. The neighbours control my emotions, they play with my emotions. They can change how I feel whenever they want to. I am helpless" 3. **Made impulse (passivity of impulse):** Here, the patient experiences that impulses (sudden drives or urges) are being imposed upon him by external forces. For example, a patient suddenly threw his coffee mug at a nurse. When asked for a reason, he replied, "an impulse came over me; this impulse was sent by CBI officers who wanted me to throw the mug. I tried resisting the impulse but could not. I am sorry." Please note that the patient with made volition experienced that an external agency controlled the movement of his hand. In contrast, the patient with made impulse experienced that the external agency put an impulse in him, and the patient himself took action on that impulse

Cont'd...

Cont'd...

The 11 SFRS can be further clubbed into subgroups:	
Three auditory hallucinations	There are three distinct types of auditory hallucinations, which are first-rank symptoms. These include: 1. **Voices heard arguing:** Here, the patient reports hearing two or more voices (the term **'voices'** is often used to describe 'auditory hallucinations') which argue about or discuss the patient. The patient is usually referred to in the third person (hence called **third-person auditory hallucination**). For example, a patient-reported hearing two voices that were having a conversation about the patient. The first voice of a middle-aged man said, "he is a strange man; he doesn't have any good qualities". The second voice of an elderly woman responded, "yes, also look how fat has he become". In this example, the patient is hearing two voices, and the voices are using the word "he" to refer to the patient. Hence the patient is being referred to in the third person 2. **Voices giving running commentary** (Voices commenting on patient's action): Here, the patient hears voices that give a running commentary on the patient's activities. For example, a patient working in the kitchen heard the following voice "she has peeled the potato, and now she is about to switch on the gas. Now, she has started to wash the potatoes". The voice usually refers to the patient in the third person, and hence this is also an example of third-person auditory hallucinations 3. **Audible thoughts (thought echo):** Here, the patient hears a voice that says the patient's thoughts aloud. For example, a patient thought, "I will have dinner at a restaurant tonight". Immediately he heard a voice of a middle-aged woman saying: "I will have dinner at a restaurant tonight". The German word **"Gedankenlautwerden"** or the French word **"echo de pensee"** are occasionally used to describe audible thoughts
Somatic passivity	Here, the patient experiences specific somatic hallucinations (such as tactile hallucinations) and believes that an external force is causing them. For example, a patient felt an intense burning sensation inside his right knee and claimed that it was because of UV rays sent by CIA agents from New York
Delusional perception	In delusional perception, a normal perception is interpreted delusionally, or in other words, a delusional explanation is attached to a normal perception. For example, a patient with schizophrenia looked at the ceiling fan and immediately understood that "all the people in the city consider him a homosexual". In this example, there was a normal perception in the first step (i.e., the patient saw a ceiling fan), and in the second step, a delusional meaning was attached to this normal perception (i.e., the delusion that everybody in the city considers the patient a homosexual). Delusional perception is a type of **"primary delusion"**

Ernst Kretschmer

Kretschmer studied the association of body types with psychiatric disorders and described that schizophrenia occurred more in persons with **asthenic** (thin, less muscular) and **athletic** (muscular) body types, whereas bipolar disorder was more likely to occur in **pyknic** (short and stocky) body type.

EPIDEMIOLOGY

- The lifetime prevalence of schizophrenia is around 1%.
- The point prevalence ranges from 0.27 to 0.83%.
- The incidence rate of schizophrenia is around 0.2/1,000/year.

Indian data: According to the **National Mental Health Survey (NMHS 2016)**, the lifetime prevalence and current prevalence of schizophrenia and other psychotic disorders were 1.41% and 0.42%, respectively. (Kindly note that the NMHS 2016 prevalence was for the entire schizophrenia spectrum disorders and not schizophrenia alone).

Schizophrenia is equally prevalent in men and women; however, the onset of illness is earlier in males and later in females. The peak age of onset is in adolescence and young adulthood (15–24 years). There is a **bimodal distribution** with a second peak in middle age in females.

If the onset is after 45 years of age, it is called **"late-onset schizophrenia"**.

Studies have found that persons who develop schizophrenia are more likely to be born in winters than in summers, although the reason for the same is unclear. Few studies found **prenatal influenza exposure** and **advanced paternal age** to be associated with the risk of the development of schizophrenia. Higher rates of birth complications and physical anomalies at birth have also been found in patients with schizophrenia.

PREVALENCE OF SCHIZOPHRENIA IN SPECIFIC POPULATIONS

- Monozygotic twin of patients with schizophrenia (**monozygotic concordance rate**): 47%
- Dizygotic twin of patients with schizophrenia (**dizygotic concordance rate**): 12%
- Non-twin siblings of patients with schizophrenia: 8%
- Children with both parents having schizophrenia: 40%
- Children with one parent having schizophrenia: 12%
- General population: 1%

DOWNWARD DRIFT HYPOTHESIS

The prevalence of schizophrenia is higher in the lower socioeconomic class. The reason for this, according to the downward drift hypothesis, is that patients with schizophrenia often face difficulties in finding meaningful employment and get estranged from their family and thus, drift down the socioeconomic class. Hence, belonging to lower socioeconomic classes does not increase the chances of developing schizophrenia; instead, developing schizophrenia leads to migration to the lower socioeconomic class.

CLINICAL FEATURES

The symptoms of schizophrenia can be divided into the following groups:

Positive Symptoms (Psychotic Symptoms)

Hallucinations and **delusions** are the two positive symptoms (psychotic symptoms) of schizophrenia. The term "positive" is used as there is an **addition of new experiences** (i.e., hallucinations and delusions) due to the disease process of schizophrenia. The predominance of positive symptoms is associated with a better prognosis in schizophrenia.

Hallucinations can occur in any five sensory modalities, the most common being auditory hallucinations. More than 70% of patients with schizophrenia experience auditory hallucinations. The content of "voices" is usually threatening, derogatory and negative (e.g., a patient-reported hearing a voice that said, "you will not be allowed to work as you are a useless person"). Certain auditory hallucinations like "voices discussing or arguing about the patient", "voices giving running commentary", and "audible thoughts" have special significance in schizophrenia. Visual hallucinations are the second most common type of hallucinations. Olfactory, gustatory and tactile hallucinations are present less often.

Delusions are also commonly present in schizophrenia, the most common being the delusion of persecution.

The positive symptoms **respond better to the antipsychotic medications** than the negative symptoms or disorganisation symptoms.

Negative Symptoms

Negative symptoms are so-called as they represent **"loss of normal functions"** of the brain in patients with schizophrenia. Negative symptoms remain more stable over the time than positive and disorganisation symptoms and are **better predictors of long-term disability** in the patients. The following are the negative symptoms:

a. **Avolition:** Avolition is the loss of will or drive to indulge in goal-directed activities (such as grooming and hygiene, educational and occupational activities)
b. **Apathy:** Apathy is the lack of concern for a task or results. For example, a student with schizophrenia failed an exam; however, he appeared totally unconcerned with the results.
c. **Anhedonia:** Anhedonia is the inability to experience pleasure in activities or relationships that were previously pleasurable. For example, a cricket enthusiast stopped playing and watching cricket entirely as he was no longer able to enjoy the game.
d. **Asociality:** Asociality is the lack of desire to socialise and an indifference to social relations, including with family and friends.
e. **Affective flattening (or blunting):** Affective flattening refers to the lack of or severe restriction of expression of emotions.
f. **Alogia:** Alogia is decreased speech output.

Disorganisation Symptoms

The disorganisation symptoms include the following:

a. **Disorganised behaviour:** It refers to **inappropriate** or odd behaviours. For example, a patient with schizophrenia would wear thick jackets and sweaters even during the peak summer and was often seen eating from the garbage bin.
b. **Disorganised thought and speech:** It refers to the disorganisation of thought processes, also called **Formal thought disorders**. The disorganised thought manifests in disorganised speech, which is difficult to understand and sometimes makes no sense.
c. **Inappropriate affect:** It refers to the disturbances of affect (emotions), such as having a burst of laughter in the middle of a serious conversation.

Motor Symptoms

Motor symptoms, also known as **Catatonic symptoms** or **symptoms of conation**, were first described by a German psychiatrist, **Karl Kahlbaum**, who also coined the term "**catatonia**". Motor symptoms are sometimes clubbed with disorganisation symptoms; however, recent research indicates that they constitute a separate symptom complex.

The motor symptoms include:

a. **Stupor:** Stupor is a state of extreme inactivity or immobility (akinesis). The patient is minimally responsive to any kind of stimulus.
b. **Excitement:** Catatonic excitement involves extreme hyperactivity, which is non-goal-directed. The patient may appear very active, even aggressive, but not indulge in any meaningful task.
c. **Mutism:** Lack of verbal response or minimal verbal response.
d. **Posturing:** It refers to the maintenance of the same posture for prolonged periods of time (e.g., a patient stood on one foot with his right hand behind his head for hours).

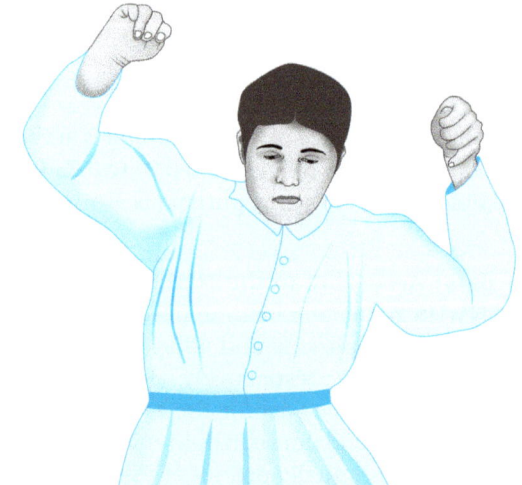

Fig. 2.1: Posturing.

e. **Waxy flexibility:** It refers to the feeling of plastic resistance, which the examiner experiences when he makes a passive movement on the patient. This feeling of plastic resistance is quite similar to when a wax candle is bent, hence the term 'waxy flexibility'.

f. **Automatic obedience:** It refers to extreme compliance with the other person's commands even if it results in unpleasant consequences for the patient. For example, a patient kept on protruding his tongue every time the examiner asked, even though his tongue would be pricked by a pin each time he protruded it.
g. **Echolalia:** It refers to the mimicking of the other person's speech. The patient repeats whatever the other person says (e.g., when a patient was asked 'what is your name? he replied with 'what is your name?).
h. **Echopraxia:** It refers to mimicking the other person's movements (e.g., While talking to the patient when the examiner scratched his forehead, the patient also started scratching his forehead immediately).
i. **Negativism:** It refers to the patient's refusal to accept the examiner's instructions or any attempt to move him without any apparent reason. For example, when asked to show his tongue, the patient did not comply. When asked to take a step forward, the patient did not move.
j. **Grimacing:** It is the maintenance of an odd facial expression by the patient.
k. **Stereotypy:** Stereotypy is the **spontaneous** repetition of odd, **purposeless** movements. For example, a patient would repeatedly and spontaneously do hand-flapping movements.
l. **Mannerisms:** Mannerism is the **spontaneous** and unusual repetition of **purposeful movements** (goal-directed behaviour). For example, a patient would repeatedly salute the people passing in front of him. Here, saluting is a goal-directed activity but was carried out in an unusual and exaggerated manner.
m. **Perseveration:** It is an **induced movement** (i.e., a movement in response to an instruction) that is senselessly repeated. For example, a patient was asked to protrude his tongue out, which he did; however, he then kept on repeating this out and in movement even though he was no longer asked to do so. It must be noted that perseveration occurs in response to an instruction, whereas stereotypy and mannerisms are spontaneous. Perseveration can be a sign of brain damage (organic brain disorders). **Logoclonia** and **palilalia** are special forms of perseveration.
    - *Logoclonia: In logoclonia, the last syllable of the last word is repeated. For example, a patient said, 'tomorrow is Monday-ay-ay-ay-ay'. Here, the last syllable 'ay' is repeated.*
    - *Palilalia: In palilalia, the patient repeats the perseverated word with increasing frequency.*
n. **Gegenhalten:** It refers to involuntary resistance offered by the patient in response to a passive movement. The strength of resistance is proportional to the strength of force applied during the passive movement.
o. **Ambitendency:** Inability to execute the desired motor movement. For example, when offered a hand for a handshake, the patient may repeatedly bring his hand forward and backwards as he cannot decide whether to shake the hand or not. Ambitendency is ambivalence in motor movements.

Cognitive Symptoms

The term cognition refers to the mental processes involved in the gaining and processing of information. The cognitive symptoms in schizophrenia include deficits in the domains of **working memory** (memory which holds information for seconds. For example, if you are told a phone number and then asked to write it down, you will have that number in the memory for a few seconds before you write it on the paper), **sustained attention, verbal declarative memory, language comprehension, information processing speed, problem-solving abilities and executive functioning** (executive functions are a set of mental skills that help in the planning and getting a task done). Cognitive symptoms are not a part of the diagnostic criteria of schizophrenia in DSM-5 yet, although the ICD-11 mentions the disturbances of cognition while describing the symptoms of schizophrenia. Cognitive symptoms have a significant impact on the patient's functioning.

Violence, Suicide and Homicide

Violent behaviour (excluding homicide) may be seen commonly in untreated patients with schizophrenia, although schizophrenia patients are much more commonly the victims of violence than the perpetrators. Also, contrary to the common belief, the rate of homicide by patients with schizophrenia is no more than a member of the general population. Suicide is the most common cause of premature death in patients with schizophrenia. Traditionally, the suicide rate in schizophrenia was put at **10%**. However, according to newer studies and DSM-5, the suicide rate is around 5–6% (around 20% of patients attempt suicide, and 5–6% of patients complete suicide).

The risk factors for suicide in a patient with schizophrenia include:
a. The most important risk factor associated with suicide is the presence of a major depressive episode and a feeling of hopelessness.
b. Also, the increased risk is associated with periods of increased symptoms (especially the presence of delusion of persecution, command hallucinations in which the hallucinatory voices give specific commands to the patient).
c. At times, patients with a better prognosis (such as lesser negative symptoms and absence of affect disturbances) have a paradoxically higher suicide risk. This may be because these patients are better able to understand the devastating effects of schizophrenia on their health and may become hopeless about the future.
d. It has been found that there is an increased risk of suicide early in the course of illness, immediately after admission and immediately after discharge from an inpatient setting.
e. Young males with comorbid substance use, and
f. Being unemployed.

DIAGNOSIS

According to DSM-5, for the diagnosis of schizophrenia, the total duration of illness should be at least six months (this 6-month period can include the period of non-specific symptoms like changes in behaviour, development of new interests, social withdrawal, etc.). This 6 month period must also include at least 1 month during which the patient has two or more of the following symptoms. At least one of these two symptoms should be (1), (2) or (3).
1. Delusions
2. Hallucinations
3. Disorganised speech (which is a result of formal thought disorders)
4. Disorganised behaviour or catatonic behaviour (symptoms)
5. Negative symptoms (i.e., diminished emotional expression or avolition)

The ICD-11 also uses similar symptoms criteria for the diagnosis of schizophrenia; however, the duration criterion of ICD-11 is **1 month** and not **6 months**.

AETIOLOGY

Schizophrenia is caused by a combination of multiple factors, which can be divided into two major groups: Genetic factors and environmental factors.

Genetic Factors

1. **Genetics:** There is a strong genetic contribution to the development of schizophrenia. It is evident by the fact that the first-degree relatives of schizophrenia patients are more likely to develop schizophrenia than the control group, and the rate of occurrence decreases in the second-degree relatives and further drops in the third-degree relatives. Since genetic sharing also decreases as one goes from first-degree relatives to third-degree relatives, it is hypothesised that genetics play an important role. This hypothesis is further strengthened by a much higher prevalence rate in monozygotic twins of schizophrenia patients (monozygotic concordance rate) in comparison to the dizygotic twins of schizophrenia patients (dizygotic concordance rate).
2. At the same time, it must be remembered that most cases of schizophrenia in the general population are sporadic and have no affected family members.
3. It appears that schizophrenia has polygenic inheritance with multiple genes involved and all adding to susceptibility by small to moderate effects. Linkage studies have found linkage to the following chromosomal sites: 1q, 2q, 5q, 6p, 6q, 8p, 10p, 13q, 15q and 22q.
4. The candidate genes for which most evidence is available include NRG1 (neuregulin 1), DTNBP1 (dystrobrevin-binding protein 1 gene, or dysbindin), DISC1 (disrupted in schizophrenia), RGS4 (regulator of G protein signalling), COMT (catechol-o-methyl transferase) and GRM3 (glutamate metabotropic receptor 3).

SCHIZOPHRENIA AND 22Q11.2 DELETION SYNDROME

22q11.2 deletion syndrome (DiGeorge syndrome, velocardiofacial syndrome) is a genetic syndrome associated with hemizygous 22q11.2 deletions (i.e., on one chromosome 22). Its manifestations include mild facial dysmorphic features, velopharyngeal insufficiency, submucous cleft palate, hypernasal speech, cardiac defects, learning difficulties and late-onset manifestations such as psychiatric disorders that commonly include schizophrenia. Around 1% of the patients with schizophrenia have 22q11.2 deletion syndrome, and this is the only genetic form of schizophrenia that is clinically recognisable and can be confirmed by genetic testing.

NATURE VERSUS NURTURE

The fact that there is a familial aggregation of schizophrenia alone does not prove that it is genetically transmitted. It has been argued that the fact that schizophrenia runs in families, could be explained in two different ways:
1. Schizophrenia is genetically transmitted and hence runs in families (nature).
2. The way of the upbringing of children is such in certain families that it results in the development of schizophrenia (nurture).

Adoption studies have helped in separating the effects of genetics from upbringing. It has been found that children who were born to mothers with schizophrenia and were adopted away soon after the birth (hence eliminating any effects of upbringing by mothers with schizophrenia) still had much higher rates of development of schizophrenia compared with children who did not have any family history of schizophrenia and were adopted away soon after birth. These studies indicate that familial aggregation is because of genetic transmission rather than the effects of upbringing. Twin study results also support the same inference.

Environmental Factors

While genetic factors increase the vulnerability to the development of schizophrenia, interaction with environmental factors appears to be necessary to precipitate the illness.

The following environmental factors are relevant:
a. **Obstetric complications:** Patients who have schizophrenia are more likely to have a history of pre and perinatal complications, such as low birth weight, prematurity, resuscitation at birth, etc., in comparison to controls. It has been hypothesised that hypoxic-ischaemic damage could be the mechanism that increases the risk of the development of schizophrenia later in life. Severe prenatal malnutrition has also been hypothesised to increase the risk.
b. **Season of birth and maternal exposure to infection:** Studies have shown that patients with schizophrenia are more likely to be born in late winter and spring. One of the hypotheses to explain this observation is that respiratory infections like influenza tend to occur in autumn and winter, and it is actually the viral infection that increases the risk of the development of schizophrenia later in life. Many studies have suggested maternal exposure to

influenza during the second trimester as a risk factor; however other studies have found no such risk. Apart from influenza, few studies have also found maternal infection with rubella to increase the risk; however, there is no conclusive evidence as yet.
c. **Childhood risk factors:** Studies have found that individuals who later develop schizophrenia are more likely to have poorer motor development, speech difficulties, delayed milestones and lower premorbid (premorbid means before the illness) IQ in their childhood than the control group. This finding supports that subtle brain abnormalities (which may be genetic or environmental in origin) mediate the development of schizophrenia.
d. **Social and geographical risk factors:** Studies have found that the incidence of schizophrenia is higher amongst those who grew up in **urban areas** than in rural areas. The underlying mechanism is yet not clear. Patients with schizophrenia are more likely to belong to lower socioeconomic status (social drift hypothesis).
e. **Immigration:** Studies have found that both first-generation migrants and second-generation migrants have an increased risk of developing schizophrenia, especially for migrants from lower socioeconomic countries and blacks moving into predominantly white societies.
f. **Drug abuse:** Use of illicit substances is much more prevalent in patients with schizophrenia than in controls. Recent research suggests that **cannabis use** can be a causal factor in some cases of schizophrenia.

Neurobiology

Abnormalities in multiple neurotransmitters have been implicated in the development of schizophrenia.
a. **Dopamine:** The most extensively investigated neurotransmitter in schizophrenia is dopamine. The current hypothesis says that the positive symptoms of schizophrenia are caused by a **hyperdopaminergic** state in the **mesolimbic tract** (a tract that connects the ventral tegmental area to the nucleus accumbens), and the negative symptoms of schizophrenia are caused by a **hypodopaminergic state** in the **mesocortical tract** (a tract that connects the ventral tegmental area to the prefrontal cortex). The efficacy of the antipsychotics, most of which are dopamine antagonists, supports the dopamine hypothesis.
b. **Serotonin:** Apart from dopamine, an excess of serotonin has also been hypothesised to be involved in the development of schizophrenia. Again, the efficacy of atypical antipsychotics, which act as serotonin antagonists in addition to dopamine antagonists, supports the serotonin hypothesis.
c. Other neurotransmitters which have shown some evidence of involvement include glutamate, GABA, norepinephrine, acetylcholine, nicotine and neuropeptides.

Neuroanatomical and Neuropathological Factors

Various anatomical structures have been found to be abnormal structurally or functionally in patients with schizophrenia; however, it has not been possible to precisely localise the neuroanatomical abnormalities in schizophrenia. Some of the findings include:
- **Cerebral ventricles:** One of the fairly consistent findings is a reduction in cortical grey matter volume and enlargement of ventricles size (especially lateral and third ventricles). However, it must be remembered that though the increase in ventricular size is statistically significant, it is not grossly enlarged in most cases. And it is still not possible to use these findings for any diagnostic purposes.
- **Limbic system:** Limbic system is a set of brain structures, which have important functions, and includes the hippocampus (memory), anterior cingulate (attention), amygdala (emotions) and entorhinal cortex. Many studies have found a reduced size of these structures in patients with schizophrenia.
- **Prefrontal cortex:** It is the most anterior part of the cortex, and many studies have found decreased blood flow and decreased glucose utilisation in the prefrontal cortex in patients with schizophrenia (known as **hypofrontality in schizophrenia**)
- **Basal ganglia and cerebellum:** These structures are involved in controlling movements. Patients with schizophrenia often have abnormal movements such as stereotypies, mannerisms, etc. It appears that basal ganglia and cerebellum disturbances are related to these motor abnormalities. Further, it must be remembered that antipsychotic-induced movement disorders (a common side effect of antipsychotics) are also caused by the blockade of dopamine receptors in basal ganglia.

Other structures in which abnormalities have been found include the thalamus (neuronal loss, especially in the medial dorsal nucleus of the thalamus) and superior temporal gyrus (superior temporal gyrus is involved in auditory processing and its disturbances appear to be the reason for the development of auditory hallucinations).

Of late, it has been hypothesised that schizophrenia is caused by disturbances of neural circuits rather than dysfunction of discrete brain areas. According to preliminary research, the neural circuit linking the prefrontal cortex and limbic system appears to be involved in the development of schizophrenia.

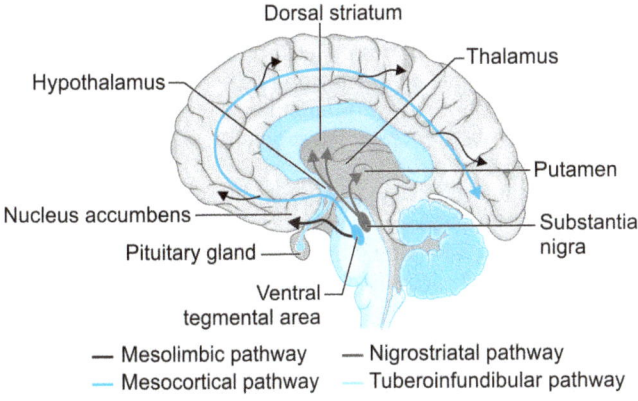

Fig. 2.2: Tracts in schizophrenia.

Electrophysiology

The study of changes in the brain's electrical activity in response to a stimulus has shown that in schizophrenia, various electrophysiological deficits are present. These deficits suggest an abnormality in information processing. Usually, in EEG, a wave called the **P300 wave** is seen about 300 milliseconds after a sensory stimulus. In patients with schizophrenia, this wave is smaller and suggests abnormal stimulus processing. Also, many patients have abnormalities in eye movement, especially smooth visual pursuit (the ability to follow a moving visual target), which again suggests abnormalities in neural pathways responsible for oculomotor control.

SOFT SIGNS IN SCHIZOPHRENIA

Soft signs are the neurological signs that do not localise the pathology and are elicited after a detailed neurological evaluation. Patients with schizophrenia often have soft signs such as astereognosis, dysdiadochokinesia, diminished dexterity and the presence of primitive reflexes.

TYPES

ICD-10 described the following types of schizophrenia.

Paranoid Schizophrenia

This clinical type is characterised by predominantly positive symptoms, i.e., hallucinations and delusions. It is the **most common type** of schizophrenia. It has a **late-onset (i.e., in the third or early fourth decade)** and a **good prognosis**. The **personality** is **usually preserved** (i.e., the person can maintain daily activities and social interactions normally).

Catatonic Schizophrenia

This clinical type is dominated by catatonic (motor) symptoms and has the **best prognosis** of all types.

Hebephrenic (Disorganised) Schizophrenia

This type is dominated by prominent disorganisation symptoms and negative symptoms. It has an **early onset (usually second decade)** and a **bad prognosis**. There is **severe deterioration of personality** (patient cannot maintain hygiene, social interactions are inappropriate, and odd behaviours such as giggling and mirror-gazing are often present).

Undifferentiated Schizophrenia

The schizophrenia not conforming to any of the above types or exhibiting features of more than one of the types is classified as undifferentiated schizophrenia.

Post Schizophrenic Depression

A depressive episode that develops after a schizophrenic illness. Some schizophrenic symptoms are still present but are no longer prominent. This disorder is associated with an **increased risk of suicide**.

Residual Schizophrenia

Residual schizophrenia is characterised by progression from an early stage (with prominent delusions and hallucinations) to a later stage where the delusions and hallucinations have become minimal and mostly negative symptoms are present.

Simple Schizophrenia

Simple schizophrenia has an insidious onset, and gradually negative symptoms develop and predominate the clinical picture. The delusions and hallucinations are not present. There is a significant behaviour change that manifests as loss of interest, idleness, aimlessness, a self-absorbed attitude and social withdrawal. These changes should be present for at least **1 year** before the diagnosis can be made.

DSM-5 AND ICD-11 CLASSIFICATION

The DSM-IV described multiple subtypes of schizophrenia similar to the above-mentioned ICD-10 subtypes. However, recent research has shown that these subtypes are not associated with different pathophysiology or prognoses and are not stable over time (e.g., a patient diagnosed with paranoid schizophrenia may show prominent motor symptoms later on and maybe diagnosed with catatonic schizophrenia later). Both ICD-11 and DSM-5 have **removed** the subtyping based on symptoms.

The types of schizophrenia that have been described in ICD-11 are according to the course of illness and include:

a. *Schizophrenia, first episode:* If a patient meets diagnostic criteria of schizophrenia and there have been no past episodes
b. *Schizophrenia, multiple episodes:* If a patient meets diagnostic criteria of schizophrenia, and there has been at least one episode in the past. Between the last and current episode, there was significant remission of symptoms
c. *Schizophrenia, continuous:* If a patient has been fulfilling the diagnostic criteria of schizophrenia for almost the entire duration of the illness (duration should be >1 year).

ICD-11 UPDATE

In ICD-11, Catatonia has been made a separate diagnostic category. The diagnosis of catatonia is made in the presence of significant motor symptoms or catatonic symptoms. It has been further divided into the following groups:
- Catatonia associated with another mental disorder (e.g., catatonia associated with schizophrenia, mood disorders or autism spectrum disorder)
- Catatonia induced by use of psychoactive substances (drugs of abuse) and medications

So, a patient who would have gotten the diagnosis of catatonic schizophrenia according to ICD-10 would get a diagnosis of Catatonia associated with schizophrenia according to ICD-11.

OTHER CLASSIFICATIONS

Apart from ICD and DSM classifications, many other classifications have been used historically, and though rarely used now, they still deserve mention.

Type I and II Schizophrenia

TJ Crow attempted to find a relation between the symptoms of schizophrenia and the underlying neuropathology. He reported two syndromes in schizophrenia, called Type I and Type II schizophrenia. The differences between the two are summarised below:

	Type I	Type II
Characteristic symptoms	Positive symptoms	Negative symptoms
Response to antipsychotics	Good	Poor
Prognosis	Good	Poor
Underlying pathology (postulated)	Increased dopamine	Structural changes in brain manifested as dilatation of ventricles

Though this distinction between Type I and Type II is currently not used, it was an important classification as it attempted to establish the neuropathological basis of symptoms.

Pseudoneurotic Schizophrenia

The diagnosis of pseudo neurotic schizophrenia was used for patients who had significant anxiety symptoms, also called **pananxiety** (i.e., persistent anxiety symptoms), many neurotic symptoms, also called **panneurosis** (neurotic symptoms such as phobia, etc.) and preoccupation with sexual problems, also called **pansexuality**. It was found that these patients may later develop psychotic symptoms. Now, this diagnosis is no longer used. In the current classificatory system, these patients would be diagnosed with borderline personality disorder.

Pfropf Schizophrenia

This diagnosis was used when schizophrenia developed in a patient with **mental retardation**. Since their intelligence was limited, these patients would not have well-developed delusions or hallucinations; instead, the presentation was mostly with behavioural symptoms like aggression etc.

Van Gogh Syndrome

This diagnosis was used for schizophrenia patients who indulged in self-mutilation (injuring self). The syndrome is named after a famous painter, Vincent van Gogh who is believed to be suffering from schizophrenia and had cut off his left ear during the active phase of his illness.

COURSE AND OUTCOME IN SCHIZOPHRENIA

Course

The course of schizophrenia varies. The studies suggest that the patients may have one of the following courses:
1. A single psychotic episode followed by complete remission (no symptoms left and no further episodes)
2. A single psychotic episode followed by incomplete remission (symptoms improve partially however no other full-fledged episode)
3. Two or more episodes with complete remission between the episodes
4. Two or more episodes with incomplete remission between the episodes
5. Continuous illness (no remission achieved ever)

Long-term Outcomes

Schizophrenia is often believed to be a chronic, deteriorating illness with invariably poor outcomes; however, the research does not support this pessimistic view. Many long term studies that involved follow-up of patients with schizophrenia for many years (in some studies for >30 years) have shown that a significant proportion of patients have favourable outcomes. Although the results vary amongst the studies, they have shown a similar trend. Around 15–25% of the patients achieve **recovery (complete cure)**, about 43% show **significant improvement** with mild residual abnormalities that did not interfere with their living, around 44% had s**ignificant symptoms** that required the patients to be hospitalised, and around 14–15% developed a severe and chronic illness.

One of the long-term follow-up studies conducted in India, called **SOFACOS (study of factors associated with the course and outcome of schizophrenia)**, had similar findings. In this study, 27% of patients had a **very favourable outcome**, 40% had a **favourable outcome**, 31% had an **intermediate outcome**, and only 2% had an **unfavourable outcome**.

The **World Health Organisation** has also carried out studies across the countries on the course and outcome of schizophrenia. These included the **International Pilot Study on Schizophrenia (IPSS), Determinants of Outcome of Severe Mental Disorders (DOSMED)** (DOSMED is also known as the 10 country study) and **International Study of Schizophrenia (ISoS)**.

One of the most interesting findings of IPSS and DOSMED was that the outcome of schizophrenia patients was **better** in developing countries compared to developed countries. It was found that the patients in developing countries had more frequent remissions, and the duration of remission was longer in comparison to patients in developed countries. The better outcome appears to be a combination of genetic factors and sociocultural factors, such as better integration of the patient into the traditional social structure that minimises social isolation in developing countries and lesser **expressed emotions** in the families in developing countries.

> **EXPRESSED EMOTIONS**
>
> Expressed emotions refer to the emotions/attitudes expressed by close relatives towards a family member who has schizophrenia or other psychiatric illnesses. The negative expressed emotions include **over-involvement, criticism** and **hostility** towards the patient. It has been found that high expressed emotions predict a poorer outcome with an increased risk of relapse.

> **DURATION OF UNTREATED PSYCHOSIS**
>
> Duration of untreated psychosis (DUP) is the duration between the onset of psychotic symptoms and initiation of the treatment. It is correlated with the outcome of the illness, with longer DUPs predicting a poorer outcome.

DIFFERENTIAL DIAGNOSIS

Psychiatric Disorders

Psychiatric disorders that can present with delusions, hallucinations or catatonic features must be carefully ruled out before making the diagnosis of schizophrenia. These include:
1. Major depression with psychotic or catatonic features
2. Bipolar disorder with psychotic or catatonic features
3. Schizoaffective disorders, schizophreniform disorders and acute psychotic disorders
4. Delusional disorders
5. Schizotypal personality disorders
6. Obsessive-compulsive disorders with poor insight/psychotic symptoms
7. Autism spectrum disorder

Medical and Neurological Disorders

Psychotic symptoms may be a feature of the intoxication/withdrawal of certain substances. Many neurological disorders can present with psychotic symptoms too.
1. Substance-induced-cannabis, amphetamines, hallucinogens, cocaine, alcoholic hallucinosis, phencyclidine, barbiturate withdrawal
2. Epilepsy (particularly temporal lobe epilepsy)
3. Other neurological disorders such as Wilson's disease, Huntington's chorea, Systemic lupus erythematosus, etc.

MANAGEMENT

Antipsychotics (neuroleptics) are the mainstay of treatment in schizophrenia. Along with pharmacological treatment, psychosocial modalities are being increasingly used to improve the outcome in patients.

The treatment of schizophrenia can be divided into three phases:
a. **Acute phase:** In this phase patient is either in the first psychotic episode or is in relapse after prior remission. There are prominent psychotic symptoms, and the patient may be aggressive and violent. The treatment focuses on controlling symptoms and ensuring the safety of the patient and others. This stage usually lasts from **4 to 8 weeks**.
b. **Stabilisation phase:** Once the patient's acute symptoms are controlled, the patient enters the stabilisation phase. The patient continues to be at risk of relapse if medications are discontinued. The focus is to consolidate the therapeutic gains. This stage may continue for around **6 months**.
c. **Stable or maintenance phase:** After the stabilisation phase, the patient enters the stable phase. In this stage, the patient is in remission, and symptoms have significantly improved. The focus is to maintain the remission and help in rehabilitation and social integration.

Pharmacotherapy

The first antipsychotic, chlorpromazine, was introduced in 1952, and since then, many newer molecules have been developed. The use of antipsychotics helps achieve remission in around 70% of patients with schizophrenia.

In the acute phase, usually, **second-generation antipsychotics** are preferred as these have a better side effect profile than the first-generation antipsychotics. However, in certain patients, such as those who had shown a good response to first-generation antipsychotics in the previous episodes, first-generation antipsychotics can be used as the first choice. Antipsychotics work better on the positive symptoms (hallucinations and delusions) and have a lesser impact on negative and cognitive symptoms.

In highly agitated patients, where the rapid onset of action is required, the **intramuscular preparations** of antipsychotics are used. Along with antipsychotics, adjunctive medications are often used in the acute phase, such as benzodiazepines for agitation management and anticholinergics like promethazine to manage extrapyramidal side effects associated with antipsychotics and beta-blockers like propranolol for management of **akathisia** (a common side effect of antipsychotics).

With the advent of effective pharmacotherapy, the role of hospitalisation has decreased; nonetheless, hospitalisation should be done in case there is—a danger to the safety of the patient or others, in the presence of extreme agitation, severe side effects of drugs or significant disturbances of biological functions such as sleep and appetite.

Once the symptoms are under control, the stabilisation phase starts. The treatment is continued with the same medication in the same dosages in the stabilisation phase, along with monitoring of side effects.

In the **stable phase**, the continuation of antipsychotics has been found to decrease the relapse rate. Most of the guidelines do not give any definitive duration till which antipsychotics should be continued. A common practice is continuing antipsychotics for one to two years after the first episode of schizophrenia (**usually 2 years**).

For patients with multiple episodes, the treatment should continue for at least five years, and treatment for an indefinite duration may be preferred in many cases.

Antipsychotics

Antipsychotics are the mainstay of treatment for psychotic disorders like schizophrenia, schizoaffective disorders, delusional disorders and others. Antipsychotics have been divided into two classes: (1) Typical antipsychotics, and (2) Atypical antipsychotics.

Typical Antipsychotics or First-generation Antipsychotics or Dopamine Receptor Antagonists (DRAs)

These were the first drugs found to be useful in treating schizophrenia. The first antipsychotic drug, chlorpromazine, was discovered accidentally in the early 1950s. Henri Laborit, a surgeon, had used chlorpromazine to decrease preoperative anxiety in his patients and found that after taking chlorpromazine, patients became quite relaxed and indifferent to the environment. Following this finding, Delay and Deniker used this molecule in patients with schizophrenia and mania and found it to be useful, and this started the journey of modern psychopharmacology.

The typical antipsychotics can be further classified according to chemical groups, as described below:
- **Phenothiazines:** Chlorpromazine, thioridazine, trifluoperazine, prochlorperazine, triflupromazine, fluphenazine, perphenazine
- **Thioxanthenes:** Thiothixene, flupenthixol
- **Butyrophenones:** Haloperidol, droperidol, penfluridol
- **Miscellaneous:** Pimozide, loxapine, molindone.

The typical antipsychotics can also be classified as **low potency (like chlorpromazine, thioridazine)** and **high potency (like haloperidol and fluphenazine)**. Apart from differing potency, the low potency and high potency antipsychotics also differ in their side effects profile.

Mechanism of action: The typical antipsychotics are effective against positive symptoms but have minimal effect on negative symptoms. The therapeutic effect of typical antipsychotics is mediated by a blockade of dopamine-2 (D2) receptors in the **mesolimbic tract (pathway which connects the ventral tegmental area to the nucleus accumbens)**. It has been found that approximately **70%** of D2 receptors need to be blocked for clinical effects to be seen. While the D2 blockade in the mesolimbic tract is therapeutic, D2 receptors blockade in **the nigrostriatal pathway (pathway from substantial nigra to striatum)** is responsible for the extrapyramidal side effects of these medications. It has been found that the optimal dose of typical antipsychotics is at the "extrapyramidal symptoms threshold", i.e., the dose at which extrapyramidal side effects start to appear. Apart from dopamine receptors, typical antipsychotics also block cholinergic, noradrenergic and histaminergic receptors, and these actions mediate many side effects of these drugs.

> The first-line treatment for catatonic schizophrenia (catatonia associated with schizophrenia) includes **intravenous lorazepam** and **electroconvulsive therapy,** unlike other types which are treated with antipsychotics.

Pharmacokinetics: The typical antipsychotics are well absorbed when administered orally and reach peak levels in around one to four hours. When administered intramuscularly, the peak levels are reached in about 30–60 minutes, and this helps in the rapid onset of action as is needed in a patient with acute agitation. The half-life of most typical antipsychotics is around 24 hours. Most typical antipsychotics are metabolised in the liver by cytochrome P450 2D6 and P450 3A.

Side effects: The common side effects of typical antipsychotics are as follows

Movement disorders: The antipsychotics can cause various movement disorders, collectively referred to as **extrapyramidal symptoms** (or **extrapyramidal side effects**). These side effects are caused by the blockade of dopamine receptors in the **nigrostriatal tract** (neural pathway from substantia nigra to striatum). The movement disorders are **more commonly** seen with typical antipsychotics than atypical antipsychotics. Amongst typical antipsychotics, high potency typical antipsychotics are **more likely to** cause these side effects. The movement disorders can be of the following types:
- **Acute dystonia:** It is the **earliest side effect** of antipsychotics and can be seen within minutes of receiving an injectable antipsychotic (oral antipsychotics can also cause acute dystonia, though it is less likely). It is characterised by a **sudden contraction** of a muscle group resulting in symptoms like **torticollis**, trismus (contraction of jaw muscles), **deviation of eyeballs** (oculogyric crisis due to contraction of extraocular muscles), laryngospasm, etc. The management includes immediate administration of parenteral **anticholinergics** like benztropine, promethazine or **diphenhydramine**. To prevent acute dystonia, prophylactic use of oral anticholinergics is suggested while prescribing typical antipsychotics.

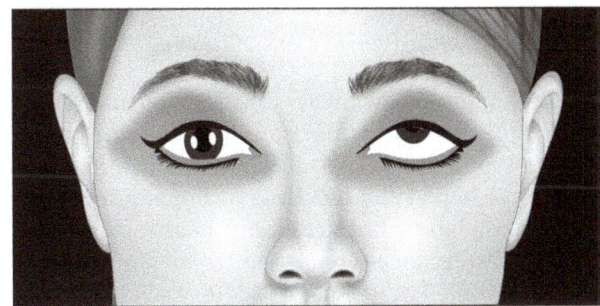

Fig. 2.3: Oculogyric crisis.

- **Acute akathisia:** It is the **commonest side** effect of antipsychotics and is characterised by an **inner sense of restlessness** along with **objective**, **observable movements** such as **fidgeting** of legs, **pacing around, and inability to sit** or **stand** in one place for a long time. The treatment options include beta-blockers such as propranolol (**drug of choice**), **anticholinergics** and **benzodiazepines**. The antipsychotic can also be changed to second-generation or low potency first-generation antipsychotics, as they are less likely to cause akathisia.
- **Drug-induced parkinsonism:** It is characterised by the triad of rigidity, bradykinesia and resting tremors.

The treatment options include using anticholinergics or a change of antipsychotics to second-generation or low potency first-generation antipsychotics. Dose reduction can also be tried. Often, the use of prophylactic anticholinergics prevents the development of drug-induced parkinsonism.

- **Tardive dyskinesia:** The term "tardive" refers to features that develop after prolonged exposure. Tardive dyskinesia develops after **long term** treatment with antipsychotics. It can present as involuntary movements of the **tongue** (e.g., twisting, protrusion), **jaw** (e.g., chewing), **lips** (e.g., smacking, puckering), trunk or extremities. Patients may also have rapid, jerky movements (choreiform movements) or slow, sinusoid movements (athetoid movements). It has been hypothesised that long term use of antipsychotics and accompanying blockade of D2 receptors results in D2 receptors up-regulation along with postsynaptic **dopamine receptor supersensitivity**, which results in the development of tardive dyskinesia. The management usually includes shifting to a second-generation antipsychotic medication. The dopamine depleting drugs which inhibit vesicular monoamine transporter (the transport protein which transports monoamines, including dopamine, into the synaptic vesicles) at the presynaptic membrane of the nerve terminal and hence result in decreased release of dopamine at the synapse are considered as first-line treatment in treating severe or disabling tardive dyskinesia. Currently, three drugs are available in this class—**Deutetrabenazine, Tetrabenazine, Valbenazine**
- **Neuroleptic malignant syndrome (NMS):** It is a fatal side effect of antipsychotics. It is characterised by **muscle rigidity, elevated temperature (>38°C), and increased CPK (creatine phosphokinase) levels**. The other symptoms include diaphoresis, tremors, confusion, autonomic disturbances, liver enzyme elevation and **leukocytosis**.

The pathophysiology involves D2 antagonism at various levels. The D2 receptors blockade in the corpus striatum causes muscle contraction and rigidity that initiates heat generation, whereas the blockade of dopamine receptors in the hypothalamus interferes with heat regulation. The autonomic disturbances are caused by dopamine blockade in spinal neurons. The increased CPK levels indicate muscle injury.

The early recognition of symptoms and prompt withdrawal of antipsychotics are of paramount importance; otherwise, the continuing muscle damage can cause **myoglobinuria** and **renal failure**.

The treatment includes skeletal muscle relaxants like **dantrolene**. Dopamine agonists such as amantadine and bromocriptine are also useful. Supportive measures, including adequate hydration, are also crucial in the management.

When drug treatment with antipsychotics needs to be restarted after recovery from NMS, second-generation antipsychotics are preferred.

Endocrine side effects: The blockage of dopamine receptors in the **tuberoinfundibular tract** results in **hyperprolactinaemia** (remember dopamine inhibits prolactin secretion, and hence dopamine blockade causes hyperprolactinaemia) and can cause galactorrhea, menstrual disturbances in females and sexual disorders including low libido and erectile dysfunction in males.

Sedation (due to blockade of histamine H1 receptors), orthostatic hypotension (due to blockade of adrenergic alpha 1 receptors) and anticholinergic side effects are usually seen with low potency typical antipsychotics such as chlorpromazine and thioridazine.

Cardiac side effects: Typical antipsychotics may cause cardiac toxicity by decreasing cardiac contractility, decreasing atrial and ventricular conduction and may cause arrhythmias, including torsades de pointes. Usually, these side effects are more common with low potency typical antipsychotics. Pimozide and haloperidol are known to cause QTc prolongation.

CNS side effects: Typical antipsychotics can lower the seizure threshold, and this side effect is more common with low potency drugs such as chlorpromazine and thioridazine

Miscellaneous: Other side effects include weight gain, hematologic side effects such as leucopenia, rarely agranulocytosis, thrombocytopenia and pancytopenia, sexual side effects like decreased libido, erectile and ejaculatory dysfunction and anorgasmia. Photosensitivity reactions can occur with chlorpromazine, and long term use of chlorpromazine may cause blue-grey discolouration of skin in areas exposed to the sun. **Chlorpromazine** use may also cause reversible corneal and lenticular deposits, and **thioridazine** may cause irreversible retinal pigmentation.

Atypical Antipsychotics or Second-generation Antipsychotics or Serotonin Dopamine Antagonists

Two clinical properties make an antipsychotic "atypical". First, low incidence of extrapyramidal side effects and second, efficacy against negative symptoms in addition to the positive symptoms.

Pharmacologically, the atypical antipsychotics differ from typical by antagonism at serotonin receptors (5HT2) along with the dopamine receptors. These drugs have a higher ratio of 5HT2 to D2 blockade compared to typicals, and the lesser D2 blockade is responsible for a lesser risk of extrapyramidal side effects and hyperprolactinaemia. The following drugs are classified as atypical antipsychotics:
- Clozapine
- Olanzapine
- Risperidone
- Paliperidone
- Iloperidone
- Quetiapine
- Ziprasidone
- Aripiprazole
- Sertindole

- Zotepine
- Lurasidone
- Asenapine
- Amisulpride
- Brepiprazole
- Cariprazine
- Pimavanserin

NEWER ANTIPSYCHOTICS

- **Brexpiprazole:** It is an atypical antipsychotic that acts as a partial agonist at D2 and 5HT1A receptors and an antagonist at 5HT2A receptor.
- **Cariprazine:** It is an atypical antipsychotic that acts as a partial agonist at D2, D3 and 5HT1A receptors and an antagonist at the 5HT2A receptor. However, unlike aripiprazole and brexpiprazole, cariprazine exhibits a higher affinity for the D3 receptor than the D2 receptor.
- **Pimavanserin:** It is the first FDA approved drug to treat delusions and hallucinations in Parkinson's disease-associated psychosis. Pimavanserin has a combination of inverse agonist and antagonist activity at 5HT2A receptors (and, to a lesser extent, at 5HT2C receptors). It does not bind to D2 receptors. It can increase the QT interval.

Apart from blocking D2 and 5-HT2 receptors (primarily 5-HT2A subtype), the atypical antipsychotics have varying actions on other dopamine receptors, serotonin receptors, muscarinic, adrenergic and histaminic receptors.

All the atypical antipsychotics are well absorbed after oral administration (asenapine is taken sublingually as when swallowed, its bioavailability is extremely poor). Metabolism in liver is by CYP1A2 (for olanzapine and clozapine), CYP2D6 (for risperidone, clozapine, olanzapine and aripiprazole) and CYP3A4 (for clozapine, quetiapine, ziprasidone, sertindole, aripiprazole and zotepine). When antipsychotics are given concomitantly with inhibitors or inducers of cytochrome P enzyme, appropriate adjustments in dosages are required. Of particular importance is the need to adjust the dosage of clozapine and olanzapine in smokers as smoking induces CYP1A2.

Side effects: The side effect profile of atypical antipsychotics is as follows:

A. **Movement disorders:** Atypical antipsychotics can cause all types of extrapyramidal side effects described earlier; however, the incidence is lesser than the typical antipsychotics. **Clozapine** is least likely to cause extrapyramidal side effects. Aripiprazole is rarely associated with acute dystonia, drug-induced parkinsonism or neuroleptic malignant syndrome, but aripiprazole can often cause akathisia.
B. **Endocrine side effects:** The incidence of hyperprolactinaemia is also lesser with atypical antipsychotics (except **risperidone** and amisulpride, which have a comparatively higher incidence).
C. Weight gain and increased risk of dyslipidaemia, diabetes and cardiovascular disease are more commonly seen with atypical antipsychotics than with typical antipsychotics. Amongst atypicals, clozapine and olanzapine have the highest incidence of metabolic side effects.
D. Other side effects include nausea, vomiting, dyspepsia, postural hypotension, sedation, **and QTc prolongation (especially with ziprasidone).**
E. FDA has given a black box warning of increased mortality in patients with dementia treated with atypical antipsychotics. FDA warned of increased risk of stroke in such patients. However, this risk appears to be small, and the benefits of antipsychotics, especially in patients with dementia with behavioural problems, outweigh any risks involved.

Clozapine

It was the first atypical antipsychotic to be developed. Clozapine is the drug of choice in treatment-resistant schizophrenia.

Clozapine has a unique mechanism of action. Unlike other antipsychotics, it has a relatively low affinity for D2 receptors. Its low affinity for D2 receptors explains the lack of extrapyramidal side effects with clozapine. Clozapine has a strong affinity for **D4 receptors** and also acts as an antagonist at 5-HT2A, D1, D3 and α (alpha) adrenergic receptors. The lack of extrapyramidal symptoms makes clozapine a preferred antipsychotic in patients intolerant to other antipsychotics because of extrapyramidal side effects, including tardive dyskinesia. Clozapine is the only antipsychotic that decreases suicidal ideation in patients with schizophrenia who have been previously hospitalised for suicidality.

TREATMENT-RESISTANT SCHIZOPHRENIA

The most widely accepted definition of treatment-resistant schizophrenia is "lack of response to at least two different antipsychotics, including at least one second-generation antipsychotic, given in adequate dosages (400–600 mg chlorpromazine equivalent) and for an adequate duration (at least 4–6 weeks)". **Clozapine** is the **drug of choice** for patients with **treatment-resistant schizophrenia.**

Treatment with clozapine is started at a very low dose (12.5–25 mg/day) and is gradually increased, with 300–600 mg/day being the effective dose for most patients. A clozapine plasma level of 250–350 ng/mL is considered a reasonable target for most patients, although few studies have found that levels >350 ng/mL are associated with better response rates.

Side effects: The common side effects of clozapine include sialorrhea, sedation, syncope, hypotension, tachycardia, nausea and vomiting. Other side effects include weight gain (clozapine causes the highest weight gain amongst all antipsychotics), constipation, and anticholinergic side effects. Clozapine can also cause life-threatening side effects, including agranulocytosis, seizures and myocarditis. Agranulocytosis and myocarditis are dose-independent side effects of clozapine, whereas seizures are dose-dependent (seen only at higher dosages).

ANC monitoring: Due to the possibility of life-threatening agranulocytosis, a minimum absolute neutrophil count (ANC) ≥1,500/µL is required to start clozapine. After starting clozapine, ANC monitoring must be regularly continued at the following intervals:
- Weekly during the first 6 months of clozapine administration
- Once in 2 weeks for the next 6 months
- Once every 4 weeks after one year, till clozapine treatment is continued

If neutropenia develops during treatment, the following action must be taken:
- **Mild neutropenia (ANC: 1,000–1,499/µL):** Continue treatment but increase ANC monitoring to three times a week
- **Moderate neutropenia (ANC: 500–999/µL):** Stop clozapine treatment, monitor ANC daily till ANC is 1,000/µL, at which point clozapine can be restarted
- **Severe neutropenia/agranulocytosis (ANC: <500/µL):** Discontinue clozapine. Clozapine can only be restarted in these cases if the benefits significantly outweigh the risks.

The contraindications to clozapine use include a **WBC count of <3,500/dL** at the time of starting clozapine, a history of agranulocytosis during clozapine treatment or use of another drug that is known to suppress the bone marrow (e.g., clozapine and carbamazepine cannot be given together as both are bone marrow suppressants)

POOR COMPLIANCE WITH ANTIPSYCHOTICS

Poor compliance with antipsychotics is common, and around 50% of patients become non-compliant within 1–2 years. In such patients, long-acting injectable antipsychotics (depot antipsychotics) can be used to improve adherence to the treatment. Patients typically receive **intramuscular injections** of antipsychotics once a month or once a fortnight. **The Z track technique** is used to give the intramuscular injection. The aim is to deposit the antipsychotic in the muscle and prevent its seepage into the subcutaneous tissue. In this technique, the skin and tissue are pulled towards one side and held firmly while the injection is given, and after removing the needle, the skin and the tissue are released. This technique prevents tracking (leakage) of the medication into the subcutaneous tissue as the track that the needle forms is zig zag, and the drug cannot come out through it.

Long-acting injectable preparations are available for the following antipsychotics:
- Flupenthixol
- Fluphenazine
- Haloperidol
- Pipotiazine
- Zuclopenthixol
- Risperidone
- Olanzapine
- Paliperidone
- Aripiprazole

Electroconvulsive therapy: Electroconvulsive therapy is one of the first-line treatments for catatonic schizophrenia **(catatonia associated with schizophrenia)**. It has similar short-term efficacy as antipsychotics in other types of schizophrenia. However, due to ease of administration, antipsychotics have become the first-line treatment and are preferred over electroconvulsive therapy. Electroconvulsive therapy is used if the patient is unresponsive/intolerant to medications.

Electroconvulsive therapy is not effective in the treatment of chronic symptoms.

PSYCHOSOCIAL TREATMENT

Apart from medications, psychological and social interventions are effective in treating schizophrenia, especially after the acute phase is treated with medications. The following psychosocial treatments can be used:

a. **Family interventions:** The patient's family is involved with a focus on illness education, coping with the illness and providing emotional support to the entire family.
b. **Supported employment:** An attempt is made to help the patient get employment while providing ongoing support.
c. **Assertive community treatment:** It involves reaching out to the patient in the community and providing necessary support.
d. **Skills training:** The focus is on improving skills, especially the patient's social skills.
e. **Cognitive behavioural therapy:** It involves the use of cognitive behavioural therapy for managing residual symptoms (the symptoms that have not responded to medicine). Another therapy, called **cognitive remediation therapy** (or cognitive enhancement therapy), focuses on the improvement of cognitive functions (such as attention and concentration, working memory, etc.) and has shown promising results in patients with schizophrenia.
f. **Token economy:** Mostly used in inpatient settings, it involves the use of tokens, which are given to patients, when they indulge in desirable behaviours (like remaining calm, taking medicines regularly etc.). Patients can redeem the tokens to get material items or privileges.

PROGNOSIS

The prognosis in schizophrenia depends on various factors. Following are the important prognostic factors:
- **Good prognostic factors:**
  - Acute or abrupt onset
  - Later onset (age >35 years)
  - Female sex
  - Prominent positive symptoms
  - Presence of affective symptoms (such as depression)
  - Family history of mood disorder.
- **Bad prognostic factors:**
  - Insidious onset
  - Early-onset (age <20 years)
  - Male sex

- Prominent negative symptoms
- Absence of affective symptoms
- Family history of schizophrenia.

OTHER PSYCHOTIC DISORDERS

Schizoaffective Disorder

Schizoaffective disorder presents with features of both schizophrenia and mood disorders and has a prominence of both psychotic and affective symptoms. The following conditions should be met to make a diagnosis of the schizoaffective disorder according to DSM-5:

1. There should be an uninterrupted period of illness during which symptoms of a major mood episode (major depressive or manic episode) are present concurrently with symptoms of schizophrenia. During this period, the patient satisfies the symptom criteria for both schizophrenia and a major mood episode (either major depression or mania)
2. There should be a period of at least **2 weeks** during which the patient has delusions or hallucinations in the absence of prominent mood symptoms. This criterion helps to differentiate schizoaffective disorder from mood disorder with psychotic symptoms, as in the latter, delusions and hallucinations are present only with prominent mood symptoms. [For example, a patient with a diagnosis of Bipolar disorder (mania with psychotic symptoms) will have symptoms of both mania and psychotic symptoms (delusions and hallucinations), but in this patient, psychotic symptoms will always accompany symptoms of mania and would never be present in the absence of manic symptoms].
3. The mood episodes should be present for the **majority of the duration** of the illness (i.e., prominent mood symptoms should be present for >**50%** of the total duration of illness). This criterion is important to be fulfilled as patients with schizophrenia can present with transient mood symptoms, and until and unless mood symptoms are present for the majority of the period, a diagnosis of schizoaffective disorder should not be made.

On a continuum of psychotic disorders with schizophrenia at one end and bipolar disorders on the other end, schizoaffective disorder lies in the middle. Patients with schizoaffective disorders have a better prognosis than schizophrenia and worse than bipolar disorder.

Subtypes

According to DSM-5, the following are the subtypes:
1. **Schizoaffective disorder (Bipolar type):** If the patient had at least one manic episode as a mood episode. Often there are depressive episodes too.
2. **Schizoaffective disorder (Depressive type):** If the patient had only depressive episodes.

ICD-11 describes the schizoaffective disorder as an **episodic illness** in which the diagnostic criteria for schizophrenia and one of the mood episodes (depression, mania or mixed episode) are met simultaneously or within a few days of each other. ICD-11 further specifies that if the mood episode is depressive, it should be either moderate or severe in intensity.

More has been discussed about mood episodes in the next Chapter.

Treatment: It involves a combination of mood stabilisers, antipsychotics and antidepressants, depending on the presentation. In schizoaffective manic type episodes, a combination of antipsychotics and mood stabilisers is commonly used. In schizoaffective depressive type episodes, a combination of antipsychotics and antidepressants is often used. While using antidepressants, the possibility of an antidepressant-induced switch from depression to mania must be taken care of.

Schizophreniform Disorder

In the DSM-5 diagnosis of schizophreniform disorder, symptoms are similar to schizophrenia, and the duration of illness is between **1 to 6 months** (To make a diagnosis of schizophrenia, the duration of illness should be >6 months). The treatment involves the use of antipsychotics for 3–6 months.

Brief Psychotic Disorders

In the DSM-5 diagnosis of brief psychotic disorder, symptoms are similar to schizophrenia, and the duration of illness is >1 day but <**1 month**. A stressor may precede the disorder, and usually, there is complete recovery. Treatment involves the use of antipsychotics. Benzodiazepines have also been found effective in the short term treatment.

Acute and Transient Psychotic Disorders

ICD-11 does not use the diagnosis of either schizophreniform disorder or brief psychotic disorder. The corresponding diagnosis in ICD-11 is acute and transient psychotic disorder. These are a group of disorders characterised by the following:

1. An **acute onset** (defined as a change from a state without psychotic features to a clearly abnormal psychotic state within a period of 2 weeks or less)
2. Presence of schizophrenia-like symptoms. Also, the clinical picture is usually polymorphic (rapidly changing and variable)
3. The presence of associated **acute stress**. Usually, an acutely stressful event such as bereavement, relationship disturbances, or other psychological trauma precipitates these disorders. However, these syndromes can arise without any associated stressor.

The duration of the episode is usually <3 months, and in most cases, it is less than a month.

Treatment

Treatment involves the use of antipsychotics. Benzodiazepines have also been found effective in the short term treatment.

Delusional Disorder

It is characterised by the presence of one (or more) delusions for a duration of at least 1 month. Other psychotic symptoms such as hallucinations, disorganisation, and negative symptoms are usually absent. If hallucinations are present, they are for a very short duration; the presence of frequent hallucinations goes against the diagnosis of delusional disorder. Apart from the direct impact of delusions, the patient's functioning is not markedly impaired in these patients. For example, a patient with a delusion of infidelity may incessantly doubt his wife and fight with her; however, he may continue to function optimally in the workplace. The following are the **risk factors** for the development of delusional disorders:
a. Advanced age
b. Social isolation
c. Sensory impairment or isolation (e.g., auditory or visual disturbances)
d. Family history of delusional disorder
e. Recent immigration
f. Certain personality features, like excessive interpersonal sensitivity (even trivial interpersonal problems cause a lot of negative emotions)

The following are the common types:
1. **Persecutory type:** The central theme is a delusion of persecution in this type.
2. **Jealous type:** In this type, the central theme is a delusion of infidelity. The delusion of infidelity may result in violence and may cause suicide or homicide in extreme cases.
3. **Erotomanic type:** In this type, the central theme is a delusion of love. Often, the patient believes that a person from a higher socioeconomic status is in love with them. The delusion persists despite clear denial by the other person, and all denials are taken as secret affirmations by the patient. In some instances, stalkers have been found to have the delusion of love.
4. **Somatic type:** In this type, the patient has a somatic delusion, such as a delusion of being infested with parasites **(delusional parasitosis)**, having misshaped body parts (delusion of dysmorphophobia) or body having a foul odour **(delusion of halitosis or olfactory reference syndrome)**.

    It is pertinent to note that DSM-5 clearly mentions that if an individual has a delusional belief of having misshaped body parts, it should be diagnosed as body dysmorphic disorder with absent insight/delusional belief and not as a delusional disorder. Similarly, olfactory reference syndrome has been included in the diagnostic category of obsessive-compulsive and related disorders. Other books continue to describe these conditions as delusional disorders.
5. **Grandiose type:** The patient has a delusion of grandiosity in this type.
6. **Mixed type:** This type is used when there is more than one delusion type.
7. **Unspecified type:** This type is diagnosed in patients when the abovementioned categories are not applicable.

Delusion of misidentification is an important example of unspecified type of delusional disorder. Delusion of misidentification can be of the following types:
- *Capgras syndrome:* The patient believes that an impostor has replaced a familiar person. For example, a patient believed that his wife has been replaced by a stranger who looks exactly like his wife.
- *Fregoli syndrome:* The patient believes that a familiar person can change their physical appearance and disguise as a stranger and can take multiple different appearances. For example, a patient saw a beggar and claimed that his brother was following him in the beggar's disguise.
- *Syndrome of intermetamorphosis:* The patient believes that people can undergo changes in physical and psychological identity and become a different person altogether.
- *Syndrome of subjective doubles:* The patient believes that he has many doubles who live their own lives.

Treatment: Antipsychotics are the drug of choice. However, the response to antipsychotics is not as good as in schizophrenia. Usually, delusional disorders persist for long periods and may become a lifelong illness.

> DSM-5 update: The DSM-4 required that to diagnose the delusional disorder, the delusions should be non-bizarre; however, DSM-5 has removed this condition.

Shared Psychotic Disorders (or Induced Delusional Disorder)

This disorder is characterised by the spread of delusions from one person to another. The individual who has the delusion (the primary case) is typically the influential member of a close relationship with a more suggestible person (the secondary case). Initially, the primary case develops a delusion and later on, the secondary case too develops the same delusion.

When two people are involved, the term **"folie a deux"** is used. Occasionally more than two individuals are involved (known as folie a trois, folie a quatre, etc.).

The treatment involves the use of antipsychotics for the primary case. Mere separation from the primary case is usually enough to treat the secondary case.

Attenuated Psychosis Syndrome

Attenuated psychosis syndrome has been included in DSM-5 as a condition that needs further study before being included as an official diagnosis. The proposed criteria for this condition include the following:
- At least one of the following symptoms is present in attenuated (less severe and transient) form, with relatively intact insight—(a) delusions (b) hallucinations, (c) disorganised speech.
- Here, attenuated means that, e.g., if delusions are present, the patient may appear suspicious at times (transient) but not always, and he may be made to question his beliefs at times (less severe, not fixed).

- Symptom(s) must have been present at least once per week for the past month.
- Symptom(s) must have begun or worsened in the past year.
- Symptom(s) is sufficiently distressing and disabling to the individual to warrant clinical attention.

CASE BASED MCQ

A 23-year-old male was brought to the outpatient department with complaints of suspiciousness towards the family members. The patient believed that the family members were poisoning his food and were controlling his activities using a machine implanted in his brain. There was also a history of disturbed sleep, poor self-care, and talking and laughing to self. His mother reported on and off episodes of agitation. The symptoms started 3 years back while he was in his final year of college. The patient was initially taken to religious leaders for treatment for a year, and when he started to worsen, he was admitted to a psychiatric hospital for 2 weeks. There is a history of occasional cannabis and alcohol use. The patient's maternal uncle had similar complaints and has been on regular medications. The most likely diagnosis is:

a. Schizophrenia
b. Substance-induced psychosis
c. Schizoaffective disorder
d. Bipolar disorder

Ans. a. The duration of illness of 3 years with symptoms of delusion of control and persecution and positive family history (in maternal uncle) suggest the diagnosis of schizophrenia.

SUGGESTED READINGS

1. American Psychiatric Association. Diagnostic and Statistical Manual of Mental Disorders. Arlington, VA: American Psychiatric Publishing, 2013.
2. Sadock B, Sadock V, Ruiz P. Kaplan & Sadock's comprehensive textbook of psychiatry. 10th ed. Philadelphia: Wolters Kluwer; 2017.
3. Tasman A, Kay J, Lieberman J, First M, Riba M. Psychiatry. 4th ed. Chichester, West Sussex: Wiley Blackwell; 2015.
4. Boland R, Verdiun M, Ruiz P. Kaplan & Sadock's Synopsis of Psychiatry. Lippincott Williams & Wilkins; 2021.
5. Rangaswamy T. Twenty-five years of schizophrenia: The Madras longitudinal study. Indian journal of psychiatry. 2012;54(2):134.
6. Geddes JR, Andreasen NC. New Oxford textbook of psychiatry. Oxford University Press, USA; 2020.
7. Oyebode F. Sims' Symptoms in the Mind: Textbook of Descriptive Psychopathology E-Book. Elsevier Health Sciences; 2018.
8. Taylor DM, Barnes TR, Young AH. The Maudsley prescribing guidelines in psychiatry. John Wiley & Sons; 2021.
9. Murthy RS. National mental health survey of India 2015–2016. Indian journal of psychiatry. 2017;59(1):21.
10. Casey P, Kelly B. Fish's clinical psychopathology: signs and symptoms in psychiatry. Cambridge University Press; 2019.
11. Stahl SM. Prescriber's guide: Stahl's essential psychopharmacology. Cambridge University Press; 2020.
12. Mwebe H. Psychopharmacology: A mental health professionals guide to commonly used medications. Critical Publishing; 2021.
13. Keepers GA, Fochtmann LJ, Anzia JM, Benjamin S, Lyness JM, Mojtabai R, Servis M, Walaszek A, Buckley P, Lenzenweger MF, Young AS. The American Psychiatric Association practice guideline for the treatment of patients with schizophrenia. American Journal of Psychiatry. 2020;177(9):868-72.

3. Mood Disorders (Depressive Disorders)

Praveen Tripathi, Priyanka Goyal

PS6.1	Classify and describe the magnitude and aetiology of depression
PS6.2	Enumerate, elicit, describe and document clinical features in patients with depression
PS6.3	Enumerate and describe the indications and interpret laboratory and other tests used in depression
PS6.4	Describe the treatment of depression including behavioural and pharmacologic therapy
PS6.5	Demonstrate family education in a patient with depression in a simulated environment
PS6.6	Enumerate and describe the pharmacologic basis and side effects of drugs used in depression
PS6.7	Enumerate the appropriate conditions for specialist referral in patients with depression

MOOD AND AFFECT

Let's revise the meaning of the two terms 'mood' and 'affect'.

Mood is the sustained (**long-term**) and internal emotional state which influences the way the world is perceived. For example, a person who has been feeling low internally for a long-time and finds everything around dull would be described as having a 'depressed mood'.

Affect is the **short-lived** and external expression of internal emotions that others can observe. For example, the person mentioned above, during the interview, avoided looking into the eyes of the examiner and started crying. The facial expression and crying are the external expressions of the underlying depressed mood. This person would be described as having a 'depressed' affect.

Mood is sometimes likened to the "climate", as it describes the long-term emotional state, whereas affect is likened to the "weather", as it describes the short-term emotional state that can fluctuate.

Mood disorders are so-called as their fundamental feature is an abnormality of mood. They are also sometimes referred to as 'affective disorders'; however, mood disorders are the preferred term.

History: The earliest description of mood disorders dates back to Hippocrates, who used the terms 'mania' and 'melancholia' to describe psychiatric disorders. Romans believed that depression is caused by black bile (melan = black, chole = bile). The modern understanding of mood disorders was heralded by the work of **Emil Kraepelin**, who differentiated Dementia praecox (the older name of schizophrenia) from manic depressive psychosis (the older name for bipolar disorder).

The observation that some patients develop only depressive episodes, whereas others have depressive episodes alternating with manic episodes, is the basis of the classification of mood disorders into unipolar disorder (with only depressive episodes) and bipolar disorder (with episodes of both depression and mania). The current classificatory systems continue to follow this classification broadly.

CLASSIFICATION

According to DSM-5, mood disorders can be classified as follows:
1. Depressive disorders (includes major depressive disorder, disruptive mood dysregulation disorder, persistent depressive disorder and premenstrual dysphoric disorder)
2. Bipolar and related disorders (includes Bipolar I disorder, Bipolar II disorder and cyclothymic disorder)

Similarly, according to ICD-11, mood disorders can be divided into depressive disorders and bipolar or related disorders.

In this chapter, depressive disorders have been discussed. Bipolar and related disorders have been addressed in the next chapter.

DEPRESSIVE DISORDERS

MAJOR DEPRESSIVE DISORDER

Major depressive disorder (ICD-11 uses the term "depressive disorder") or unipolar depression (or simply depression) is one of the commonest psychiatric disorders. It presents with one or more major depressive episodes without any manic, hypomanic or mixed episodes.

Epidemiology

Major depressive disorder is a common psychiatric disorder with a lifetime prevalence ranging from 4.9 to 17.1% across different studies. One of the largest epidemiological studies, the National Comorbidity Survey Replication, conducted in the USA, found the lifetime prevalence of major depressive disorder to be 16.6%. In other words, every sixth person develops major depressive disorder at least once in their lifetime.

According to DSM-5, the 12-month prevalence of the major depressive disorder in the USA is around 7%. The rates of major depressive disorder in India were found to be lower.

In the **National Mental Health Survey 2016,** the lifetime prevalence of depression was found to be 5.3%, whereas point prevalence was found to be 2.7%. Amongst psychiatric disorders, depression is associated with maximum disability-adjusted life years (DALYs).

> According to WHO's World Mental Health Survey, depression is the second most prevalent mental disorder globally (the most prevalent mental disorder is specific phobias). According to National Mental Health Study (NMHS-2016), carried out by NIMHANS, Bangalore, depression is the **most common mental illness** in India (excluding tobacco use disorders).

The prevalence of the major depressive disorder in females is twice as compared to males. Multiple reasons have been proposed for the same, including more emotional expressiveness, hormonal factors, effects of childbirth, and higher psychosocial stresses that females experience compared to males.

The most common age of onset of major depressive disorder is in the middle-ages, the mean age being 40 years. However, recent studies have shown that the incidence is increasing in the 20s. In fact, the DSM-5 says that in the USA, the incidence of depression appears to peak in the 20s. This shift towards the younger age of onset may be explained by increasing substance use in this age group.

The prevalence of major depressive disorder is more in separated, divorced or widowed than married individuals. There is no correlation between the prevalence of major depressive disorder and socio-economic class or race.

Clinical Features and Diagnosis

Major depressive disorder can present with single or recurrent major depressive episodes. Major depressive episodes usually present with disturbances in mood, psychomotor activity, cognition and biological functions.

A. **Mood disturbances:** Mood disturbances are considered the most important feature of major depressive episodes. These include:
   1. **Depressed mood:**
      - Patients may report sadness, feeling empty or mournful. The 'sadness' has a distinct quality and is often described as '**painful**', giving it a somatic description like physical pain.
      - The sadness is also '**persistent**' (i.e., present for most of the time) and '**pervasive**' (i.e., present in most activities, patients often say that they can't feel good irrespective of what they do).
      - Children and adolescents may complain of 'irritable mood' rather than sadness. Others may observe the depressed mood state in patients' facial expressions, way of talking, or physical appearance.
      - In a few so-called "**masked depression**" cases, the patient refuses the feeling of sadness and instead complains of physical symptoms like headache, body ache, or heaviness in the chest. However, careful questioning and observation reveal the presence of depressive symptoms.
   2. **Anhedonia and loss of interest:**
      - Anhedonia is "loss of interest in and withdrawal from regular and pleasurable activities".
      - Patients report a lack of enjoyment in the activities, and there may be distinct changes in their behaviour. For example, a cricket enthusiast may stop playing cricket, or an avid music learner may start being absent from the music classes.

B. **Biological functions:** The biological functions of sleep, appetite and sexual drive are often disturbed and the following symptoms may be presented:
   1. **Weight and appetite changes:** Patients may present with significant weight loss or gain, (i.e., a change of more than 5% body weight in a month). Similarly, the appetite may either decrease or increase significantly. There may be a craving for specific foods such as sweets and other high carbohydrate foods. Children may present with failure to have expected weight gains.
   2. **Sleep disturbances:** Sleep disturbances are quite distressing for the patients and are the reason for seeking consultation in many. Patients may present with insomnia or hypersomnia. Insomnia is typically either early morning insomnia, (i.e., waking up too early in the morning with an inability to go back to sleep, also called terminal insomnia) or middle insomnia (i.e., waking up during the night multiple times with difficulties in going back to sleep). Some patients may present with initial insomnia (difficulty in falling asleep). Some patients present with hypersomnia and report that they do not feel refreshed despite sleeping for long hours.

      The sleep architecture is also often disturbed, with a decrease in NREM III and IV stages, an increase in REM sleep, as well as a **shortening of REM latency** (the period between sleep onset to the first REM period).

      Apart from sleep and appetite disturbances, loss of libido is another example of disturbed biological functioning.

C. **Psychomotor disturbances:** The term "psychomotor disturbances" refers to both motor and cognitive (thinking) disturbances due to an underlying psychological cause. Patients with depression may present with the following symptoms:
   1. **Psychomotor agitation or retardation:** Patients may present with psychomotor agitation, (i.e., increased psychomotor activity such as restlessness, pacing around, continuous hand movements etc.,) or psychomotor retardation, (i.e., decreased psychomotor

activity such as decreased spontaneous movements, slumped posture with a downward gaze, slowed speech etc.).

In extreme cases, psychomotor retardation may present as stupor (stupor is a state of markedly decreased level of consciousness in which the patient can be aroused only by persistent and vigorous stimulation. It is a stage of consciousness before coma).

Apart from agitation and retardation, in severe cases, psychomotor disturbances may manifest in the form of special facial features. These facial features are caused by changes in tone of corrugator and zygomatic facial muscles and result in two clinical signs:

a. **Veraguth fold:** It is a triangular fold in the nasal corner of the upper eyelid and was described by Swiss psychiatrist Otto Veraguth.

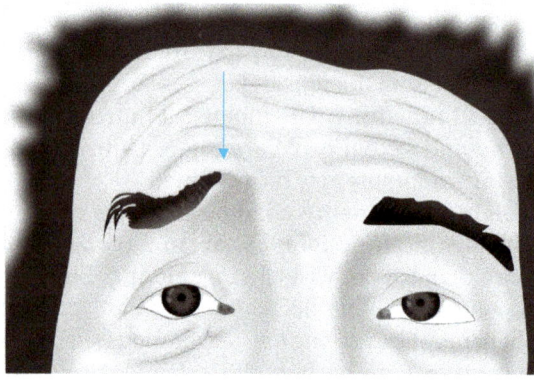

Fig. 3.1: Veraguth fold.

b. **Omega sign:** It is an omega (Ω) shaped fold of skin just above the root of the nose. It consists of vertical skin folds over the glabella along with horizontal folds in the forehead, which together resemble the Greek alphabet omega.

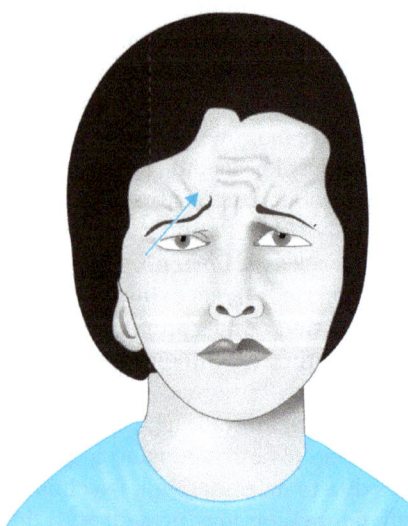

Fig. 3.2: Omega sign.

2. **Fatigue and loss of energy:** Patients may complain of low energy levels, getting tired quickly, and even basic daily chores may seem difficult.

3. **Poor concentration and diminished ability to think:** Patients may report slowness of thinking, difficulty concentrating, distractibility, forgetfulness and indecisiveness. In elderly patients, memory disturbances may be marked along with the slowing of other mental functions. This may lead to an erroneous diagnosis of dementia in elderly patients with depression. Sometimes, the term '**pseudodementia**' is used to refer to depression in elderlies with significant memory disturbances.

D. **Cognitive disturbances:** It refer to faulty thinking patterns. These include:
   1. **Negative thinking:** The patients often get negative thoughts, including negative views about self, others, and the future. The patient may believe that they are worthless or have excessive guilt about minor issues (called pathological guilt, e.g., a patient-reported that he is a cruel person as he had once slapped his son).

   Some patients may develop psychotic symptoms, such as delusions and hallucinations.

   The psychotic symptoms can be classified as:
   - **Mood congruent psychotic features:** Here, the content of delusions or hallucinations is understandable in the context of the prevailing mood state. For example, a severely depressed patient developed a delusion that he is the poorest person alive and his children will die of starvation (delusion of poverty). Another patient with severe depression had a delusion that his internal organs had decayed (nihilistic delusions), and he also heard "voices", which told him that he was a pathetic human (auditory hallucinations with accusing content). The content of these delusions and hallucinations "matches" with the depressed mood; hence, these are "mood-congruent" psychotic features.
   - **Mood incongruent psychotic features:** Here, the content of delusions and hallucinations does not "match" with the prevailing mood state. For example, a patient with severe depression developed a delusion that he is the richest man on the earth (delusion of grandeur).

   2. **Suicidal thoughts:** Patients may have suicidal thoughts, which may range from **passive death wishes** (I wish I was dead) to **suicidal intent** (I would kill myself) to suicidal intent with a definite plan (I would kill myself by jumping from a building). It has been found that almost two-thirds of patients with depression have suicidal thoughts, and around 10–15% of depression patients die by suicide.

> **Paradoxical suicide:** It is the phenomenon wherein the risk of suicide increases as the patient starts to improve, hence the term paradoxical suicide. When patients are severely depressed, even if they have suicidal thoughts, they are unlikely to act on them as they lack the motivation and energy levels to take any step. However, when patients start to improve, the energy levels improve before the decrease in suicidal thoughts, and in that window of increased energy levels, while still having suicidal thoughts, the chances of suicide may actually increase.

> The symptoms of depression can be remembered with a mnemonic: **SIGECAPSS**
> - **S**adness of mood
> - **I**nterest (loss of)
> - **G**uilt
> - **E**nergy (lack of)
> - **C**oncentration (poor)
> - **A**ppetite (disturbances)
> - **P**sychomotor agitation or retardation
> - **S**uicidal thoughts
> - **S**leep disturbances

Diagnosis

According to DSM-5, for the diagnosis of a major depressive episode, at least five of the above nine symptoms should be present for at least 2 weeks, and at least one of the symptoms should be either (1) depressed mood or (2) loss of interest or pleasure. The symptoms should cause clinically significant distress or impairment in social, occupational or other important areas of functioning. ICD-11 also uses similar diagnostic criteria with some variations.

Specifiers

When the diagnosis is made, the presence of any characteristic symptoms or features is described using certain 'specifiers'. These include:

a. **Severity:** The severity of a major depressive episode is described as 'mild', 'moderate' or 'severe' depending on the number of symptoms present and the impairment in the patient's functioning.
b. **With psychotic features:** If delusions and/or hallucinations are present, the specifier of "psychotic features' is added. Sometimes, the term psychotic depression" is used for a major depressive episode with psychotic features. For example, a patient with a major depressive episode with all the symptoms of depression and delusions and marked functional impairment would be diagnosed with a "severe major depressive episode with psychotic features" Further, the specifier, mood-congruent or incongruent, is added to psychotic features.
c. **With seasonal pattern:** This specifier is added if the patient develop depressive episodes in a particular season (usually winter or fall) and achieves complete remission in a particular season (usually spring). These seasonal depressive episodes often present with hypersomnia, increased appetite, craving for carbohydrates and weight gain.
d. **With catatonia:** This specifier is used if catatonic features such as stupor or negativism are present
e. **With peripartum onset:** This specifier is used if the onset of the depressive episode is during pregnancy or within 4 weeks postpartum
f. **With anxious distress:** This specifier is used if the patient has significant anxiety symptoms during the major depressive episode.
g. **With mixed features:** This specifier is used if patients meet the full criteria for major depressive episodes and also have a few symptoms of mania/hypomania. Mixed features are a risk factor for developing bipolar disorder later during the course of the illness.
h. **With melancholic features:** Major depressive episodes with melancholic features are usually seen in elderly patients. This specifier is used in the presence of the following features:
   - Prominent biological symptoms: (1) early morning awakening (waking up at least **2 hours** before the usual time) (2) significant anorexia and weight loss.
   - Significant psychomotor agitation or retardation.
   - Anhedonia and lack of mood reactivity, (i.e., the patient's mood does not respond to events, mood doesn't become better even if some positive event occurs).
   - A distinct quality of intensely depressed mood often referred to as a state of despondency or despair or empty mood. The patient reports feeling miserable
   - Depression is worse in the morning.
   - Excessive guilt

   The melancholic features are usually seen in severe major depressive episodes and are more likely to be seen in the presence of psychotic features. Patients with depression with melancholic features are at a higher risk for suicide.
i. **With atypical features:** The specifier of atypical features is used in the presence of the following features:
   - **Reversed biological symptoms:** (1) hypersomnia, (2) increased appetite and weight gain
   - Leaden paralysis (feeling that limbs have become heavy and difficulty in moving the limbs)
   - Presence of 'mood reactivity' (i.e., the patient's mood improves in response to a positive event)
   - A long-standing pattern of interpersonal rejection sensitivity, (i.e., the person is quite sensitive to events where he feels that he is being rejected/disliked by others)
j. **In remission:** DSM-5 provides the criterion for both 'partial remission' and 'full remission'.
   - *Full remission*: An immediately previous depressive episode is said to be in full remission when no significant symptoms are present for a period of at least **2 months.**
   - *Partial remission*: This specifier is used if some symptoms of an immediately previous depressive episode are present but full criteria are no longer met. Or, it has been less than 2 months since no significant symptoms are left.

> ICD-11 uses the diagnosis of single episode depressive disorder when there is a single depressive episode, and there is no past history of any depressive episodes. The diagnosis of recurrent depressive disorder is used when there are more than one depressive episodes.

> **Endogenous versus exogenous (reactive) depression:**
> In the older classificatory system, two subtypes of depression were described.
> **If a stressor preceded the depressive episode, it was called exogenous or reactive depression.** On the other hand, in the absence of a stressor, the diagnosis of endogenous depression was made. The two types were believed to differ on the basis of aetiology too. It was considered that reactive depression is a 'reaction' to a negative life event and is due to a psychological cause, whereas endogenous depression is because of a 'biological cause'.
> This classification is no longer used. The current concept of depression is unitarian, (i.e., depression is a single illness). The hypothesis that endogenous and reactive depression have different biological underpinnings was also found to be untrue.

Aetiology

Genetic factors, biological factors and psychosocial factors contribute to the development of the major depressive disorder.

Genetic Factors

Major depressive disorder is known to have a strong genetic contribution, as evidenced by family, twin and adoption studies. A meta-analysis found that the first degree relatives of patients with the major depressive disorder had a three-fold increased risk of developing the major depressive disorder compared to the general population.

The twin studies have suggested that the heritability of major depressive disorder is around 35–50%. Similarly, adoption studies have also suggested significant genetic contributions in the development of the major depressive disorder.

Linkage studies have not been able to provide any consistent findings, though there is evidence of linkage to the loci for cAMP response element-binding protein (CREB 1), which is located on chromosome 2.

Further, a study on the interaction between stressful circumstances, major depressive disorder and polymorphism in the serotonin transporter gene showed interesting results. The promoter region of the serotonin transporter gene, known as **5-HTTLPR**, has two variants, the short (s) allele and the long (l) allele. It was found that amongst those who were exposed to a major life stressor, the chances of development of depression were lower and the levels of depressive symptoms that developed were lowest amongst those who had l/l genotype, intermediate amongst those who had s/l genotype and highest among those with s/s genotype. Further, it was found that the presence of short alleles (s) is associated with poorer antidepressant response to SSRIs (selective serotonin reuptake inhibitors) in comparison to individuals with homozygous long alleles.

Neurobiology

In the past, the theories on the aetiology of depression were primarily focused on psychological and social factors. In the last few decades, with an improved understanding of brain functioning, various biological theories have been proposed, ranging from changes in neurotransmission to structural changes in the brain. Researchers are trying to integrate all these theories and develop an integrated model of the neurobiology of depression.

1. **Neuroanatomy of depression:** Limbic system (a system of emotions) is central to the processing of emotions and includes the cingulate gyrus, hippocampus, hypothalamus, and anterior thalamic nuclei. Apart from these, it is now known that the prefrontal cortex and some other structures are also responsible for the normal emotional experiences and disturbances in these structures can result in the development of depression. In patients with depression, the studies have consistently shown structural and functional changes in the following brain structures:

   a. *Prefrontal cortex:* The prefrontal cortex is situated anteriorly to the premotor cortex (involved in the planning of motor actions) and the primary motor cortex (involved in conscious motor actions) of the frontal lobe.

   The prefrontal cortex can be further subdivided into:
   - *Dorsolateral prefrontal cortex (DLPFC):* It is involved in cognitive functions such as executive functioning, problem-solving and working memory
   - *Orbital prefrontal cortex (OFC):* It is involved in the regulation of emotions and behaviours
   - *Ventromedial prefrontal cortex (VMPFC):* It is involved in the generation of emotions and also regulates pain sensations, sexual and eating behaviours, autonomic responses, neuroendocrine responses and aggression.
   - *Anterior cingulate cortex:* It is involved in selective attention and also the regulation of emotions.

   > Executive functions are the 'higher level' cognitive functions that control and coordinate other cognitive functions and behaviours to achieve desired goals.

   Magnetic resonance studies have shown a reduction in the prefrontal cortex volume (all four areas) due to reduced neuronal and glial density in patients with depression. Further, the functional imaging studies (which measure regional blood flow and glucose metabolism) have shown increased abnormal activity in VMPFC and OFC and decreased activity in the DLPFC. The low activity in DLPFC corresponds to deficits in various mental functions seen in patients with depression.

   b. *Amygdala:* Amygdala, located medially in the temporal lobe, is the structure most closely related to emotions and emotional learning and memory (formation of memories of emotional events). Studies have shown that in patients with depression, the amygdala's volume is reduced, and there is an abnormal **activation** of the amygdala.

   c. *Hippocampus:* It is involved in learning and memory. It is connected to the hypothalamus and provides inhibitory feedback to the HPA axis (hypothalamic-pituitary-adrenal axis). It must also be remembered that the hippocampus is one of the two brain areas (the other being the olfactory bulb) where new neuronal growth continues even in adulthood. Patients with depression have been found to have a lower volume as well as disturbed functioning of the hippocampus.

The neural network connecting the prefrontal cortex to the amygdala and the hippocampus has further connections to multiple brain regions, including midbrain/brainstem structures.

Usually, the prefrontal cortex has an inhibitory action on the limbic system. It has been hypothesised that in depression, due to decreased prefrontal cortex activity, there is poor regulation of limbic system structures. The resulting overactivity of the limbic system causes the emotional symptoms of depression (remember that the limbic system is associated with emotions). Further, since the limbic system structures have extensive connections with the hypothalamus and midbrain, its abnormal functioning results in neuroendocrine and neurotransmission abnormalities (described below).

2. **Hormonal dysregulation:** The disturbance of the hypothalamic pituitary adrenal (HPA) axis in depression is well studied. Around 50% of patients with depression have HPA axis dysfunction, which manifests as cortisol hypersecretion (as measured by urinary free cortisol levels, salivary cortisol levels, plasma cortisol levels). HPA overactivity can also be elicited by the more definitive dexamethasone suppression test (DST).

   Elevated HPA activity is a characteristic response to stress and shows that stress plays a vital role in the development of depression. Apart from HPA axis dysregulation, other hormonal disturbances include:
   a. **Subclinical hypothyroidism**, which is associated with depressive symptoms; both increased TSH response and decreased TSH response to TRH infusion have been seen in patients with major depressive disorder.
   b. Also, low estrogen and low testosterone levels are associated with depression, and correction improves depressive symptoms.
   c. Blunted secretion of growth hormone during sleep has also been found in patients with depression.

3. **Immunological mechanisms:** It has been found that in depression, the concentration of proinflammatory cytokines is raised. The proinflammatory cytokines influence the serotonergic and noradrenergic systems and stimulate the HPA axis. The brain may perceive such changes as a stressor, which may further increase HPA activity.

4. **Neurochemistry:** The '**monoamine hypothesis of depression**' states that the deficiency of monoamines, serotonin and norepinephrine causes depression. Apart from serotonin and norepinephrine, low dopamine activity has also been hypothesised to play a role.

   The efficacy of antidepressant drugs, which act by blocking the reuptake of norepinephrine, serotonin and dopamine, further gives credence to this theory. Few studies have found lower levels of gamma-aminobutyric acid (GABA) activity in patients with depression. Also, glutamatergic and cholinergic disturbances have been found. However, recent research suggests that neurotransmitter disturbances may not be directly responsible for the development of depressive symptoms. Instead, wider disturbances in the neural circuits that cause depression may also result in neurotransmitter disturbances.

   It must be remembered that both noradrenergic and serotonergic pathways start from the midbrain nuclei (raphe nuclei for serotonergic pathways and locus ceruleus for noradrenergic pathways) and project to limbic areas, prefrontal areas as well as the hippocampus.

5. **Brain-derived neurotrophic factor:** Recent studies have focused on the role of brain-derived neurotrophic factor (BDNF) in depression. BDNF plays an essential role in neurogenesis, especially in the hippocampus. Chronic and severe stress has been postulated to decrease BDNF, which can result in neuronal loss/decreased neurogenesis in the hippocampus. It has been found that patients with depression have lower levels of BDNF and these levels tend to become normal with antidepressant treatment.

6. **Final neurobiological model of depression:** Based on the evidence available so far, it appears that genetic vulnerability and stress play a major role in the development of depression. Even mild stress may precipitate an episode in patients with high genetic susceptibility. Chronic stress (psychological or physical) results in raised cortisol levels, which, if persistent, may damage hippocampal neurons. Further, chronic stress is also related to low BDNF levels, which again has an adverse effect on hippocampal neurogenesis. The resulting impaired hippocampal function, abnormal regulation of the HPA axis (remember hippocampus provides negative feedback to the HPA axis), result in sustained hypercortisolaemia.

   Apart from HPA axis overactivation, other mechanisms also play important roles. The reduced regulation of the limbic system by the prefrontal cortex results in emotional disturbances seen in depression. Further, decreased activity in noradrenergic and serotonergic transmission and increased pro-inflammatory cytokines contribute to the development of depression.

> **Dexamethasone suppression test in depression:**
> Cortisol releasing hormone (CRH) released from the hypothalamus stimulates the release of adrenocorticotropic hormone (ACTH) from the pituitary, which in turn results in the secretion of cortisol from adrenals, and cortisol exerts negative feedback on CRH. Also, there is a circadian rhythm, with a cortisol surge in the early morning.
> In the dexamethasone suppression test, a high potency glucocorticoid is administered at night. In healthy subjects, it should suppress the release of CRH and ACTH, and also, the next morning cortisol surge should be suppressed. However, in patients with depression, the cortisol surge does not get suppressed, suggesting an HPA axis overactivity.

Psychosocial Theories of Depression

1. **Life events and environmental stress:** As discussed above, stress plays an important role in the development of depression. Stressful life events such as losing a loved

one or job loss may trigger a depressive episode. Further, early life experiences, such as the loss of parents at a young age and parental neglect or abuse, may predispose an individual to the development of depression later in life. It has been found that stressful events are usually present before the first depressive episode; however, in subsequent episodes, the role of stress becomes less and less important. It appears that every depressive episode makes a person more vulnerable to future episodes by producing long-term changes in the brain, and the subsequent episodes may be precipitated by minimal stress or even in the absence of a stressor. The **'kindling'** hypothesis of depression is that every depressive episode makes the person vulnerable to another episode by decreasing the stress threshold required to precipitate the episode.

2. **Cognitive theory:** The cognitive theory of depression was proposed by **Aaron T Beck**. According to this theory, negative thoughts (or negative cognitions) play a primary role in the development of depression. Of particular importance are the three negative cognitions (Beck's cognitive triad) that include: (1) negative view of self, (e.g., I am not good at anything), (2) negative view of the world (e.g., my friends won't ever accept me, they will laugh at me) and (3) negative view of the future (e.g. I won't pass the exams and if I did by fluke, I would never get a job).

   Further, it has been found that patients with depression process information in a biased manner. They often have '**cognitive distortions**' (explained in the Chapter 20 'Psychological Theories and Interventions')

3. **Theory of learned helplessness:** According to this theory, if a person experiences adverse events repeatedly, he may start believing that he has no control over events happening around him. This may lead to a loss of motivation to take any action and a loss of self-esteem. According to this theory, depression results from a real or perceived loss of control over the situations.

4. **Psychodynamic theory:** Psychodynamic theory of depression, as described by Sigmund Freud and Karl Abraham, tries to explain the development of depression by taking into account the childhood experiences of the patient and the unconscious mental processes. According to this theory, a disturbed relationship with the mother during infancy predisposes the patient to depression. Later in life, there is an **object loss** (object loss refers to a significant separation such as the death of a loved one or loss of a relationship). To deal with the loss, introjection of the lost object is used as a defence mechanism, (i.e., the patient internalises an image of the lost object within himself). And finally, since the patient had a combination of love and hatred towards the lost object (which has since been internalised), the feelings of anger and aggression are directed towards self, resulting in depression. Nowadays, psychodynamic theories are considered to be outdated.

Differential Diagnosis

Major depressive episodes should be differentiated from mixed episodes, mood disorders due to another medical condition, e.g., Hypothyroidism, Parkinson's disease, Alzheimer's disease and poststroke), substance-induced depressive disorders, (e.g., cocaine-induced depressive disorders), attention deficit hyperactivity disorder, adjustment disorder and grief.

Comorbidities

The major depressive disorder often presents with comorbidities, most commonly substance use disorders, panic disorders, obsessive-compulsive disorders, social anxiety disorders, eating disorders and borderline personality disorders. The presence of comorbidities worsens the prognosis.

Course and Prognosis

An untreated depressive episode has an average duration of 6–13 months, whereas the average duration comes down to about 3 months with treatment. Around 75% of patients experience more than one episode of depression, and the risk of recurrence increases with each new episode.

The **good prognostic factors** include advanced age at onset, mild episodes, absence of any psychotic symptoms, stable family and social functioning and absence of any comorbid psychiatric disorder.

The **bad prognostic factors** include a history of previous depressive episodes, comorbid anxiety disorder, coexisting dysthymia, coexisting substance use disorder and a longer duration of untreated illness. The more the treatment is delayed, the lesser is the likelihood of achieving remission, underscoring the need for early initiation of treatment.

Treatment

Ensuring the patient's safety is the most crucial task of treatment. A detailed assessment of the suicide risk must be done. It should include an evaluation of suicidal thoughts and behaviour, including the suicide plan and the availability of means for suicide. The factors known to increase suicide risk include the history of past suicide attempts, presence of psychotic symptoms, severe anxiety, impulsivity, use of psychoactive substances and panic attacks. However, it has been found that the prediction of suicide risk remains poor despite best efforts. Apart from suicide, the risk of violence towards others, including homicide, must also be assessed.

Although most patients with depression are treated on an outdoor basis, in certain cases, hospitalisation is required. The **inpatient treatment** is considered in the presence of the following:
1. Risk of suicide or homicide
2. Significant disturbances in biological functions, including grossly reduced oral intake
3. Severe illness with lack of family and social support
4. Presence of complicating comorbid psychiatric or medical conditions
5. Lack of response to outpatient treatment

The use of measurement tools, including clinician-rated and/or self-rated scales, helps in determining the severity of the illness and provides an objective indication of the effectiveness of the treatment provided.

The commonly used scales in depression include **HAM-D (Hamilton Rating Scale for Depression)**, **MADRS (Montgomery Asberg Depression Rating Scale)**, **Beck Depression Inventory (BDI)** and **Patient Health Questionnaire (PHQ-9)**.

The treatment is divided into three phases:

1. **Acute phase:** The acute phase of treatment lasts for around 6-12 weeks. During this phase, the goal is to achieve complete remission of symptoms with a full return to the patient's baseline level of functioning. It must be remembered that it is important to achieve complete remission because the presence of any residual symptoms predicts relapse of the depressive episode. The treatment options include:

    a. *Pharmacotherapy:* Antidepressant medications have been grouped into different classes based on their mechanism of action. These include:
    - Selective serotonin reuptake inhibitors (SSRIs) such as fluoxetine, escitalopram, sertraline etc.
    - Serotonin-norepinephrine reuptake inhibitors (SNRIs) such as venlafaxine, desvenlafaxine, duloxetine, milnacipran etc.
    - Tricyclic antidepressants (TCAs) such as imipramine, amitriptyline, desipramine etc.
    - Monoamine oxidase inhibitors (MAOIs) such as phenelzine, tranylcypromine, isocarboxazid, etc., and
    - Other antidepressants such as bupropion, mirtazapine, etc.

    When psychotic symptoms are present, a combination of antidepressants and antipsychotics is used.

    The available antidepressants have similar efficacy, speed of response and effectiveness. The choice of antidepressant is largely based on the least objectionable **side effect profile** in a given patient. Cost of medications, history of prior treatment response and the patient's preference should also be considered while choosing an antidepressant.

    Selective serotonin reuptake inhibitors are usually well-tolerated and are recommended as the **first-line pharmacological treatment** for depression.

    The effect of antidepressant treatment is usually observable as early as the first 1-2 weeks of treatment; however, the maximum therapeutic effect is achieved after at least 4-6 weeks of continuous treatment. An antidepressant should be given for at least 4-6 weeks before it can be concluded that it is ineffective. In case there is no response, it is recommended that a different antidepressant be used (either belonging to the same class or a different class). In case of partial response, increasing the dose of antidepressant, switching to another antidepressant or augmenting (addition of) with another antidepressant, lithium, thyroid hormone or second-generation antipsychotics, can be done.

    b. *Other somatic therapies:*
    - **Electroconvulsive therapy:** Electroconvulsive therapy (ECT) uses electric currents to produce brief seizures and is used to treat various psychiatric disorders. Electroconvulsive therapy has the highest rate of response and remission among all the treatment modalities for depression, with around a 70-90% improvement rate. Electroconvulsive therapy is the **first-line treatment** for (i) severe major depressive episode with high suicide risk (ii) severe major depressive episode with psychotic symptoms (iii) severe major depressive episode with catatonia (iv) in patients who refuse food leading to nutritional compromise (v) in patients where a rapid response is required (vi) in patients who have not responded to pharmacotherapy/psychotherapy
    - **Transcranial magnetic stimulation:** Transcranial magnetic stimulation (TMS) uses a magnetic coil that is applied to the head to generate rapidly changing magnetic fields, resulting in the production of small electric currents (known as **eddy currents**) in superficial cortical neurons. High frequency transcranial magnetic stimulation over the left dorsolateral prefrontal cortex is approved for use in patients with major depressive disorder who have not responded satisfactorily to at least one antidepressant trial.
    - **Vagal nerve stimulation:** Left vagal nerve stimulation using an electronic device planted in the skin has been found to be effective and has been approved for patients with treatment-resistant depression based on its potential benefit with long term treatment. However, there is no evidence of any acute efficacy of this treatment modality.
    - **Sleep deprivation:** Sleep deprivation is another modality known to have a significant but temporary antidepressant effect. The positive results of sleep deprivation are usually reversed by the next night of sleep. Few studies have suggested that total and partial sleep deprivation followed by immediate treatment with an antidepressant or lithium may sustain the antidepressant effect of sleep deprivation. However, more evidence is required before this modality can be used clinically.
    - **Phototherapy:** Phototherapy has been used primarily in patients with seasonal depression. These patients who usually have a depressive episode in the winter seasons can benefit from phototherapy that involves exposing the patient to bright light in the range of 1,500 to 10,000 lux for 1-2 hours before dawn each day for around a week. The evidence for phototherapy is, however, not robust enough.

c. *Psychotherapy:* Various psychotherapeutic techniques have been found useful in the treatment of depression. These include:
- *Cognitive behavioural therapy (cognitive therapy):* Cognitive behavioural therapy primarily focuses on identifying and challenging negative thoughts and developing alternative ways of thinking. It also involves using behavioural techniques such as activity scheduling (planning what activities need to be done in a day), role-playing, etc. It is one of the most commonly used therapy and has been found effective in multiple studies.
- *Interpersonal therapy:* Interpersonal therapy focuses on the patient's current interpersonal problems responsible for the depressive episode.
- *Behavioural therapy:* Behavioural therapy is based on the hypothesis that maladaptive behavioural patterns result in the development of depression. This therapy uses behavioural techniques like activity scheduling, social skill training, problem-solving etc., to alleviate the symptoms of depression.
- *Psychoanalytically oriented therapy:* The goal of psychoanalytic psychotherapy is to make changes in the personality or character of the patient and not to focus on current symptoms only. These therapies may continue for years and are rarely used nowadays.
- Other therapies include family therapy (treating the entire family as a unit) and group therapies.

The choice of a specific treatment modality depends on various factors. Medications are the preferred treatment modality in patients with moderate-to-severe symptoms (can be used in the mild depressive episode, too), significant sleep or appetite disturbances, a history of prior positive response to antidepressant medications and patient's preference.

Psychotherapy as treatment can be used in patients with mild to moderate symptoms, in the presence of significant psychosocial stressors, comorbid personality disorder and a history of prior positive response to psychotherapy.

A **combination of pharmacotherapy and psychotherapy** has been found to be more effective than either alone in many studies.

2. **Continuation phase:** The continuation phase follows the acute phase, and its duration is between 4–9 months. This phase aims to prevent relapse in the period immediately following remission. In this phase, the treatment given during the acute phase is continued at the same dose, intensity and frequency.

3. **Maintenance phase:** Patients with chronic and/or recurrent major depressive disorder are given maintenance treatment after the continuation phase. Other candidates for maintenance therapy include those with residual symptoms, in the presence of ongoing psychosocial stressors, a history of severe episodes in the past and a family history of mood disorders.

At least 2 years of maintenance treatment is recommended for patients who have had three or more depressive episodes. The treatment that was effective in the acute and continuation phases should be continued in the maintenance phase.

After 2 years, the decision to continue or stop the treatment is taken after considering risk versus benefit.

ANTIDEPRESSANTS

Tricyclic and tetracyclic antidepressants (TCAs): These were the first class of antidepressants widely used in clinical practice. They act by blocking the reuptake transporters of **serotonin** and **norepinephrine** and hence increase the levels of these neurotransmitters in the synapses. Secondary effects of TCAs include antagonism of muscarinic, histamine H1, alpha 1 and alpha 2 adrenergic receptors and blockage of cardiac sodium channels. These secondary effects are responsible for the side effects of these drugs.

TCA toxicity

A patient with TCA toxicity (after unintentional or intentional overdosage) presents with cardiovascular manifestations that include hypotension, chest pain and palpitations; CNS manifestations including **altered sensorium, respiratory depression and seizures;** and peripheral autonomic manifestations such as dry mouth, blurred vision, urinary retention, etc. **Metabolic acidosis** can be present secondary to tissue hypoxia caused by cardiovascular abnormalities/TCA induced seizures.

ECG findings include sinus tachycardia, **prolongation of PR, QRS and QT interval**s, AV block and **right axis deviation**.

The mainstay of treatment is serum alkalinisation, using **intravenous sodium bicarbonate**. A QRS interval of >100 ms is the criterion for this treatment. Gastric lavage and activated charcoal are only beneficial if administered immediately after the overdosage.

❖ **The class TCAs include the following drugs:**
  ➤ Imipramine, desipramine, trimipramine, amitriptyline, nortriptyline, protriptyline, amoxapine, doxepin, maprotiline and clomipramine.
  ➤ The TCAs differ in their affinity for transporters, with clomipramine being the most serotonin selective and desipramine the most norepinephrine selective of TCAs.

❖ **The side effects of TCAs include the following:**
  ➤ **Anticholinergic side effects** like **constipation**, **urinary retention**, blurred vision, dry mouth, decreased sweating and delirium. Due to significant anticholinergic side effects, TCAs should be avoided in **patients with glaucoma** and prostate hypertrophy.
  ➤ Side effects due to blockade of α (alpha) receptors, like postural hypotension (rarely **hypertension**) can also be seen.
  ➤ *Cardiac side effects:* TCAs can cause tachycardia, flattened T waves, prolongation of QT interval and ST-segment depression. Severe side effects like cardiac **arrhythmias** and hypotension can occur due to the blocking of cardiac sodium channels.

Cont'd...

Cont'd...

> - *Neurological side effects:* Fine, rapid **tremors** can occur. Excessive blockade of serotonin and norepinephrine receptors can cause seizures.
> - Sedation due to blockage of H1 histamine receptors.
> - *Other side effects*: Weight gain is common. TCAs (especially amoxapine) have also been found to be associated with Hyperprolactinaemia and may cause Amenorrhoea, **gynaecomastia**, impotence, galactorrhea etc.
- **Important properties of individual drugs:**
  > - **Amoxapine has D2 blocking properties and can cause extrapyramidal side effects like antipsychotics.**
  > - **Imipramine** is used in the treatment of nocturnal enuresis.
  > - Clomipramine is one of the first-line treatments in OCD; however, SSRIs are preferred over clomipramine due to better side effect profile.

Selective serotonin reuptake inhibitors (SSRIs): These are the most commonly prescribed antidepressants. They act by blocking the reuptake of serotonin and do not have the problematic side effects of TCAs. The SSRIs include fluoxetine, fluvoxamine, citalopram, escitalopram, sertraline, paroxetine and **vilazodone**. The SSRIs are the first-line drugs for depression, obsessive-compulsive disorder, post-traumatic stress disorder, panic disorder, generalised anxiety disorder and phobias.
- **Side effects:** The side effects of the SSRIs include the following:
  > - *GI side effects:* Gastrointestinal side effects are the **most common** side effects and include nausea (most common), diarrhoea, anorexia and constipation (constipation is seen with paroxetine). Gastrointestinal side effects are usually short-lasting and improve with time.
  > - *Sexual dysfunction:* Sexual dysfunctions (including anorgasmia, decreased libido, and inhibited orgasm) are the **most common** side effects associated with long-term SSRI treatment.
  > - **QTc interval prolongation**
  > - *CNS side effects:* Anxiety, insomnia, sedation, vivid dreams, nightmares, emotional blunting, seizures, extrapyramidal symptoms, sweating
  > - *Anticholinergic side effects:* Mostly associated with paroxetine
  > - *Haematologic adverse effects:* Functional impairment of platelet aggregation, hyponatraemia
  > - *Miscellaneous:* Weight gain is a common side effect; rarely Hyperprolactinaemia and allergic rashes can be present.

Serotonin syndrome
Concurrent administration of an SSRI with MAO inhibitors, L-tryptophan or lithium, can significantly increase the plasma serotonin concentration and cause serotonin syndrome. It is a potentially fatal syndrome and presents with the following features:
- Diarrhoea, restlessness
- **Hyperreflexia**, agitation and autonomic instability
- **Myoclonus**, hyperthermia, rigidity, seizures
- Delirium, coma and death
- It is treated using cyproheptadine and supportive care

Vortioxetine: It is a recently introduced antidepressant that works as an inhibitor of serotonin reuptake but also has other actions like agonism at 5HT1A receptor, partial agonism at 5HT1B receptor and antagonists at 5HT3, 5HT1D and 5HT7 receptors.

Serotonin norepinephrine reuptake inhibitors (SNRIs): These drugs block neuronal serotonin and norepinephrine uptake transporters and hence are also referred as dual reuptake inhibitors. They include venlafaxine, desvenlafaxine, duloxetine, milnacipran, and levomilnacipran. The side effect profile is quite similar to SSRIs. In addition, SNRIs can cause hypertension at higher dosages.

Discontinuation syndrome
Sudden discontinuation or rapid reduction of the dosage of antidepressants can cause a **discontinuation syndrome**. It is characterised by the following symptoms: (mnemonic **FINISH**)
- **F**lu-like symptoms (lethargy, fatigue, aches)
- **I**nsomnia
- **N**ausea
- **I**mbalance (dizziness, vertigo)
- **S**ensory disturbances (paraesthesias)
- **H**yperarousal (anxiety, irritability)

  All antidepressants can cause discontinuation syndrome. **Venlafaxine** is most commonly associated with a discontinuation syndrome. Short-acting SSRIs (paroxetine and fluvoxamine) are also commonly associated with a discontinuation syndrome.

Monoamine oxidase (MAO) inhibitors: These drugs act by inhibiting the metabolism of monoamines. There are two isoforms of the enzyme, monoamine oxidase (MAO), MAO-A (metabolism of serotonin, norepinephrine and dopamine) and MAO-B (preferential metabolism of dopamine). The nonselective MAO inhibitors, including tranylcypromine, phenelzine and isocarboxazid, inhibit both the isoforms irreversibly, leading to increased levels of these neurotransmitters. However, MAO Inhibitors are rarely used because of their adverse side effects profile, including the possibility of hypertensive crisis.

Cont'd...

Cont'd...

- **Cheese reaction:** Cheese, red wine, and beer contains tyramine (which is an indirectly acting sympathomimetic). Normally, when these items are consumed, the MAO-A present in the gastrointestinal tract degrades the tyramine. However, when MAO inhibitors are used, the tyramine escapes the degradation and gets absorbed. This may lead to a dangerous elevation of blood pressure and a hypertensive crisis (also called cheese reaction). Hence these food items are restricted in a patient who is on MAO inhibitors. **Phentolamine** is the drug of choice for cheese reaction.

MAOIs (and SSRIs) were found to be more effective than TCAs in the treatment of atypical depression.
Atypical antidepressants: There are many other antidepressants with novel mechanisms of action. These include:
- **Trazodone and nefazodone**: These drugs are classified as SARI (serotonin antagonist and reuptake inhibitors). The mechanism of action is weak inhibition of serotonin reuptake and strong antagonism at 5 HT2A and 5 HT2C receptors. Trazodone can cause **priapism** as a side effect.
- **Mirtazapine:** Mirtazapine belongs to a class called NSSA (noradrenergic and specific serotonergic antidepressant). The mechanism of action is the antagonism of the central presynaptic α2 (alpha2) receptors. This results in increased firing of norepinephrine and serotonin neurons. The other important action is the antagonism of postsynaptic 5 HT2 and 5 HT3 receptors. Mirtazapine causes sedation and weight gain but **does not cause problematic sexual side effects**. Other side effects include dry mouth, constipation, myalgia and disturbing dreams.
- **Bupropion:** Bupropion belongs to a class called NDRI (norepinephrine dopamine reuptake inhibitors). The mechanism of action is inhibition of the reuptake of both **norepinephrine and dopamine**. The advantage of bupropion is a benign side effect profile with a low risk of sexual side effects, weight gain or sedation. The common side effects are insomnia, tremors, restlessness and nausea. A particular worrisome side effect is **seizures** (usually seen at higher dosages). Bupropion is also used for **smoking cessation**.
- **Tianeptine and amineptine:** These antidepressants work by **enhancing** the reuptake of serotonin (serotonin reuptake enhancer).

Esketamine
In 2019, the FDA approved **nasal spray of esketamine** (the S-enantiomer of ketamine) for treatment-resistant depression. The important points to be noted are:
- Esketamine has a novel mechanism of **action of glutamate receptor modulation**, and is claimed to have a much **faster onset of action** in comparison to the currently available antidepressants
- Esketamine is approved for use in patients with treatment-resistant depression (defined as a lack of response to two different antidepressants, given in adequate dosages and for an adequate period)
- Esketamine is used as a **nasal spray** and is given along with an oral antidepressant.
- Because of the risk of misuse, it is administered in the office of a certified medical doctor. The patient self-administers the nasal spray under the supervision of a doctor

DYSTHYMIA OR DYSTHYMIC DISORDER (PERSISTENT DEPRESSIVE DISORDER)

Dysthymia is characterised by the presence of depressed mood for a period of more than **2 years** (1 year for children or adolescents). There may be symptoms of low self-esteem, lack of interest, withdrawal from society, sleep and appetite disturbances and poor concentration; however, the symptoms are never severe enough to make a diagnosis of even mild depressive episode. Also, the **socio-occupational dysfunction is lesser** than in patients with depression. Usually, the onset is insidious and is in childhood or adolescence. Patients often report that for as long as they can recall, they were always sad and depressed.

Treatment is similar to major depressive disorder, and a combination of pharmacotherapy and psychotherapy is usually most effective.

In DSM-5, the diagnoses of dysthymia and chronic major depressive episode, (i.e., major depressive episode continuing for more than 2 years), have been combined under the newer diagnosis of "persistent depressive disorder". The ICD-11, on the other hand, continues to have the diagnostic entity of 'dysthymic disorder.'

> **Double depression:** If a patient with dysthymia has worsening of symptoms, and a diagnosis of a depressive episode can be made, it is called as double depression. In other words, a depressive episode superimposed on dysthymia is called double depression.

RECURRENT DEPRESSIVE DISORDER

Recurrent depressive disorder is characterised by a history of more than one depressive episode. in the absence of any manic, hypomanic or mixed episodes (in the presence of any of these, the diagnosis would be bipolar disorder).

PREMENSTRUAL DYSPHORIC DISORDER

The premenstrual dysphoric disorder is caused by changing levels of sex hormones during the menstrual cycle. The symptoms manifest in the final week of the menstrual cycle, before the onset of menses; they start to improve with the onset of menses and become minimal or absent in the week post menses. The symptoms can be divided into three categories—mood symptoms (mood swings, irritability, depressed mood, anxiety), behavioural symptoms (decreased interest, poor concentration, changes in appetite and sleep) and physical symptoms (breast swelling or tenderness, joint or muscle pain, bloating and weight gain). The symptoms are severe enough and cause clinically significant distress in occupational, personal and social activities.

It is important to differentiate premenstrual dysphoric disorder from **premenstrual syndrome (PMS)**. Though the symptoms are quite similar, however, both the number as well as the severity of symptoms is lesser in premenstrual syndrome, and so is the degree of dysfunction.

The treatment of the premenstrual dysphoric disorder is symptomatic and involves analgesics for pain symptoms, diuretics (for fluid retention), SSRIs and benzodiazepines for affective symptoms and insomnia; fluid retention is at times treated using diuretics.

DISRUPTIVE MOOD DYSREGULATION DISORDER

The diagnosis of disruptive mood dysregulation disorder has been added to DSM-5 for children up to the age of 18 years. Earlier, the children with this disorder would get a diagnosis of bipolar disorder; however, studies have established DMDD as a separate entity. This disorder is characterised by recurrent episodes of severe temper outbursts (either verbal aggression or physical aggression towards people or property) along with persistent irritable or angry mood even between the episodes. DMDD is frequently comorbid with other psychiatric disorders, with ADHD being the most common comorbidity.

Since this diagnosis has recently been introduced, the evidence-based treatment approach is unclear. However, medications like SSRIs, stimulants and antipsychotics have been found useful in certain cases. Cognitive behavioural therapy (CBT) has also been found to be effective in preliminary studies.

CASE BASED MCQ

A 27-year-old male was brought to the emergency department after he attempted suicide by hanging. According to the father, the patient had put the noose around his neck, and if he had not reached in time, he might have hanged himself. During the interview, the patient said he lost his job 6 months back, after which his marriage was also called off. Since then, he has always felt sad and lost his appetite and sleep. He didn't feel like going out or talking to friends. He also reported having frequent thoughts of ending his life and finally decided to die by hanging, but his father entered his room just before he could take the final step. There is no history of any psychiatric illness in the past. What is the next best step in the management?

a. Start antidepressants on an outpatient basis
b. Admit the patient and start antidepressants
c. Cognitive behavioural therapy
d. Admit the patient and plan for electroconvulsive therapy

Ans. d. Given the high risk of suicide, the patient should be admitted, and electroconvulsive therapy should be the preferred treatment modality.

SUGGESTED READINGS

1. American Psychiatric Association. Diagnostic and Statistical Manual of Mental Disorders. Arlington, VA: American Psychiatric Publishing, 2013.
2. Sadock B, Sadock V, Ruiz P. Kaplan & Sadock's comprehensive textbook of psychiatry. 10th ed. Philadelphia: Wolters Kluwer; 2017.
3. Tasman A, Kay J, Lieberman J, First M, Riba M. Psychiatry. 4th ed. Chichester, West Sussex: Wiley Blackwell; 2015.
4. Caspi A, Sugden K, Moffitt TE, Taylor A, Craig I, Harrington H et al. Influence of Life Stress on Depression: Moderation by a Polymorphism in the 5-HTT Gene. Science. 2003;301(5631): 386-9.
5. Palazidou E. The neurobiology of depression. Br Med Bull. 2012;101:127-45.
6. Clinical practice guidelines for the treatment of depression across three age cohorts. American Psychological Association. 2019.
7. Taylor D, Barnes T, Young A. The Maudsley Prescribing Guidelines in Psychiatry. 14th ed. Chichester, West Sussex: Wiley Blackwell; 2021.

4 Mood Disorders (Bipolar and Related Disorders)

Praveen Tripathi, Priyanka Goyal

PS7.1	Classify and describe the magnitude and aetiology of bipolar disorders
PS7.2	Enumerate, elicit, describe and document clinical features in patients with bipolar disorders
PS7.3	Enumerate and describe the indications and interpret laboratory and other tests used in bipolar disorders
PS7.4	Describe the treatment of bipolar disorders including behavioural and pharmacologic therapy
PS7.5	Demonstrate family education in a patient with bipolar disorders in a simulated environment
PS7.6	Enumerate and describe the pharmacologic basis and side effects of drugs used in bipolar disorders
PS7.7	Enumerate the appropriate conditions for specialist referral in patients with bipolar disorders

Mood disorders can be broadly divided into depressive disorders (unipolar depression) and bipolar disorders.

In DSM-5 and ICD-11, bipolar and related disorders have been further classified as:
- Bipolar I disorder (presence of both manic and depressive episodes),
- Bipolar II disorder (presence of depressive episodes and hypomanic episodes but never any episode of mania) and
- Cyclothymic disorders (presence of subsyndromal hypomanic and depressive symptoms without ever fulfilling the criteria for an episode of mania, hypomania or major depression).

BIPOLAR I DISORDER

For the diagnosis of bipolar I disorder, a patient must have had at least one manic or mixed episode. Though not required for the diagnosis, the vast majority of patients with bipolar I disorder also experience major depressive episodes during the course of the illness. Apart from manic and depressive episodes, these patients may also experience hypomanic episodes.

Clinical Features

Manic episode: A manic episode presents with disturbances in mood, psychomotor activity, cognition and biological functions, as described below:

A. **Mood disturbances:** Mood disturbances are considered the most important feature of manic episodes. The abnormal mood usually manifests as—
   1. **Elevated or irritable mood:** The patient classically presents with elevated mood (excessive cheerfulness), associated with laughter and excessive enthusiasm. In some patients, the predominant mood may be irritability. These patients may become hostile, especially when their wishes are not fulfiled. The mood state may also fluctuate rapidly, e.g., a patient who was cheerful may suddenly burst into tears. This is called 'lability of mood'. If irritability and hostility dominate the clinical picture, the episode is called 'dysphoric mania' (in contrast to the classical 'euphoric mania', where excessive cheerfulness is the prominent feature).

> **Elevated mood:** The patients may present with different grades of elevation of mood, as defined below:
> 1. **Euphoria:** Euphoria is a state of excessive happiness without any reason.
> 2. **Elation:** Elation is euphoria, along with increased psychomotor activity.
> 3. **Exaltation:** Exaltation is euphoria, with increased psychomotor activity and the presence of delusions of grandiosity.
> 4. **Ecstasy:** Ecstasy is a state of extreme happiness or blissfulness.
>
> Euphoria can be seen in patients with mania or hypomania; the rest of the stages are seen in patients with mania.

B. **Biological functions:** These include—
   1. **Decreased need for sleep:** Patients with mania may sleep significantly less than their usual sleep duration but still feel energetic and rested. Hence, they rarely complain about decreased sleep. In comparison, patients with depression who have decreased sleep bitterly complain about it as they often feel tired and not fresh when they get up.

Often, a decrease in the need for sleep heralds the onset of a new manic episode.

Apart from sleep, sexual functioning too is disturbed. Hypersexuality is often seen in manic patients; however, it has not been included separately as a diagnostic criterion by DSM-5 or ICD-11. The appetite is usually not disturbed significantly; however, neglect of nutrition and increased activity levels may cause weight loss.

C. **Psychomotor disturbance:** The term "psychomotor disturbances" refers to the motor and cognitive (thinking) disturbances due to an underlying psychological cause. These include–
   1. **Increased talkativeness or pressured speech:** The speech may become excessive, loud and difficult to interrupt. The term 'pressured speech' refers to rapid and fast speech that is difficult to interrupt and understand. The patient may speak continuously, intrude in other's conversations and crack jokes and puns, often inappropriately.
   2. **Flight of ideas or subjective experience that thoughts are racing:** Patients may have a 'flight of ideas' wherein the thoughts flow rapidly (externally expressed by an increased rate of speech) and abruptly shift from one topic to another due to attention being diverted by external stimuli or because of internal superficial associations. The patient may subjectively report that thoughts are racing in their mind or that thoughts are so crowded that it is difficult to even speak.
   3. **Distractibility:** Patients are often quite distractible, and irrelevant stimuli catch their attention (such as the clothes of the interviewer, activities of passers-by, background noise and images). It may be difficult to hold long conversations with these patients due to the distractibility.
   4. **Increased goal-directed activities or psychomotor agitation:** Patients frequently have increased goal-directed activity in professional (e.g., starting multiple new projects with little knowledge, entering new businesses), social (excessive socialisation, making new friends), and personal (increased religious involvement, increased sexual drive) domains. Patients may also have psychomotor agitation (purposeless or non-goal directed activity) such as restlessness and pacing around.
   5. **Excessive involvement in activities that have a high potential for painful consequences:** As patients have elevated mood, a subjective feeling of increased physical and mental efficiency, as well as poor judgement, they may end up doing activities that may result in painful consequences such as making wrong business investments, excessive spending, sexual misadventures, gambling, making sudden trips, giving away possessions, etc.

D. **Cognitive disturbances:** The thought process in patients with mania is excessively positive and optimistic. The following features may be present:
   1. **Inflated self-esteem or grandiosity:** The patients may have increased self-confidence, maybe boastful, and may make big claims. Patients often overestimate their capabilities and may make claims of knowing influential people and celebrities. Some patients may develop delusions such as delusion of grandiosity (e.g., a patient claimed that he is so powerful that he can change the weather). The delusions can be mood-congruent or mood incongruent. Similarly, hallucinations can be present and may be congruent or incongruent to the mood.

Though not included in the criteria, lack of insight and poor judgment are common features of manic episodes. The patients may harm themselves or others, due to either poor judgement or delusions (e.g., a patient who believed that he was so strong that he could catch hold of an electric wire without getting injured got electrocuted when he attempted to do so). Substance use is often initiated or increases significantly during the manic episode. Further, patients during manic episodes are often overdressed, may wear excessive makeup, and have a flamboyant style.

Diagnosis

According to DSM-5, for the diagnosis of a manic episode, there should be a distinct period of abnormally and persistently elevated or irritable mood (symptom 1) and abnormally and persistently increased goal-directed activity or energy, along with at least three (or more) of the symptoms 2–8 (mentioned above) (four symptoms from 2–8 are required if the mood is only irritable instead of elevated) for at least a period of one week (or any duration if hospitalisation is necessary).

The symptoms should be severe enough to cause marked impairment in social and occupational functioning or necessitate hospitalisation to prevent harm to oneself or others.

The ICD-11 mentions a similar criterion for the diagnosis of a manic episode.

Hypomanic Episode

The symptoms of hypomanic episodes are similar to those described for a manic episode. However, the symptoms are **not** severe enough to cause marked impairment in social or occupational functioning or to necessitate hospitalisation. Further, the duration criterion for a hypomanic episode is **four days** (in comparison to seven days for a manic episode). Finally, if psychotic features (delusions or hallucinations) are present, it indicates a severe episode, and hence by definition, it is a manic episode. In other words, there is no diagnosis like a hypomanic episode with psychotic features, as the presence of psychotic features in itself implies that the episode is severe enough to be diagnosed as a manic episode.

Major Depressive Episode

The symptoms of a major depressive episode in a patient with bipolar disorder are the same as those in major depressive disorder. Hence, as far as depressive episodes are concerned, the differential diagnosis between major depressive disorder and bipolar disorder is made on the basis of longitudinal history (i.e., presence or absence of manic/hypomanic episodes in the past).

> **Major depressive disorder versus bipolar disorder:**
> Say a patient presents with a depressive episode. If this patient never had any hypomanic/manic/mixed episode in the past, the diagnosis would be a major depressive disorder (or depressive disorder). However, if the patient later develops a manic/hypomanic/mixed episode, the diagnosis would change to bipolar disorder.
>
> Is it possible to identify whether this first depressive episode belongs to a major depressive disorder or bipolar disorder? Although not with certainty, **certain features predict future bipolarity**. These include:
> 1. Early age at onset
> 2. Psychotic depression before the age of 25 years
> 3. Rapid onset and offset of the depressive episode with a short duration of the episode
> 4. Recurrent episodes (>5)
> 5. Marked psychomotor retardation
> 6. Mood lability as a trait in the patient
> 7. Family history of bipolar disorder

Specifiers for Bipolar and Related Disorders

When the diagnosis is made, the presence of any characteristic symptoms or features is described using certain 'specifiers'. These include:

a. **Severity:** The severity of a major depressive episode/manic episode is described as 'mild', 'moderate' or 'severe' depending on the number of symptoms present and the impairment in the patient's functioning.
b. **With psychotic features:** If delusions and/or hallucinations are present during manic/depressive episodes, the specifier of 'psychotic features' is added. Further, it is mentioned whether the psychotic features are 'mood congruent' or 'mood incongruent'.
c. **With seasonal pattern:** This specifier is added if at least one type of episode (either mania, hypomania or depression) develops in a particular season and also achieves remission in a specific season.
d. **With catatonia:** This specifier is used if catatonic features such as stupor or negativism are present in the manic/depressive episode.
e. **With peripartum onset:** This specifier is used if the onset of the manic episode/hypomanic episode/depressive episode occurs during pregnancy or within four weeks postpartum.
f. **With anxious distress:** This specifier is used if the patient has significant anxiety symptoms during the major depressive episode/manic episode/hypomanic episode.
g. **With mixed features:** This specifier can apply to manic/hypomanic/depressive episodes. If full criteria are met for a manic/hypomanic episode and alongside few depressive symptoms are also present, the diagnosis becomes manic or hypomanic episode with mixed features. Similarly, if full criteria are met for a major depressive episode and few manic/hypomanic symptoms are also present, the diagnosis becomes a depressive episode with mixed features.

> **Mixed episode:**
> Apart from manic episodes, hypomanic episodes, and depressive episodes, a diagnosis of 'mixed episode' can be made according to ICD-11. According to ICD-11, a mixed episode is characterised by a mixture of manic and depressive symptoms or a very rapid alteration between prominent manic and depressive symptoms.
>
> In contrast, DSM-5 mentions 'with mixed features' as a 'specifier'.

h. **With melancholic features:** Melancholic features are usually seen in elderlies with a major depressive episode. Melancholic features have already been described in the Chapter 3 'Mood Disorders (Depressive Disorders)'.
i. **With atypical features:** The specifier of atypical features is used in patients with major depressive episodes. Atypical features have already been described in the Chapter 3.
j. **In remission:** DSM-5 provides the criteria for both 'partial remission' and 'full remission'.
   - **Full remission:** An immediately previous episode of mania/hypomania/depressive episode is said to be in full remission when no significant symptoms are present for a period of at least two months.
   - **Partial remission:** This specifier is used if some symptoms of an immediately previous manic, hypomanic or depressive episode are present, but the full criterion is no longer met. Or, it has been <2 months since no significant symptoms were left.
k. **With rapid cycling:** In the context of bipolar type I or bipolar type II disorder, if there are **four or more mood episodes** (manic, hypomanic or depressive episodes) in the previous 12 months, the diagnosis of 'rapid cycling' bipolar disorder is made. The individual mood episodes should be demarcated from each other by full remission or by a switch in polarity (e.g., a depressive episode followed immediately by a manic episode would be considered a separate episode).

> **Akiskal** has proposed many other types of bipolar disorders beyond the ICD and DSM classifications. A 'bipolar spectrum' has been proposed, which consists of the following types:
>
> **Types of bipolar disorders:**
> - **Bipolar 1/2:** Schizobipolar disorder (schizoaffective disorder)
> - **Bipolar I:** Mania with depression (or mania alone)
> - **Bipolar I 1/2:** Depression with protracted hypomania
> - **Bipolar II:** Depression with discrete hypomanic episodes
> - **Bipolar II 1/2:** Depression superimposed on cyclothymia
> - **Bipolar III:** Depression plus induced hypomania (e.g., hypomania occurring solely in association with antidepressants or other somatic treatment)
> - **Bipolar III 1/2:** Bipolar disorder associated with substance use
> - **Bipolar IV:** Depression superimposed on hyperthymic temperament

Epidemiology

The estimates of lifetime prevalence of bipolar I disorder range between 0–2.4%. A large epidemiological study in the

United States, the National Comorbidity Survey Replication, found a lifetime prevalence of 1%. The prevalence of bipolar I disorder is slightly more in men than women, with the lifetime male to female prevalence ratio being 1.1:1. In contrast, bipolar II disorder is more common in women. Manic episodes are more common in men, and depressive episodes are more common in women.

According to **NMHS 2016 (National Mental Health Survey)** in India, the point prevalence of bipolar disorders is 0.3%, and the lifetime prevalence of bipolar disorders is 0.5%. Males were found to have a slightly higher prevalence than females.

The mean age of onset for bipolar I disorder is around 18 years, and for bipolar II disorder in the mid-20s. However, onset in childhood or in the elderly population can be seen. Bipolar I disorder is more common in single, separated, divorced or widowed individuals than married individuals. The prevalence is not different in different races. Bipolar I disorder is more commonly seen in upper socio-economic groups.

Aetiology

Genetics

Bipolar disorder has a strong genetic component. The first degree relatives of patients with bipolar disorder have an increased risk of developing bipolar disorder (and also unipolar depression) in comparison to the general population. Twin studies have shown that the concordance rate for mood disorder in the monozygotic twin of a patient with bipolar disorder is around 60%, whereas the concordance rate in dizygotic twins is around 20%. This indicates a clear role of genetics as monozygotic twins share the entire genome, which is not the case with dizygotic twins. The heritability in bipolar disorder has been estimated to be **very high, around 85%**.

It appears that multiple genes have a small size and cumulative effect on the development of bipolar disorder, the so-called polygenic inheritance.

The results of linkage studies have been variable. The strongest data is available for linkage to chromosomes 18q and 22q. Genome-wide association studies have found a significant association with CACNA1C, which encodes a subunit of the L-type calcium channel.

Environmental

The fact that even the monozygotic concordance rate is not 100% shows that environmental factors also play a role in developing bipolar disorder in addition to genetics. Some important environmental factors whose role has been established are described here.

Stressful life events (such as loss of job, academic setback, relationship problems, etc.) can precipitate both manic and depressive episodes. This is probably because of disruption of the sleep cycle and other circadian rhythms.

A history of childhood sexual abuse increases the likelihood of later development of bipolar disorder (and other psychotic disorders).

Also, like in schizophrenia, high levels of expressed emotions may increase the chances of relapse in patients with bipolar disorder.

Neurobiology

1. **Neurochemistry**: It has been hypothesised that mania is caused by a **hyperdopaminergic state**. This hypothesis is supported by the efficacy of antipsychotics (dopamine receptor antagonists) in the treatment of mania. Few studies have also found increased glutamate levels in patients with bipolar disorder.
2. **Hormonal dysregulation:** Similar to major depression, a hyperactive hypothalamic–pituitary–adrenal axis with hypersecretion of cortisol has been found in patients with bipolar disorder.
3. **Neuroimaging:** Imaging studies have found decreased cerebral volume and hippocampal volume in patients with bipolar disorder. Abnormalities in white matter tracts, predominantly in frontal and temporal white matter regions, have also been found. Neuropathological studies have found a reduction in neuronal and glial cell density in the prefrontal cortex.

Functional neuroimaging studies have shown elevated neural responses in the amygdala and reduced response in the regulatory prefrontal cortex in response to negative emotional cues.

However, all these findings need to be replicated in further studies before they can be used for diagnostic purposes.

Patients with bipolar disorder also show **soft neurological signs** such as abnormalities of executive function, verbal memory, attention and processing speed.

Comorbidity

The most common comorbidity is anxiety disorders (panic disorder, social anxiety disorder, specific phobias). Other common comorbidities include substance use disorders, obsessive-compulsive disorders, and eating disorders.

Differential Diagnosis

Bipolar I disorder should be differentiated from major depressive disorder based on the presence of manic episodes. Other important differential diagnoses include bipolar II disorder, substance/medication-induced bipolar disorder, anxiety disorders, personality disorders (especially borderline personality disorder), schizophrenia spectrum disorders (especially in cases of bipolar disorder with psychotic features), attention deficit hyperactivity disorder (especially in children and adolescents in whom hyperactivity and distractibility may be confused with manic symptoms) and disorders with prominent irritability (especially in children in whom irritability may be mistaken for manic symptoms).

Course and Prognosis

Both bipolar I and II disorders are chronic illnesses, and recurrence of episodes is quite likely. In both subtypes, the first episode is usually depressive. Long-term studies show that patients spend much more time in depressive periods than in manic/hypomanic periods in both subtypes. Further, as the illness progresses, the time interval between the successive episodes tends to decrease and finally stabilises. Frequently the episodes have incomplete remission, and some residual symptoms are left.

Stressful factors act as precipitants in the initial episodes; however, later, their role decreases and illness takes an autonomous course. The **kindling effect**, wherein every episode increases the likelihood of another episode, is seen in bipolar disorders. The prognosis is worse than the major depressive disorder. The rate of completed suicide in bipolar disorder is **10–15%**. Suicide is usually seen during a depressive episode or in the presence of mixed features.

In patients with bipolar I disorder, shorter duration of manic episodes, late-onset, and lesser comorbidities (both medical and psychiatric) were associated with better outcomes. On the other hand, depressive symptoms, psychotic symptoms, inter episodic depressive symptoms, comorbid alcohol dependence, male gender and poor premorbid occupational functioning were the predictors of worse outcomes.

Treatment

While treating a patient with bipolar disorder, the immediate goal is to ensure the patient's safety. A detailed assessment of suicide risk must be done that includes evaluating suicidal thoughts and behaviour, any plans for suicide, and the availability of means for suicide. During a manic episode, the patient may cause harm to self due to poor judgement and secondary to underlying psychopathology. Apart from suicide, the risk of violence towards others must also be assessed.

The clear **indications for admission** in a patient with bipolar disorder include:
1. Risk of suicide or homicide
2. Significant disturbances in biological functions, including grossly reduced oral intake
3. Severe illness with lack of family and social support
4. Presence of complicating comorbid psychiatric or medical conditions
5. Lack of response to outpatient treatment

The use of measurement tools, including clinician-rated and/or self-rated scales, helps in determining the severity of the illness and provides an objective indication of the effectiveness of the treatment provided. The commonly used scales in depression include Hamilton Rating Scale for Depression (HAM-D), Montgomery Asberg Depression Rating Scale (MADRS), Beck Depression Inventory (BDI) and Patient Health Questionnaire (PHQ-9). The commonly used rating scale in mania is the **Young Mania Rating Scale (YMRS).**

The treatment of bipolar disorder depends on the phase.
A. **Treatment of acute mania or hypomania:** The treatment of acute mania focuses on rapid symptom control and returning to the usual functioning levels. Pharmacotherapy involves the use of mood stabilisers, antipsychotics and benzodiazepines.

American Psychiatric Association guidelines suggest the following:
1. To treat a severe manic episode, a **combination** of lithium with an antipsychotic or valproate with an antipsychotic should be used. Usually, due to a better side effect profile, second-generation antipsychotics (atypical antipsychotics) are preferred over typical antipsychotics.
2. For treatment of less ill patients, monotherapy with either lithium, valproate or an antipsychotic (preferably a second-generation antipsychotic) can be used.
3. Short term use of benzodiazepines as an adjunctive treatment, especially for control of agitation and insomnia, can be helpful.
4. In patients with mixed features (mixed episodes), valproate is preferred over lithium.
5. In patients with refractory illness, clozapine can be used.
6. In patients with psychotic symptoms (delusions and/or hallucinations), an antipsychotic (preferably a second-generation/atypical antipsychotic) must be added to the treatment regimen.
7. Electroconvulsive therapy can be used in patients who are treatment-resistant, in case of severe mania during pregnancy or otherwise in patients who are severely ill.

Since the average duration of a manic episode is around 6 months, treatment should be continued for at least 6 months; if stopped earlier, symptoms may reappear. The treatment of hypomania is similar to the treatment of acute manic episodes.

B. **Treatment of acute depression**: The treatment of acute depression in a patient with bipolar disorder is challenging, and guidelines differ regarding the preferred treatment.
1. According to American Psychiatric Association (APA) guidelines, the first-line pharmacological treatment is the initiation of either **lithium or lamotrigine**. (Other guidelines have recommended the use of valproate too as first-line treatment.). Although recommended by APA, recent studies have shown that lithium is much more effective in the prevention of depression in bipolar disorders than in the treatment of acute depression.
2. **Quetiapine** has also been found to be particularly effective in the short term and long-term treatment of bipolar depression. Apart from quetiapine, lurasidone and olanzapine + fluoxetine combination are effective too. These three agents are also considered first-line treatment in bipolar depression.
3. In severely ill patients, a combination of mood stabilisers with antidepressants can be considered, although the use of antidepressants in a patient with bipolar depression increases the risk for manic switches (i.e., a patient may switch from a depressive episode to a manic episode after administration of an antidepressant) as well as a risk of inducing rapid cycling. The risk of a manic switch is more with TCAs and SNRIs than with SSRIs. If at all used, antidepressants should be combined with mood stabilisers.

4. Antidepressants should never be used alone in bipolar depression because of the aforementioned reasons.
5. Electroconvulsive therapy can be used in patients with high suicide risk or who are not responding to or are intolerant of medications.

C. **Maintenance treatment/prophylaxis in bipolar I disorder:** Given that bipolar disorder is a highly recurrent illness (over 90% of patients have another mood episode within 5 years), the prophylaxis should be given after two or more acute episodes in bipolar I disorder or after a single manic episode if it was severe and was associated with significant risk.

The **first-line treatment** includes lithium, divalproex, and lamotrigine. However, it must be remembered that lamotrigine has limited efficacy in the prevention of manic episodes, and it may not be a good choice in patients with predominantly manic episodes. Atypical antipsychotics have also been used, although most of them (except quetiapine and olanzapine) are more effective in the prevention of manic episodes and not depressive episodes. The prophylaxis should be continued for at least 2 years; however, in patients who have had multiple episodes, it may be continued indefinitely.

Although pharmacotherapy is the mainstay of treatment in bipolar disorders, psychotherapy also plays a role. **Psychoeducation** (individual or group based) has been found to improve compliance with treatment and reduce the risk of relapse in a patient with bipolar disorders. In psychoeducation, patients (and family members) are educated about the nature of the illness, the need for medications, the possible side effects, the role of maintaining a regular lifestyle (including a regular sleep cycle), and the need to abstain from substance abuse.

CYCLOTHYMIC DISORDER

Cyclothymic disorder can be considered a milder form of bipolar disorder. It is characterised by a chronic, fluctuating mood disturbance involving numerous distinct periods of hypomanic and depressive symptoms.

The diagnosis is made in the presence of the following:
1. For at least **2 years** (1 year in children and adolescents), the patient experiences distinct periods of hypomanic symptoms and depressive symptoms; however, these symptoms are never severe enough/not present for enough duration to make the diagnosis of a major depressive, manic or hypomanic episode.
2. The symptoms are persistent, and DSM-5 requires that the symptoms should be present for at least half the time out of 2 year period and that the patient should never be without symptoms for >2 months at a time

The age of onset is usually between 15–25 years of age, and it's more common in females.

Treatment: Mood stabilisers such as lithium, valproate, and carbamazepine are the first-line treatment. Antidepressants should be used with caution because of the risk of antidepressant-induced manic/hypomanic switches.

Lithium:
Lithium is used for the treatment of acute episodes (both mania and depression) as well as for prophylaxis in bipolar disorder. **John FJ Cade**, an Australian psychiatrist, was the first person to establish the effectiveness of lithium in the treatment of mania.

Lithium is a monovalent cation and gets **rapidly and completely absorbed** after oral administration. The plasma half-life is initially **1.3 days** and gets increased to **2.4 days** after continued administration for >1 year. Lithium does not bind to plasma proteins, is not metabolised in the body and gets excreted unchanged through the **kidney**.

Indications:
Acute manic episode: Lithium is an effective treatment for acute mania; however, since its onset of action is delayed (1–3 weeks), an antipsychotic, benzodiazepine or valproate, is usually added in the initial treatment period. Lithium is also effective for prophylaxis against future manic episodes.

Bipolar depression: Lithium is effective in the treatment of bipolar depression and prophylaxis of the same; however, the antimanic efficacy of lithium is more than its antidepressive efficacy.

Maintenance treatment: Maintenance treatment with lithium decreases the frequency, severity and duration of manic and depressive episodes in patients with bipolar disorders.

Lithium is an effective **antisuicidal** agent and decreases the risk of suicide by 80% in patients with bipolar disorder.

Lithium is also used in patients with schizoaffective disorders as well as an adjuvant to antidepressants in major depressive disorder.

Other indications for which lithium has been used, but is not the first-line treatment include obsessive-compulsive disorder, aggression, **headache (cluster, migraine)**, gout, epilepsy, movement disorders, **neutropenia**, and ulcerative colitis.

Correlates of lithium responsiveness: Response to lithium in patients with bipolar disorder is better in the following clinical conditions:
- **Euphoric (elated) mania** (wherein patients' predominant mood state is euphoria) (In patients with dysphoric mania, where the predominant mood state is irritability, valproate is a better choice over lithium).
- Three or fewer episodes (patients who have had four or more manic/depressive episodes respond poorly to lithium)
- MDI sequence (it means that patients in whom sequence of mood episodes has been mania→ depression→ interval respond better to lithium)
- Absence of rapid cycling
- Family history of bipolar disorder
- Absence of comorbidities like substance use
- Lithium has a narrow therapeutic index and thus requires therapeutic drug monitoring. The effective serum concentration of lithium in the treatment of acute mania is **1.0–1.5 mEq/dL**. The serum concentration required for maintenance treatment is **0.6–1.2 mEq/dL**

Cont'd...

Cont'd...

Side effects:
- **Neurological:** Lithium can cause **postural tremors** (usually treated with beta-blockers **like propranolol**), lack of spontaneity and memory disturbances; rarely, it can cause raised intracranial tension and peripheral neuropathy.
- **Endocrine: Hypothyroidism**, rarely hyperthyroidism, hyperparathyroidism.
- **Renal:** Most common is polyuria, at times progressing to diabetes insipidus, which is treated with thiazide diuretics or potassium-sparing diuretics (like amiloride, spironolactone or triamterene). Rarely nephrotic syndrome, renal tubular acidosis or interstitial fibrosis can be seen.
- Others include dermatological side effects such as **acne, psoriasis, hair loss, and rashes**. Nausea, vomiting, diarrhoea, weight gain and benign T wave changes can also occur.
- **Teratogenic effects:** Lithium, if taken in pregnancy, can cause malformations in the cardiovascular system of the fetus, most commonly **Ebstein's anomaly** of tricuspid valves. The teratogenic risk of lithium is lower than that of valproate and carbamazepine.

Lithium toxicity: The risk factors for lithium toxicity include renal impairment, **dehydration** and a low **sodium diet**. Usually, the sign of toxicity starts to appear at levels above **1.5 mEq/dL**. As the levels of lithium associated with toxicity are not much different from levels required for therapeutic effect, hence lithium has a **narrow therapeutic index**. The early signs of toxicity include **gastrointestinal symptoms** like abdominal pain, vomiting and neurological symptoms like **coarse tremors, ataxia,** and **dysarthria**. The later signs and symptoms include impairment of consciousness, muscular fasciculations, increased **deep tendon reflexes,** and convulsions. There might be circulatory failure and death. The management involves stopping lithium, correcting dehydration, and use of polyethylene glycol (not activated charcoal) to remove unabsorbed lithium from the gastrointestinal tract. In severe cases, haemodialysis may be required.

PSYCHIATRIC ASPECTS OF PREGNANCY (TABLE 4.1)

1. **Postpartum blues (baby blues):** In the postpartum period, most women develop **transient** depressive symptoms like tearfulness, emotional lability (frequent mood changes), sadness and, at times, sleep disturbances. These symptoms may last for days to weeks and need no professional treatment. The support of family members usually helps the new mother deal with postpartum blues.
2. **Postpartum depression:** If the depressive symptoms are severe and prolonged, a diagnosis of 'postpartum depression' is made. According to DSM-5, a depressive episode can develop after childbirth or may develop before the delivery. These episodes are referred to as depressive episodes with peripartum onset (or peripartum depressive episodes).

Table 4.1: Differences between postpartum blues and postpartum depression.

	Postpartum blues	Postpartum depression
Incidence	30–75% of women who give birth	10–15% of women who give birth
Time of onset	3–5 days after childbirth	Within 3 months of childbirth
Tearfulness	Yes	Yes
Emotional lability	Yes	Yes
Anhedonia	No	Common
Sleep disturbances	Occasional	Common
Suicidal thoughts/ thoughts of harming the baby	No	Sometimes
History of mood disorder	No association	Usually present
Family history of mood disorder	No association	Usually present
Guilt	Rare	Common
Increased risk of development of future episodes of depression	No	Yes
Treatment	Support to mother	Pharmacotherapy plus psychotherapy

Brexanolone:
In 2019, US FDA approved brexanolone IV infusion (60 hours continuous IV infusion), the first-ever drug approved specifically for the treatment of postpartum depression.
Brexanolone is chemically identical to endogenous allopregnanolone, a hormone that decreases after childbirth. Brexanolone acts as a positive allosteric modulator of GABAA receptors (which become dysregulated in the postpartum period).

3. **Postpartum psychosis (puerperal psychosis):** Postpartum psychosis is usually seen within 2–3 weeks of delivery.

The following are the important characteristics of postpartum psychosis:
- Initially, the patient presents with symptoms like insomnia, tearfulness and emotional lability, followed by the development of delusions and hallucinations.
- The content of delusion may involve thoughts that 'baby is dead' or that patient did not give birth to the baby or some other persecutory belief. Hallucinations may have similar content. Postpartum psychosis is considered a psychiatric emergency as the patient may act on hallucinations and delusions and harm herself or the baby. Postpartum psychosis is essentially an

episode of bipolar disorder (or depressive disorder) that was triggered by the stress of childbirth (and accompanying hormonal changes).
- Two-thirds of patients develop another mood episode (manic, depressive or mixed episode) within 1 year of childbirth.
- About 50-60% of affected women had given birth to the first child, and in 50% of cases, delivery was associated with a non-psychiatric perinatal complication.
- 50% of affected women have a family history of mood disorder.

Subsequent pregnancy carries a high risk of another episode of postpartum psychosis, the risk being around 50%.
- In most cases, recovery is complete from acute illness.

Treatment involves the use of antipsychotics, often in combination with lithium and, in some cases, antidepressants.

Pregnancy and Use of Mood Stabilisers

The following points must be remembered:
- The risk of relapse of bipolar disorder is increased during pregnancy and even more during the postpartum period. If a patient is on a mood stabiliser and it is stopped abruptly, the risk of relapse becomes quite high.
- Relapse during pregnancy has an adverse effect on the health of both mother and child.
- **No mood stabiliser is entirely safe.** A risk versus benefit assessment must be done, and the decision to continue (or not) the treatment should be taken after careful evaluation.
- **Lithium use in pregnancy:** Lithium use during pregnancy can cause **Ebstein's anomaly**; however, the risk of the same is very low (1:1,000). Lithium use can also cause atrial and ventricular septal defects. If lithium is used during pregnancy, high-resolution ultrasound and echocardiography should be done at 6th and 18th weeks of gestation. At the end of pregnancy, rapid changes in the total body water occur and may predispose the mother to lithium toxicity. To prevent this, fluid balance monitoring is needed.
- **Valproate use in pregnancy:** Valproate is the most teratogenic among mood stabilisers and should be avoided. The use of valproate can cause **neural tube defects** (i.e., spina bifida). Valproate must be given only if all other treatment methods have failed. In such a case, folate supplements must be given to the patient. The use of folate for at least 1 month before conception decreases the chances of development of neural tube defects.

Few studies have reported that in utero exposure to valproate may adversely impact the cognitive development of the child. A study found that children of mothers who took valproate during pregnancy had low IQ scores in comparison to control subjects.
- **Carbamazepine use in pregnancy:** Carbamazepine is a teratogenic drug and should be avoided. The use of carbamazepine can cause **neural tube defects (i.e., spina bifida)**, although the risk is lesser than valproate. The use of folate for at least one month before conception decreases the chances of development of neural tube defects. If carbamazepine is used, prophylactic Vitamin K should be given to the mother and to the baby after delivery to prevent haemorrhagic disease in the newborn.
- Limited studies have suggested that lamotrigine is safer than valproate and carbamazepine in pregnancy.
- **Antipsychotics are safer than mood stabilisers** and less likely to cause any teratogenic effects. So, antipsychotics should be preferred over mood stabilisers for prophylaxis during pregnancy.
- If a patient develops an acute manic episode in pregnancy, **antipsychotics are again preferred** over mood stabilisers.

SUICIDE

As suicide is most commonly due to mood disorders, this topic has been covered in this Chapter.

Suicide is death caused by injuring oneself with the intent to die. As clearly mentioned in this definition, while injuring oneself, the person intends to die as a consequence of the act.

If an individual tries to harm self with the intent to die but survives, it is called a suicide attempt.

Suicide is a serious public health problem with grave consequences for families and society. According to NCRB (national crime records bureau), suicide numbers in India reached an all-time high in 2021, with a suicide rate of **12.0 per lakh of the population**.

In India, the most common method of suicide is **hanging**, the second most common being use of poison. Globally too, the most common method of suicide is hanging.

Risk Factors

Suicide is difficult to predict precisely. Some people have had suicidal thoughts for years but never act on them. In other cases, suicide may be an impulsive act without any prior planning. Nonetheless, certain factors are known to increase the suicide risk, and these include:

1. **Previous suicide attempt:** A past suicide attempt is the **single most important risk factor** that indicates an increased risk of suicide.
2. **Signs of suicidal intent:** Certain actions such as giving away personal property, transferring money to the account of loved ones, writing a will, and writing a suicide note, are suggestive of imminent risk of suicide and must be taken seriously. Most people who die by suicide communicate their intention to their loved ones or the doctors.
- **Hopelessness:** The presence of **hopelessness** increases the risk of suicide.
- **Gender differences:** The suicide rate in men is higher than the suicide rate in women, although women are much more likely to attempt suicide than men. This is primarily because men tend to use more lethal methods such as firearms or hanging.
- **Age:** The suicide rate increases with age and peaks after 45 years in men and after 55 years in women. Older persons attempt suicide less often than younger persons but are more likely to be successful. The suicide rate is rising in youths too. Suicide is rarely seen before puberty.

- **Marital status:** Single, never married and divorced individuals have a higher rate. Being married and having kids decreases the risk of suicide
- **Physical health:** History of a chronic illness, chronic pain, loss of mobility, and disfigurement increase the risk of suicide.
- **Mental health:** Suicide is almost always a result of a mental illness. Nearly 95% of persons who die by suicide had a mental illness, most commonly depression. Other psychiatric disorders associated with an increased risk of suicide are schizophrenia, dementia, alcohol dependence (and other substance dependence), and personality disorders (especially borderline personality disorder and antisocial personality disorder). Patients suffering from depression with delusions are at the highest risk of suicide. For admitted patients, the risk of suicide is highest in the first week after admission. The period after discharge is also a high-risk period. The presence of delusions or hallucinations also increases the suicide risk.
- Family history of suicide, poor social support and unemployment are other risk factors.

Aetiology

1. **Sociological factors: Emile Durkheim** divided suicide into three social categories:
   a. *Egoistic suicide:* It applies to those who are not strongly integrated into any social group. For example, unmarried individuals with a lack of family integration have a higher risk of suicide than married individuals who have kids and are integrated with family.
   b. *Altruistic suicide:* It applies to those who are excessively integrated into a social group. For example, a soldier sacrifices his life for the love of the nation.
   c. *Anomic suicide:* It applies to those whose integration into society gets disturbed. For example, an individual who faces massive economic losses and a loss of social status.
2. **Biological factors:**
   a. **Genetic factors:** Both twin studies and adoption studies have shown that suicide has a strong genetic component. It has been hypothesised that the genetic factor may impact the ability to control impulsive behaviour and hence the vulnerability for suicide.
      Tryptophan hydroxylase (TPH) is an enzyme involved in serotonin synthesis. *TPH* gene has two alleles: U and L. The L allele is associated with reduced capacity to hydroxylate tryptophan to 5-hydroxytryptophan (a step in serotonin synthesis). Lower levels of 5-hydroxyindoleacetic acid (5-HIAA) were found to be associated with LL and UL genotype. Suicide attempts were seen most often in individuals with LL genotype followed by UL genotype. The L allele of tryptophan hydroxylase was associated with increased suicide risk.
   b. **Biological factors:** Multiple studies have found that low levels of the serotonin metabolite **5-HIAA** in cerebrospinal fluid (CSF) are associated with an increased risk of suicide.

Management

It is important to assess the suicide risk and take appropriate measures. If the risk is high, inpatient treatment with regular supervision is recommended.

In many cases with high suicide risk, electroconvulsive therapy is considered the treatment of choice because of its rapid onset of action.

Depending on the diagnosis, appropriate pharmacotherapy and psychotherapy are used. Supportive psychotherapy may help alleviate some of the symptoms.

> - **Parasuicide:** The term parasuicide is used when a person indulges in self-injurious behaviour (e.g., making superficial cuts on the skin) but doesn't have the intention to kill self.
> - **Physician suicide:** The suicide rate of doctors is one of the highest of any profession and significantly more than the general population. Female physicians are at even higher risk than their male counterparts for suicide. Anaesthetists and psychiatrists have the highest suicide rate of all the branches.
> - **Copycat suicide:** There have been reports where adolescents belonging to the same group have committed suicide one after another. It is believed that suicide by one member influences the behaviour of others; this is called copycat suicide. Some studies have found an increased rate of adolescent suicides after the release of a television program/movie that shows suicide by an adolescent or after the suicide by some popular figure like a pop star.

CASE BASED MCQ

A 22-year-old unmarried female started behaving strangely for the last 2 months. She would spend hours dressing and grooming and appeared excessively cheerful. She would sleep for <3 hours at night and start practising playing the piano in the early morning, disturbing other family members. She was calling everyone she knew and would insist on talking for hours even when the other person was not interested. One year back, she had an episode characterised by sadness of mood, negative thoughts, poor sleep and appetite. What is the likely diagnosis?
a. Recurrent depressive disorder
b. Bipolar disorder (current episode, mania)
c. Bipolar disorder (current episode, depression)
d. Schizophrenia

Ans. b. The history of euphoria, increased activity levels, over-talkativeness, and decreased sleep for the last 2 months is suggestive of a manic episode. In addition, there is a history of a depressive episode 1 year back. Hence the diagnosis is bipolar disorder (current episode, mania).

SUGGESTED READINGS

1. American Psychiatric Association. Diagnostic and Statistical Manual of Mental Disorders. Arlington, VA: American Psychiatric Publishing, 2013.
2. Sadock B, Sadock V, Ruiz P. Kaplan & Sadock's comprehensive textbook of psychiatry. 10th ed. Philadelphia: Wolters Kluwer; 2017.
3. Tasman A, Kay J, Lieberman J, First M, Riba M. Psychiatry. 4th ed. Chichester, West Sussex: Wiley Blackwell; 2015.
4. Boland R, Verdiun M, Ruiz P. Kaplan & Sadock's Synopsis of Psychiatry. Lippincott Williams & Wilkins; 2021.
5. Murthy RS. National mental health survey of India 2015–2016. Indian journal of psychiatry. 2017;59(1):21.
6. Geddes JR, Andreasen NC. New Oxford textbook of psychiatry. Oxford University Press, USA; 2020.
7. World Health Organization. International classification of diseases for mortality and morbidity statistics (11th Revision).
8. https://www.cdc.gov/suicide/facts/index.html#:~:text=Suicide%20is%20death%20caused%20by,suicide%20or%20protect%20against%20it
9. https://ncrb.gov.in/sites/default/files/adsi2020_Chapter-2-Suicides.pdf
10. Dutheil F, Aubert C, Pereira B, et al. Suicide among physicians and health-care workers: A systematic review and meta-analysis. *PLoS One*. 2019;14(12):e0226361.

5 Anxiety or Fear-related Disorders

Praveen Tripathi, Priyanka Goyal

PS8.1	Enumerate and describe the magnitude and aetiology of anxiety disorders
PS8.2	Enumerate, elicit, describe, and document clinical features in patients with anxiety disorders
PS8.3	Enumerate and describe the indications and interpret laboratory and other tests used in anxiety disorders
PS8.4	Describe the treatment of anxiety disorders including behavioural and pharmacologic therapy
PS8.5	Demonstrate family education in a patient with anxiety disorders in a simulated environment
PS8.6	Enumerate and describe the pharmacologic basis and side effects of drugs used in anxiety disorders
PS8.7	Enumerate the appropriate conditions for specialist referral in anxiety disorders

ANXIETY

Anxiety is a commonly experienced human emotion. It is characterised by a sense of "nervousness" along with associated autonomic symptoms such as palpitations, perspiration, heaviness in the chest, etc.

SYMPTOMS OF ANXIETY

A. Physical symptoms:
a. Palpitations
b. Tremors
c. Sweating
d. Hyperventilation
e. Heaviness in the chest
f. Dry mouth
g. Cold, clammy skin
h. Restlessness
i. Diarrhoea
j. Increased urinary frequency and urgency
k. Mydriasis
l. Hyperreflexia

B. Psychological symptoms:
a. Feeling of nervousness, vague sense of apprehension
b. Fearfulness and irritability
c. Confusion
d. Hyperarousal

Anxiety is not always abnormal. In fact, it has been found that anxiety (arousal) has an **'inverted U shaped'** relationship with performance. When anxiety is too low, the performance is poor. As anxiety increases, the performance also increases to a certain level, after which any further increase in anxiety decreases the performance. This relationship is commonly experienced in day-to-day life too. For example, if a student is entirely relaxed about an upcoming exam, his performance may remain sub-optimal. Some level of anxiety for exams is needed to work hard and get a good result. However, if the student becomes too anxious, it will hamper the performance.

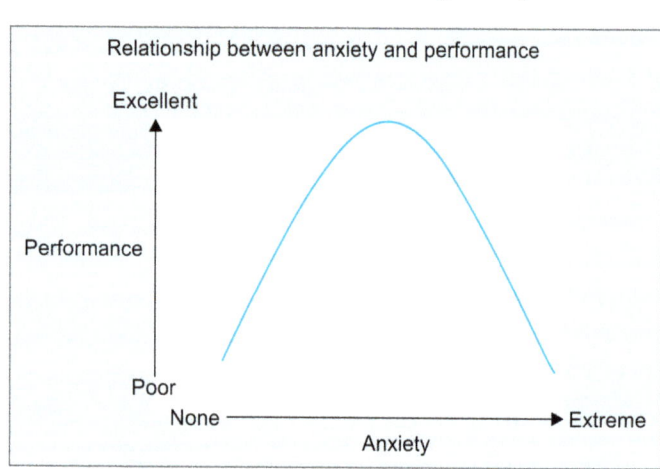

Anxiety and Fear

Both anxiety and fear are alerting signals and warn the person of an impending danger. However, there are finer differences. Fear is a response to an external, well-defined and known threat, whereas anxiety is a response to an internal, vague and unknown threat. The emotional response to an approaching tiger (external and known threat of getting killed) is fear, whereas the emotional response while going on the stage for public speaking (internal and vague threat of possibly getting humiliated) is anxiety.

CLASSIFICATION OF ANXIETY DISORDERS

The ICD-11 and DSM-5 have classified the following as anxiety disorders:
- Panic disorder
- Agoraphobia
- Specific phobia
- Social anxiety disorder (social phobia)
- Generalised anxiety disorder (GAD)
- Separation anxiety disorder
- Selective mutism

PANIC DISORDERS

Panic attack: It is an acute attack of intense anxiety associated with a **feeling of impending doom**.

According to DSM-5, at least four of the following symptoms should be present to make the diagnosis of a panic attack:
1. Palpitations, pounding heart or accelerated heart rate
2. Sweating
3. Trembling or shaking
4. Shortness of breath
5. Feeling of choking
6. Chest pain or discomfort
7. Nausea or abdominal distress
8. Feeling dizzy or light-headed or faint
9. Chills or heat sensations
10. Numbness or tingling sensations (paraesthesia)
11. Derealisation (feeling of unreality) or depersonalisation (feeling of being detached from oneself)
12. Fear of losing control or "going crazy"
13. Fear of dying

During the attack, anxiety increases rapidly and peaks in around 10 minutes. The attack usually lasts for about 20–30 minutes and can sometimes last for hours. During the attack, patients are focused on the somatic symptoms and may believe that they are about to die of cardiac or respiratory causes; others may feel that they will 'go mad'. Patients also believe that they are incapacitated and feel a strong need to escape from their current situation and reach a place of safety, such as the home.

Due to its frightening nature, the patient fears the possibility of more panic attacks. This worry about the possibility of having another panic attack is called **anticipatory anxiety**. Patients also start worrying about the consequences of panic attacks. They may believe that panic attacks suggest a life-threatening illness like cardiac or respiratory disease or a severe psychiatric disorder.

Patients also often develop a fear of situations associated with the previous panic attacks and may avoid those situations (**avoidance**). Patients may develop fear and avoidance of situations from which escape is difficult and where help might not be available (as during attacks, patients want to escape from the situation; and believe that they can not control themselves and need external help). This results in symptomatology that is quite similar to agoraphobia (explained later in this chapter). If the symptoms are severe enough, a separate diagnosis of agoraphobia should be made in these patients.

Usually, panic attacks are unexpected (out of the blue); however, they may occur in particular situations (called **situational panic attacks**). Some patients may have panic attacks in a particular situation on some occasions, but not always (called **situationally predisposed panic attacks**). Many patients have panic attacks at night, which wake them up from the sleep (called **nocturnal panic attacks**).

Panic attacks may be a feature of many psychiatric disorders such as specific phobias (where panic attacks are usually seen only in the presence of the phobic stimulus), social phobias (usually panic attacks are limited to the social situations), obsessive-compulsive disorder (usually in the context of obsessional concerns such as contaminations), depression, etc. However, in all these disorders, panic attacks occur in particular situations and hence are called **expected panic attacks**.

A diagnosis of **panic disorder** is made in the presence of recurrent and **unexpected** panic attacks. Also, according to DSM-5, to make a diagnosis of panic disorder, at least one of the panic attacks should be followed by a month of one of the following symptoms: (1) excessive concerns about additional panic attacks (anticipatory anxiety) or their consequences; (2) maladaptive changes in behaviour related to attacks (such as avoidance).

Epidemiology

According to DSM-5, the 12-month prevalence of panic disorder across the United States and several European countries is about 2–3% in adults and adolescents. Panic disorders are rarely seen in children, and females are more commonly affected than males. According to NMHS 2016, panic disorder has a 0.50% lifetime prevalence and 0.28% current prevalence in India.

Differential Diagnosis

- **Medical disorders:** The following table lists the medical conditions with a panic attack-like presentation **(Table 5.1)**.
- **Psychiatric disorders:** As discussed above, panic attacks may be present in many psychiatric conditions such as

Table 5.1: Medical conditions that can present with panic-like symptoms.

Cardiovascular disorders	Myocardial infarction. Angina, arrhythmias (especially supraventricular tachycardia), mitral valve prolapse, congestive heart failure
Respiratory disorders	Asthma, chronic obstructive pulmonary disease (COPD), hyperventilation syndrome
Neurological disorders	Seizures, cerebrovascular diseases, migraine, vestibular diseases
Endocrine disorders	Hyperthyroidism, hypoparathyroidism, hypoglycaemia, pheochromocytoma, carcinoid syndrome, Cushing's disease, Addison's disease
Substance-induced	Caffeine, cocaine, cannabis, nicotine, hallucinogens, amphetamines
Substance withdrawal	Alcohol, sedatives, and hypnotics
Haematological	Anaemia

specific phobias, social phobias, post-traumatic stress disorder, and obsessive-compulsive disorder, and therefore, a distinction needs to be made. Further, panic disorder with accompanying anticipatory anxiety may also resemble GAD; however, it must be remembered that in GAD, the anxiety is about most of the aspects of life, whereas in panic disorder, the anxiety is about the possibility of the next panic attack.

Aetiology

Neurobiological Factors

Anxiety and fear are normal adaptive responses to threats. It is believed that the dysregulation in brain circuits that mediate fear and anxiety results in panic disorder. This circuit involves the amygdala, hypothalamus, locus ceruleus, anterior cingulate, periaqueductal gray, insula and the prefrontal cortex. This dysregulation results in severe anxiety response (panic attacks) to non-threatening stimuli.

Neurotransmitters: Neurotransmitters and neuromodulators that have been hypothesised to be involved in the development of panic disorder include norepinephrine, serotonin, GABA, and cholecystokinin. Recently endogenous opioids have also been found to play a role. Increased noradrenergic activity (increased sympathetic tone) has been found in patients with panic disorders. Noradrenergic agents like yohimbine and isoproterenol can cause panic attacks by increasing noradrenergic activity (hence called panicogens).

Deficient serotonergic activity has also been found in patients, and the effectiveness of selective serotonin reuptake inhibitors (SSRIs) in treating panic disorders provides evidence for the same.

The most robust evidence of the involvement of GABA is provided by the effectiveness of benzodiazepines in the management of panic disorder. Another evidence is the ability of GABA antagonists (like flumazenil) and reverse benzodiazepine agonists (like beta-carboline) to induce panic attacks (panicogens).

Cholecystokinin and pentagastrin (an agonist of cholecystokinin receptor) are also known to induce panic attacks.

Apart from the above mentioned neuroendocrine panicogens, certain substances cause panic attacks by causing respiratory stimulation. These so-called respiratory panicogens include carbon dioxide (5–35% mixtures), sodium lactate and bicarbonate.

Genetics: The genetic contribution to the development of the panic disorder is suggested by a four to eight times higher risk of development of the panic disorder in the first degree relatives of patients compared to control and a higher monozygotic concordance rate than dizygotic concordance rate.

Psychological Theories

Psychoanalytic theory: According to the psychoanalytic theory, unconscious internal conflicts are responsible for the development of the symptoms. Sigmund Freud proposed that anxiety signals that certain unconscious and unacceptable thoughts or impulses (such as unacceptable sexual thoughts) are trying to reach the conscious mind. On getting this signal, the ego (the part of the mind that maintains equilibrium) uses a defence mechanism called "repression" and prevents these unacceptable thoughts/impulses from reaching the conscious mind. If this defence fails, anxiety may appear with an overwhelming sense of apprehension and somatic symptoms (presents as a panic attack). Psychoanalytic theories have few practical applications in patient management, and they have been described in this book primarily because of their historical significance.

Cognitive theory: According to cognitive theory, panic attacks develop due to **catastrophic misinterpretation of benign sensations** (e.g., a person who has tachycardia after fast walking may misinterpret it as a sign of impending heart attack). This misinterpretation further increases the arousal (in this case, further increase in heart rate) and may set in motion a vicious cycle that ends in a panic attack.

Comorbidities

Panic disorders frequently present with comorbid psychiatric disorders. Common comorbidities include other anxiety disorders (especially agoraphobia), major depression, bipolar disorders and substance use disorders. Identifying panic disorder with comorbid depression is especially important because of the high suicide risk in this subset of patients.

Treatment

Both pharmacotherapy and psychotherapy are effective in the treatment of panic disorder.

Pharmacotherapy: The effective medications include benzodiazepines, SSRIs, serotonin-norepinephrine reuptake inhibitors (SNRIs), tricyclic antidepressants and monoamine oxidase inhibitors (MAOIs). Of these, the most commonly used are benzodiazepines and SSRIs. A widely used approach is to start a benzodiazepine (like alprazolam or clonazepam) along with an SSRI (like paroxetine, escitalopram, etc.). The benzodiazepines provide immediate relief from symptoms and are gradually tapered off and stopped while the SSRIs are continued for a longer duration. Pharmacotherapy is generally continued for at least 8–12 months and may continue for a longer period.

Psychotherapy: Cognitive behavioural therapy is the most commonly used therapy and focuses on challenging the catastrophic interpretations of benign stimuli. In case any avoidance behaviour is present, it is discouraged.

Family therapy and group therapy are also used in some patients. Other modalities like psychodynamic psychotherapy (which works on principles of psychoanalysis) are rarely used nowadays.

Few studies have shown that combining pharmacotherapy with cognitive behavioural therapy provides better results than either alone, although evidence is conflicting.

AGORAPHOBIA

Agoraphobia is defined as a fear of places from which **"escape is difficult".** According to DSM-5, for a diagnosis of agoraphobia, the patient should have marked fear or anxiety about two (or more) of the following situations:
1. Using public transportation (e.g., buses, trains, etc.)
2. Being in open spaces (e.g., parking lots, bridges, etc.)
3. Being in enclosed places (e.g., theatres, shops, etc.)
4. Being in crowded places or standing in line
5. Being outside of the home alone

The patients are fearful or anxious about these situations (agoraphobic situations) as they have thoughts that if they were to develop panic-like symptoms or some other embarrassing symptoms (such as vomiting, etc.), they would not be able to escape or get any help. Patients actively avoid the agoraphobic situations and may insist that someone accompany them while going to any of the feared situations (the presence of a companion reassures them that help would be available if something were to happen). Due to this strong avoidance, patients may become homebound. Further, they may change their behaviours significantly to avoid the feared situation (e.g., a patient may take an apartment near the workplace to avoid using public transport).

Researchers in the USA believe that agoraphobia develops due to panic attacks. According to them, a patient who has unexpected panic attacks becomes fearful of situations where he believes escape or getting help would be difficult. On the other hand, researchers in Europe (as reflected in ICD) believe that agoraphobia is dominant over panic attacks. Now, it is agreed that both diagnoses should be made if the symptom criteria of both are met.

Aetiology

As mentioned earlier, most the researchers believe that agoraphobia is a consequence of panic disorder, and hence researchers have studied the two conditions together with a focus on panic disorder. The aetiology of panic disorder has already been discussed.

Epidemiology

According to DSM-5, the 12-month prevalence rate of agoraphobia is 1.7% in adolescents and adults, with a much lesser prevalence in children and the elderly. Females are twice as likely to develop agoraphobia as males. According to NMHS, agoraphobia has a 1.62% current prevalence in India.

Differential Diagnoses

Agoraphobia should be differentiated from conditions that manifest with anxiety symptoms and avoidance, such as social phobia, specific phobias, separation anxiety disorder, major depressive disorder, paranoid personality disorder, schizophrenia, avoidant personality disorder and dependent personality disorder.

Treatment

Both pharmacotherapy and psychotherapeutic techniques are used.

Pharmacotherapy: Similar to panic disorder, benzodiazepines and SSRIs are the first-line agents. Benzodiazepines provide immediate symptom control, whereas SSRIs are more useful for long-term treatment. Tricyclic antidepressants are also effective but not as commonly used because of their adverse side effects profile.

Psychotherapy: Cognitive behavioural therapy has been found to be useful. It focuses on behavioural techniques such as systematic desensitisation (graded exposure to stimuli while using relaxation techniques), graded exposure (to the feared situation) and relaxation techniques, along with cognitive techniques with a focus on correcting faulty thinking patterns. These techniques have been explained in detail in the section on specific phobias.

Behavioural therapy, which uses only behavioural techniques without using cognitive techniques, is also helpful.

Other treatment modalities like psychodynamic psychotherapy, group therapy and family therapy are at times used.

SOCIAL ANXIETY DISORDER (SOCIAL PHOBIA)

Social anxiety disorder (or social phobia) is the fear of **'humiliation or embarrassment'** in social or performance situations. The individual fears that he might behave in an embarrassing manner or show anxiety symptoms. And that others would evaluate him negatively, resulting in humiliation and embarrassment. It must be remembered that the patient is not afraid of social situations per se; instead, the fear is that of embarrassment or humiliation in the social situations.

Some anxiety is 'normal' in social and performance situations (such as interviews, public speaking, meeting new people, eating or drinking in public), which involve potential evaluation by others. However, in patients with social anxiety disorder, the situations mentioned above result in incapacitating levels of anxiety, often associated with escape (leaving the anxiety-provoking situation) and avoidance (not going to such situations in the first place). The anxiety symptoms that these patients experience include blushing (hallmark symptom), trembling, sweating, dryness of mouth, and stumbling over words. When these symptoms occur, the patient gets further convinced that others will notice these, and the anxiety increases even more. Escape and avoidance may provide temporary relief but reinforces the belief of incompetence in social functioning.

Epidemiology

According to DSM-5, the 12-month prevalence rate of social anxiety disorder in the United States is approximately 7%. Females are more commonly affected than males. The mean age of onset is 13 years.

Comorbidity

Most patients with social anxiety disorder have another comorbid anxiety disorder. Apart from this, depression and alcohol use disorders are also common.

Aetiology

Certain traits in childhood have been linked to the later development of social anxiety disorder. The most important ones are extreme shyness and behavioural inhibition (a tendency to withdraw from new people or settings). It has been suggested that these traits may be an early manifestation of social anxiety disorder.

- **Genetic factors** also contribute, as suggested by higher rates of social anxiety disorder in relatives of individuals with the disorder in comparison to relatives of individuals without the disorder. Further evidence of genetic role is provided by a higher monozygotic concordance rate than the dizygotic concordance rate.
- **Neurochemical factors** involved include serotonin, dopamine and norepinephrine dysregulation.

Differential Diagnosis

Other psychiatric disorders that may present with social avoidance, such as agoraphobia, panic disorder, avoidant personality disorder, major depressive disorder and schizoid personality disorder, should be differentiated from social anxiety disorder.

Treatment

Both pharmacotherapy and psychotherapy are effective in the treatment of social anxiety disorder, and a combination of the two may be more effective than either alone.

Pharmacotherapy: SSRIs are considered the **first-line treatment** for social anxiety disorders. Due to their rapid onset of action, benzodiazepines are frequently used in the short term; however, the possibility of dependence on benzodiazepines should be kept in mind. For performance situations such as stage performance or exams, beta-blockers like propranolol or atenolol are frequently used immediately before exposure.

Other medications that can be used include SNRIs, MAOI, RIMA (reversible inhibitors of monoamine oxidase A), buspirone and pregabalin.

Psychotherapy: Cognitive behavioural therapy that focuses on exposure techniques alone or exposure techniques along with cognitive restructuring has the best evidence in the management of social anxiety disorder. Exposure involves confronting the feared situation in a graded manner, starting from situations that cause lesser anxiety and gradually moving to situations that cause more anxiety. Cognitive restructuring is based on cognitive theory, according to which the patients tend to overestimate the risk and underestimate their own coping skills in feared situations. Cognitive restructuring involves challenging this faulty thinking pattern and dysfunctional belief system. Other techniques that can be used include relaxation training, social skill training, group therapy, etc.

■ SPECIFIC PHOBIA (TABLE 5.2)

Specific phobia is the persistent, marked and excessive or unreasonable fear of a specific object or a situation.

Table 5.2: Types of phobias.

Phobias	
Claustrophobia	Fear of closed spaces
Acrophobia	Fear of heights
Algophobia	Fear of pain
Thanatophobia	Fear of death
Ailurophobia	Fear of cats
Cynophobia	Fear of dogs
Mysophobia	Fear of dirt and germs
Xenophobia	Fear of strangers

The exposure or anticipation of exposure to the feared stimuli leads to physiological and psychological symptoms of anxiety, at times causing a panic attack. These patients get anxious only in response to exposure/anticipation of exposure to the particular phobic stimulus; otherwise, they do not show any anxiety symptoms. Additionally, patients usually show avoidance (behaviours to avoid the phobic stimulus) and escape behaviours.

The DSM-5 classifies specific phobias into the following subtypes:
1. Animal (e.g., dogs, spiders)
2. Natural environment (e.g., storms, heights, water)
3. Blood-injection-injury (e.g., needles, medical procedures)
4. Situational (e.g., elevators, aeroplanes, enclosed spaces)
5. Others

Patients with animal, natural environmental, and situational phobias usually show a sympathetic response on exposure to the feared stimuli; on the other hand, patients with a blood-injection-injury phobia are more likely to have a biphasic, **vasovagal response,** wherein initially there is a brief acceleration of heart rate and elevated blood pressure, followed by a drop in both that may result in fainting.

Epidemiology

According to DSM-5, the 12-month prevalence rate for specific phobias in the USA is approximately 7–9%. The prevalence in females is about twice that in males, although the blood-injection-injury subtype is equally prevalent in both sexes. The mean age of onset for specific phobias is between 7 and 11 years, although situational phobias have a later onset, usually in the early 20s. According to NMHS, phobic anxiety disorders have a 1.91% current prevalence in the Indian population.

Comorbidity

The vast majority (>80%) of patients with specific phobias have another psychiatric comorbidity, common ones being depression, bipolar disorder, other anxiety disorders and substance use disorders.

Aetiology

The evidence for genetic transmission is provided by higher rates of specific phobia in first degree relatives of persons with specific phobia in comparison to first degree relatives of persons without specific phobias. Further evidence is provided by a higher concordance rate in monozygotic twins than in dizygotic twins. Neurobiologically, hyperactivation of the amygdala (amygdala is involved in fear processing) and the insula has been found in patients with phobic disorders. Studies have shown that children with 'behavioural inhibition' are predisposed to the development of phobias.

Two important psychological theories on the aetiology of phobias are as follows:

1. **Behavioural theory:** According to this theory, phobias develop by classical conditioning and are maintained by operant conditioning (for details about classical and operant conditioning, refer to the chapter, Psychological theories and interventions). Phobia of a neutral stimulus may develop if this neutral stimulus gets repeatedly paired with a frightening (anxiety-provoking) stimulus.
   a. For example: Say, a young boy is shown a white rat toy, and immediately afterwards, a loud and scary sound is made. The boy's response to the loud sound would be that of fear. If repeatedly the white rat toy is paired with the loud sound, after some time, the mere sight of the white rat toy will be enough to cause anxiety in the young boy. This is the first stage in the development of phobia, mediated by classical conditioning.
   b. If the white rat toy is no longer paired with the loud sound, the boy will gradually stop being fearful of the white rat toy (called the extinction of response). This extinction of response doesn't happen in phobia due to avoidance.
   c. If the child starts avoiding the white rat toy, he will never know that now the white rat toy is no longer linked with any loud sound. Since avoidance helps the child to reduce anxiety, it reinforces the avoidance behaviour (negative reinforcement, a concept of operant conditioning). The avoidance helps in reducing the anxiety in the short term, but in the long term, the phobia becomes stable. This is the second stage in the development of phobia mediated by operant conditioning.
2. **Psychoanalytical theory:** Freud proposed that phobias are caused by an unresolved Oedipus complex (for details, refer to the chapter 'psychoanalysis'). According to this theory, the unconscious incestuous sexual desire tries for conscious expression, resulting in anxiety. To control the anxiety, the ego uses the defence mechanism of repression. However, if repression fails to be entirely successful, other defence mechanisms are used. The primary defence mechanism used is displacement, in which the anxiety is displaced from the person evoking it to a less relevant object or situation. The chosen object may have some association with and symbolises the primary source of anxiety (hence defence mechanism of symbolisation is also involved). Finally, the defence mechanism of avoidance is used to avoid this new anxiety-causing stimulus, and a complete picture of phobic disorder develops.

Differential Diagnosis

Specific phobias should be differentiated from panic disorders, agoraphobia and anxious (avoidant) personality disorders, paranoid personality disorders, obsessive-compulsive disorders.

Treatment

Psychotherapy

1. **Behaviour therapy:** It is the **most effective therapy** in treating specific phobias. The therapy is based on the behavioural theory that phobias are learned behaviours and hence can be unlearned by using behavioural techniques. The treatment focuses on exposure-based techniques, wherein the patient is intentionally confronted with the feared object or situation. The following are the exposure-based techniques that are commonly used:
   a. **Systematic desensitisation:** Here, a list of anxiety-provoking stimuli is made, from the least anxiety-provoking stimulus to the most anxiety-provoking stimulus (e.g., in a patient with claustrophobia, the least anxiety-provoking stimulus may be bolting the door of the bathroom, and the most anxiety-provoking stimulus may be getting stuck in a lift with power failure and no lights, with a number of other situations in between). Also, the patient is trained in relaxation techniques, such as progressive muscle relaxation. Finally, the patient uses relaxation techniques in the presence of the least anxiety-provoking stimulus so that the anxiety-provoking stimulus no longer elicits any anxiety response (desensitisation to stimuli). Once desensitisation occurs, the patient moves to the subsequent stimuli in the list, and the process is repeated till complete desensitisation is achieved.
   b. **In vivo exposure:** Here, a hierarchy of anxiety-provoking stimuli is made, and the patient is made to confront the feared object in a graded manner. However, no relaxation techniques are used, and instead, the patient is allowed to get habituated to the feared object till it no longer elicits any anxiety response. Once habituation occurs, the patient is exposed to the next stimuli in the hierarchy, and the process is repeated
   c. **Imaginal exposure:** Here, instead of using the actual stimulus, the patient is made to imagine the feared stimulus, and habituation is attempted. Of late, VRE (virtual reality exposure) has been developed in which a three-dimensional simulation of the feared stimulus is used to increase the efficacy of exposure.
   d. **Modelling (participant modelling):** Here, the patient sees other patients or therapists contact the phobic stimulus and learns by observation.
   e. **Flooding (implosion):** In this technique, the patient is exposed to the phobic stimulus in its severe form, and the accompanying anxiety is gradually allowed to subside by habituation. For example, a patient who is afraid of heights is taken to the roof of a 50-floor

building, where the patient is likely to experience intense anxiety. As the patient remains there, the anxiety should gradually decrease due to habituation. This technique is rarely used as sudden exposure to a strong stimulus may result in a panic attack.

Along with the exposure-based techniques, the addition of cognitive restructuring (that focuses on phobia specific irrational thoughts and reinforces that phobic situation is, in reality, safe) is efficacious.
2. **Insight oriented psychotherapy:** It uses the principles of psychoanalysis for the treatment and is rarely used nowadays.
3. Other modalities include relaxation techniques, supportive therapy and family therapy.

Pharmacotherapy

In the treatment of specific phobias, pharmacotherapy has a limited role. The medications that have shown some efficacy include benzodiazepines and beta-blockers (both provide short term symptomatic relief). Other drug classes that have been found effective in the studies include SSRIs and d-cycloserine.

GENERALISED ANXIETY DISORDER

It is characterised by **excessive worries** and anxiety about minor and everyday issues (hence the term 'generalised anxiety' or '**free-floating anxiety**') such as work, relationships, health, etc. The patient finds it difficult to control the worries and experiences distress and impairment in functioning. The worry and anxiety are associated with somatic symptoms such as tremulousness, muscle tension, heaviness in the chest, irritability, insomnia, increased urinary frequency and diarrhoea.

According to DSM-5, the 12-month prevalence of GAD is 2.9%, with the women to men ratio being 2:1. Generalised anxiety disorder is often comorbid with other anxiety disorders such as social phobia, social phobia and panic disorder, and major depressive disorder is a common comorbidity. According to NMHS, generalised anxiety disorder has a 0.57% lifetime prevalence and 0.57% current prevalence in the Indian population.

Aetiology

- **Genetic factors:** Higher rates in first degree relatives of patients with GAD than controls suggest a genetic contribution to the development of GAD. A higher concordance rate in monozygotic twins than in dizygotic twins, too, suggests a genetic contribution.
- **Neurobiological factors:** In patients with GAD, resting levels of catecholamines are normal; however, studies have found a reduced density of alpha-2 adrenergic receptors in platelets as well as a subnormal response to both stimulation as well as blockade of alpha-2 adrenergic receptors. This suggests the downregulation of alpha-2 receptors due to prior higher levels of noradrenaline (norepinephrine). The efficacy of benzodiazepines to relieve anxiety symptoms suggests abnormalities in GABA functioning. Studies have found abnormalities in benzodiazepine receptor binding and distribution. Some studies have shown abnormalities in serotonin transmission, too, but any strong evidence is still elusive.
- **Psychological factors:** Patients with GAD and other anxiety disorders have a diminished '**sense of control**', i.e., they believe that they would not be able to control difficult situations in their lives and may inaccurately perceive a neutral situation as threatening by focusing selectively on negative details. Early life experiences have been hypothesised to result in the development of a diminished sense of control. In particular, if parents are overprotective and do not express encouragement and warmth towards the child's attempts to explore the world, it may develop a sense of inefficacy in the child, which may later predispose him to anxiety disorders like GAD. Patients with GAD also have 'an intolerance of uncertainty, i.e., they have a negative reaction to uncertain situations and events. Excessive worry, a cardinal feature of GAD, is an ineffective attempt to assert control over uncertain future events. Patients who have excessive worries report that by worrying, they can prepare for negative outcomes and minimise their emotional responsiveness to negative outcomes. Therefore, worrying is an attempt to get a feeling of control over future outcomes.

Differential Diagnosis

The GAD must be differentiated from various medical and psychiatric disorders with similar presentations. The differentials of GAD are quite similar to panic disorders.

Comorbidity

Patients with GAD often have other anxiety disorders such as panic disorders, phobias, OCD and PTSD as comorbidities. Particularly, major depressive disorder is a common comorbidity.

Treatment

Psychotherapy

- **Cognitive behavioural therapy:** It is the **most effective** psychotherapy in GAD and consists of both cognitive techniques such as cognitive restructuring (in which faulty thinking patterns are identified and corrected) and behavioural techniques such as exposure and relaxation training.
- **Supportive psychotherapy**, wherein the patient is provided reassurance and support, can also be used, but its long-term efficacy is not proven.
- **Insight oriented psychotherapy:** It uses the principles of psychoanalysis for the treatment and is rarely used nowadays.

Pharmacotherapy

Benzodiazepines and SSRIs are most commonly used for the pharmacological treatment of GAD. Benzodiazepines provide immediate anxiolytic effects, and apart from anti-anxiety, they also have effects such as muscle relaxation and a general sense of well-being. However, benzodiazepines should be avoided in the longer term because of their dependence potential. A good strategy is to start benzodiazepines and SSRIs together, gradually taper down the benzodiazepines in the next 2–3 weeks and then stop them while continuing the SSRIs for a longer period of time.

Azapirones like buspirone, which are 5-HT1A receptor partial agonists, are also effective, but unlike benzodiazepines, they take around 2–3 weeks to show an anxiolytic effect.

Venlafaxine, a serotonin-norepinephrine reuptake inhibitor, has also been found to be effective. Recently, pregabalin has also shown efficacy in treating symptoms of GAD.

Beta-blockers can also be used specifically for somatic symptoms of anxiety, such as performance associated anxiety.

MIXED ANXIETY AND DEPRESSIVE DISORDER

This diagnosis is used when symptoms of both anxiety and depression are present, but they are not severe enough to meet the criteria of either an anxiety disorder or a depressive disorder. To make the diagnosis of mixed anxiety and depressive disorder, some autonomic symptoms (such as tremors, palpitations, etc.), should be present in the patient. The treatment is symptomatic.

SEPARATION ANXIETY DISORDER

Separation anxiety disorder is characterised by excessive fear or anxiety regarding separation from home or from those to whom the individual is attached (such as a mother or other primary caregivers). It is more commonly seen in children and is comparatively less common in adolescents and adults.

Separation anxiety is universally seen in infants and usually peaks between 9–18 months of age, followed by a gradual decline and diminishment by 2.5 years. Separation anxiety disorder is diagnosed when the separation anxiety is excessive and developmentally abnormal, as suggested by the following:

- There is a persistent and excessive fear of separation from prominent attachment figures, which manifests in the form of reluctance to go to school, work, or away from home, or sleep in a separate room. In case separation happens or is anticipated, there is significant distress. There may be physical symptoms such as headaches or abdominal pain when separation happens (e.g., in school). There may be recurrent nightmares on the theme of separation too.
- There is a persistent and excessive worry that something untoward will happen to the attachment figures, such as an accident or a grave illness that will result in the separation. There is also an excessive worry of something untoward happening to self, such as kidnapping or an accident that will result in the separation.

For diagnosis, the symptoms must persist for at least 4 weeks in the case of children and adolescents and at least 6 months in adults.

Treatment: The **combination** of CBT (cognitive behavioural therapy) and SSRI is more effective than CBT alone or SSRIs alone. Other psychotherapy modes such as family therapy and psychoeducation can also be used.

SELECTIVE MUTISM

Selective mutism is an anxiety disorder that is more commonly seen in children than adolescents or adults. As the name suggests, it is characterised by consistent failure to speak in one or more specific social situations (usually the school setting) while speaking fluently in other more familiar situations, such as at home. Some children with selective mutism may only whisper or use gestures or single-syllable words for communication. These children are at greater risk of delayed onset of speech or language abnormalities. Children with selective mutism almost always have social anxiety.

The treatment usually involves the use of CBT, SSRIs, and psychoeducation of the family.

CASE BASED MCQ

A middle-aged man presented with complaints of fear of travelling alone for the last three years. He would always insist that a family member accompany him whenever he went outside. The patient also lost his job as he insisted on working from home and refused to come to the office when his company asked for it. Prior to the consultation, he had left his house only on two occasions in the last one year, and that too when his younger brother accompanied him. When asked why, the patient said, 'I am afraid that if something were to happen to me, someone should always be there to help me. What is the likely diagnosis?
a. Agoraphobia
b. Panic disorder
c. Social anxiety disorder
d. Generalised anxiety disorder

Ans. a. The history is suggestive of fear of travelling alone, which is a feature of agoraphobia.

SUGGESTED READINGS

1. American Psychiatric Association DS, American Psychiatric Association. Diagnostic and statistical manual of mental disorders: DSM-5. Washington, DC: American psychiatric association; 2013.
2. Geddes JR, Andreasen NC. New Oxford textbook of psychiatry. Oxford University Press, USA; 2020.
3. Boland R, Verdiun M, Ruiz P. Kaplan & Sadock's Synopsis of Psychiatry. Lippincott Williams & Wilkins; 2021.
4. Tasman A, Kay J, Lieberman JA, First MB, Riba M, editors. Psychiatry, 2 Volume Set. John Wiley & Sons; 2015.
5. Simon N, Hollander E, Rothbaum BO, Stein DJ, editors. The American Psychiatric Association Publishing Textbook of Anxiety, Trauma, and OCD-Related Disorders. American Psychiatric Pub; 2020.

6. Obsessive-compulsive and Related Disorders

Praveen Tripathi, Priyanka Goyal

Obsessive-compulsive and related disorders have been introduced as a separate diagnostic category in both DSM-5 and ICD-11. The disorders that constitute this diagnostic category are characterised by **repetitive and intrusive thoughts and/or repetitive behaviours** and include the following:
- Obsessive-compulsive disorder (OCD)
- Body dysmorphic disorder (BDD)
- Hoarding disorder
- Body focused repetitive behaviour disorders (Trichotillomania and Excoriation disorder)
- Olfactory reference disorder
- Hypochondriasis

OBSESSIVE-COMPULSIVE DISORDER

Obsessive-compulsive disorder is a common psychiatric disorder characterised by the presence of obsessions and/or compulsions.

Obsessions are:
1. Recurrent and intrusive (enter the individual's mind repeatedly) thoughts, images or impulses.
2. Individual recognizes obsessions are a product of their own mind. In other words, the patient identifies obsessions as their 'own thoughts/images/impulses'. This criterion helps in differentiating obsessions from thought insertion. A patient with thought insertion also gets repetitive thoughts; however, he identifies them as someone else's thoughts that are being forced into his mind.
3. Obsessions are usually distressing (because of their violent or obscene content), and the patient finds them absurd and senseless.
4. The patient usually tries to resist obsessions, and obsessions lead to anxiety.

Compulsions are behaviours (or mental acts) that usually follow obsessions and reduce the anxiety associated with obsessions.

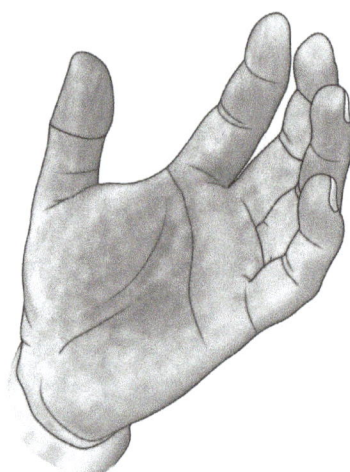

Fig. 6.1: Dry hands due to OCD.

The patient experiences both obsessions and compulsions as irrational and hence **ego-dystonic** (thoughts/behaviours which are not agreeable to self, i.e., unwanted thoughts/behaviours). The obsessions and compulsions are time-consuming (take >1 hour/day) and cause socio-occupational dysfunction. Also, patients often show **avoidance behaviours** and avoid stimuli that may trigger obsessions or compulsions (e.g., a patient who has obsessive thoughts about germs avoids using public toilets). Patients with OCD may have good or fair insight (i.e., they understand that their OCD beliefs are definitely or probably not true or that they may or may not be true), poor insight (they think that their OCD beliefs are probably true) or absent insight/delusional beliefs (they are convinced that their OCD beliefs are true).

The symptoms of obsessions and compulsions must be present for at least **2 weeks** to diagnose OCD.

Symptom pattern: Around 3/4th of the patients with OCD have both obsessions and compulsions, and most patients have multiple obsessions and compulsions. Symptoms can change over time, and there are four major symptom patterns:

1. **Contamination:** This is the most common pattern wherein patients have an obsession of contamination (e.g., the thought that hands are contaminated with dust or germs; the body is unclean; the household items are contaminated with urine and should not be touched etc.) followed by compulsion of washing. For example, a patient repeatedly had the thought that his hands were dirty; this thought would intrude in his mind again and again, even when he was trying to study or meditate. The thought would make him anxious; he would realize that the thought is senseless and try to stop it, but would usually be unsuccessful (obsessional thought). To decrease the anxiety and discomfort, the patient would feel compelled to wash his hands (compulsive behaviour) repeatedly. The washing would stop the thoughts for some time, and later the same cycle would get repeated. He would also avoid potentially unclean areas, such as using a public toilet, or travelling by train, as, in those places, the thoughts and associated anxiety would become unbearable (avoidance).
2. **Pathological doubt:** This is the second most common pattern where patients have obsessions of doubt followed by compulsions of checking. For example, a shopkeeper would have repeated doubts about whether he locked his shop properly or not at closing down. He would check the lock multiple times and made a ritual of checking the lock seven times before leaving. He had to drive back from midway to home on some occasions to check the lock. The repeated doubts are obsessions, and the repetitive checking is a compulsion.
3. **Intrusive thought:** This is the third most common pattern, characterised by repetitive, intrusive thoughts without any overt compulsions. The obsessive thoughts are usually about religion or aggression or sex and cause significant guilt and distress to the patient. For example, a patient repeatedly had the thought of having sex with a family member. The thought made him extremely anxious and ashamed of himself. The patient understood that the thought was senseless and would try to stop it but was unsuccessful (obsessional thought). To decrease the anxiety, the patient would chant prayers in his mind and beg for forgiveness from god. This would temporarily decrease the anxiety (**mental compulsions**).
4. **Symmetry:** In this fourth most common pattern, patients have an extreme need for symmetry or precision along with the compulsion of slowness (e.g., a patient would try to put all the pens on the table at the same distance from each other and at a precisely 180° angle. If even a single pen was not properly aligned, the patient would feel anxious and uncomfortable, and hence it would take hours for him to set up the table before doing any work

- The most common obsession is the obsession of contamination.
- The most common compulsion is the compulsion of washing.

> **MAGICAL THINKING**
>
> Patients with OCD may believe that just because they thought about an event, it will happen in reality. This is referred to as magical thinking. For example, a patient would repeatedly have a thought, "If I do not knock on the door four times, the house will catch fire". Hence the patient would always knock on the door four times before entering the house. Magical thinking is a common symptom of OCD.

Epidemiology

According to DSM-5, the 12-month prevalence of OCD in the United States is 1.2%, and the international prevalence rates vary from 1.1 to 1.8%. According to NMHS, OCD has a 0.76% current prevalence in India. Females have a slightly higher prevalence than males in adulthood, whereas males are more commonly affected in childhood. The mean age of onset is around 20 years, with males having an earlier age of onset than females.

Aetiology

Neurobiology

It has been hypothesised that the neural circuit involved in OCD is the **cortico-striatal-thalamic-cortical (CSTC) circuit**. It is a neural circuit that starts in the cortex (primarily orbitofrontal cortex and anterior cingulate cortex) and projects to the striatum, from the striatum to the thalamus and back to the cortex. This circuit controls automated behaviours like grooming and other habits, and dysfunction in the circuit can result in excess of such behaviours. Structural and functional neuroimaging findings have corroborated this hypothesis. Studies have also found a **bilaterally small caudate nucleus** in patients with OCD.

Neurotransmitters: Neurotransmitter systems involved in the development of OCD include serotonergic, dopaminergic, glutamatergic and GABAergic systems. The efficacy of serotonin reuptake inhibitors (SSRIs and clomipramine) and dopamine antagonists (antipsychotics) provides indirect evidence of the involvement of these neurotransmitters.

Neuroimmunology: The role of autoimmune factors in OCD is suggested by the presence of obsessive-compulsive symptoms in patients with Sydenham chorea, a feature of rheumatic fever. It has been hypothesised that antibodies against basal ganglia may cause symptoms of OCD.

Genetics

Genetic contribution is suggested by a higher monozygotic concordance rate than the dizygotic concordance rate and higher rates of OCD in family members of patients with OCD compared to control groups.

Psychological Theories

1. **Behavioural theory:** According to the learning theory, obsessions develop when a neutral object or thought gets

paired with an anxiety-provoking object/event so that the previously neutral object/thoughts start provoking anxiety, too (e.g., a person with a regular concern for hygiene and thought that 'hand hygiene must be maintained for a good health', witnessed a friend develop severe food poisoning. Later the thought that 'The hands must be clean; otherwise a serious illness may develop' started causing excessive anxiety). Compulsions develop when the person discovers that certain actions can reduce the anxiety caused by obsessional thoughts. Since these actions reduce anxiety, they get reinforced and are repeated by the patient (e.g., washing hands, in the above-mentioned case, would reduce anxiety). Similarly, avoidance of anxiety-provoking stimuli also reduces anxiety and hence gets reinforced (e.g., avoiding going to public toilets or touching anything that is perceived to be 'dirty').

2. **Cognitive theory:** According to this theory, patients with OCD tend to misinterpret their thoughts. Most people have random thoughts and do not give importance to those thoughts; however, patients with OCD may give exaggerated importance to such thoughts and treat them as a real threat. For example, most parents may have a random thought of harming their child, but they dismiss it as a senseless thought. However, patients with OCD may take that thought as a real danger and indulge in neutralising behaviours (e.g., hiding all sharp objects in the house etc.).

3. **Psychodynamic theory:** According to Sigmund Freud, a regression from the oedipal phase to the anal phase of psychosexual development is seen in OCD. The defence mechanisms involved in the development of OCD include reaction formation, isolation of affect and undoing. (Kindly refer to the Chapter, Psychoanalysis, for details). According to this hypothesis, the following events happen.

During early childhood, patients have some unacceptable impulses, which are managed using the defence mechanism of reaction formation (e.g., a patient with unacceptable sexual impulses uses reaction formation and becomes sexually prudish), resulting in the development of obsessional personality traits. Later, the use of 'isolation of affect' results in the development of obsessions. In 'isolation of affect', the affect (emotions) associated with an anxiety-provoking idea is removed from that idea. This free "anxiety" gets attached to some neutral idea which now becomes anxiety provoking, resulting in the formation of obsessions. Finally, 'undoing' leads to the development of compulsions. In undoing, an act is done to neutralize a previous act/thought. For example, washing hands when a thought comes that the hands are dirty). It must be remembered that psychodynamic theory and treatment are rarely used nowadays.

Comorbidity

The most common comorbidity in patients with OCD is a major depressive disorder. Other common comorbidities include anxiety disorders such as panic disorder, generalised anxiety disorder, social anxiety disorder and specific phobias. Tic disorder is another common comorbidity that is most commonly seen in males with childhood-onset OCD. Obsessive-compulsive personality disorder (OCPD) is also a common comorbidity.

Differential Diagnosis

Other psychiatric disorders: OCD may resemble anxiety disorders that present with repetitive thoughts and avoidant behaviours, such as generalised anxiety disorders. However, the repetitive thoughts in generalised anxiety disorder are excessive worries about real-life concerns, whereas obsessions usually do not involve real-life concerns. Also, compulsions are usually a feature of OCD and are not seen in generalised anxiety disorder.

In depression, the patient may present with ruminations (meaningless chain of thoughts); however, the content of thinking is usually mood-congruent (i.e., matches with the depressive mood), and these thoughts are not considered senseless or distressing (unlike in OCD).

Psychotic disorders like schizophrenia can sometimes be difficult to differentiate from OCD with absent insight/delusional beliefs. The absence of obsessions and compulsions and the presence of typical delusions and hallucinations in psychotic disorders help in the differentiation. OCD may be present as a comorbidity in schizophrenia, and both the diagnosis should be made if the criteria for both are met.

Neurological disorders: Disorders of basal ganglia like Sydenham chorea and Huntington's disease can present with symptoms similar to OCD. A detailed neurological assessment and imaging are required to rule out the neurological causes, especially in patients with a late onset of obsessions and compulsions.

Tic disorders: The presentation of complex tics may be quite similar to compulsions. However, tics are preceded by sensory urges, whereas obsessions precede compulsions.

Course and Prognosis

Around 50% of patients with OCD have a sudden onset of symptoms. The course is usually chronic and variable. Around 20–30% of patients have significant improvement in their symptoms, around 40–50% have moderate improvement, and the remaining 20–40% have no improvement or further deterioration.

> **PANDAS:** Paediatric Autoimmune Neuropsychiatric Disorders Associated with Streptococcal infection.
> In a small number of cases, OCD in children may be precipitated/worsened after infection with Group A β-hemolytic *Streptococcus* (GABHS). It has been hypothesised that the infection triggers an autoimmune response in the basal ganglia and leads to the rapid development of OCD and tics. These cases of infection triggered OCD are referred to as PANDAS.

Treatment

A **combination** of pharmacotherapy and psychotherapy is the preferred approach.

A. ***Pharmacotherapy:*** The standard approach is to start treatment with an SSRI. It has been found that higher dosages of SSRIs are associated with better results, although the likelihood of side effects increases too.

Clomipramine, a Tricyclic antidepressant with potent serotonin uptake blocking property, is also considered a first-line treatment; however, it is rarely used as the first drug due to its adverse effect profile.

With serotonergic agents (SSRIs and clomipramine), around 50-70% of patients respond to the treatment. If treatment with SSRIs or clomipramine provides only partial results, augmentation with antipsychotics (such as **haloperidol**, quetiapine, risperidone and olanzapine) is used. Other drugs that can be used include venlafaxine, lithium, valproate and **carbamazepine**. Benzodiazepines are also often used in the short term as anxiolytics.

B. *Psychotherapy*: Cognitive behavioural therapy relying primarily on the behavioural technique of **exposure and response prevention** (ERP) has the best evidence among all the psychotherapeutic techniques. Exposure and response prevention involves exposure of the patient to a stimulus known to produce obsessional thoughts (**exposure**), followed by asking the patient to not indulge in compulsive behaviour (**response prevention**). This technique reduces the frequency of compulsive behaviour, and later a decrease in the frequency of obsessional thoughts also occurs.

Other behavioural therapies such as **desensitisation, thought stopping, flooding,** and **aversive conditioning** have also been used.

Psychodynamic psychotherapy has not been found effective. Family therapy can be used and helps the family members understand the illness and reduces discord amongst the members.

C. *Other treatment modalities*: Deep brain stimulation has been used in a few intractable cases of OCD. In extreme cases that are treatment-resistant, electroconvulsive therapy and psychosurgery can be considered. The psychosurgical techniques usually include **cingulotomy** and **capsulotomy** (also known as sub **caudate tractotomy**).

BODY DYSMORPHIC DISORDER

This diagnosis was described under 'somatoform disorders' in DSM-IV; however, in DSM-5 and ICD-11, it has been included in 'obsessive-compulsive and related disorders' due to its similarities with the OCD. The onset of BDD is usually in adolescence, and it is more common in females than males. Body dysmorphic disorder (also known as dysmorphophobia) is characterised by:

1. Preoccupation with an **imagined defect in the physical appearance**. If a slight physical anomaly is actually present, the concern regarding it is clearly excessive.
2. Presence of **repetitive behaviours** (e.g., mirror checking, excessive grooming) or mental acts (e.g., comparison with others appearance) and reassurance seeking from others about the appearance.

Excessive preoccupation causes significant distress and socio-occupational dysfunction. Patients are preoccupied with their appearance and believe that they are ugly and unattractive. The preoccupation may be about more than one body part, and the most common sites are **hair, skin and nose**.

Muscle dysmorphia is a particular type of BDD almost exclusively seen in males and is characterised by the preoccupation that one's body is insufficiently muscular.

Patients with BDD may develop ideas of reference (that others are noticing their defects or discussing them) and may start hiding the body parts by clothing or become homebound to avoid being laughed at. They may also avoid all reflective surfaces to stop seeing their presumed deformities.

The degree of insight into illness may vary, and the following are the grades of insight:

1. *Good or fair insight*: The patient recognizes that his beliefs about defects in physical appearance are probably not true
2. *Poor insight*: The patient thinks that beliefs about defects in physical appearance are probably true
3. *Absent insight/delusional beliefs*: The patient is completely convinced about beliefs, and the belief is firm, fixed and unshakeable (belief is delusional in intensity)

Comorbidity

More than 90% of patients with BDD experience a major depressive episode. Anxiety disorders are another common comorbidity. Around 20% of patients with BDD attempt suicide.

Treatment

SSRIs are usually the first-line treatment, along with cognitive behavioural therapy. Cosmetic surgeries are usually unsuccessful in decreasing dissatisfaction with body appearance, and many a time, these patients end up suing their plastic surgeons.

HOARDING DISORDER

Hoarding disorder was earlier considered a subtype of OCD; however, in DSM-5 and ICD-11, it has been made a separate diagnostic entity. It is characterised by:

1. An inability to discard items (discarding includes throwing away, selling or giving to others) that are of little or no value because of a fear that the item may be needed later in future or because of extreme emotional attachment to the item.
2. This inability to discard useless items results in cluttering of the house and a lack of living space.

Most of these patients have poor insight and accumulate items such as newspapers, magazines, old clothes, books etc. There have been reports of the accumulated items catching fire or being infested by pests and, in some cases, patients getting crushed under the possession.

Treatment

Hoarding disorder is quite resistant to treatment. The most effective treatment is cognitive behaviour therapy, in which the patient is helped in decision making (e.g., which items can be discarded and which ones are really useful) and exposure and habituation to discarding (patient is taught to handle the emotions that develop after discarding). SSRIs have been found to be useful in some cases.

BODY-FOCUSED REPETITIVE BEHAVIOUR DISORDER

As the name suggests, these disorders are characterised by repetitive actions directed at the body, specifically integument. The patient tries to stop these behaviours unsuccessfully, and the behaviours have dermatological sequelae such as hair loss and lesions of the skin.

The two important types include:
1. Trichotillomania and
2. Excoriation disorder

Trichotillomania (Hair-pulling Disorder)

It is characterised by repetitive hair pulling, resulting in hair loss. The hair loss is usually visible, but patients may sometimes conceal the hair loss by using make-up or wigs.

Prior to pulling, patients have an impulse to pull out their hair and try to resist the impulse. However, there is an increasing feeling of tension, which drives the patient to do the act of hair-pulling. The act of hair pulling is associated with a sense of relief and, at times, even pleasure. Similar to patients with OCD, patients with trichotillomania consider their behaviour undesirable. The most commonly involved areas are the scalp, eyebrows or eyelashes. Around 35–40% of patients with trichotillomania, at some time during the course of illness, chew or swallow the hair they pull (trichophagy). Trichophagy can cause complications like trichobezoars (hairball accumulations in the intestine), intestinal obstruction and malnutrition.

The mean age at onset is early teenage, and it is more commonly seen in females than males.

Two types of hair pulling have been described:
1. **Focused pulling:** In this type, there is an urge to pull followed by an intentional act of pulling the hair
2. **Automatic pulling:** In this type, the pulling occurs without the person becoming aware of it. The patient reports that they do not even realize when they are pulling the hair.

The treatment mainly involves psychotherapy. Studies have found the effectiveness of behavioural therapy using habit reversal techniques (in habit reversal technique, the patient learns to identify and be aware of the urge that precedes hair pulling and then replaces the act of hair-pulling with some other voluntary acts such as making a fist). Cognitive behavioural therapy has also been found to be effective. Few studies have found SSRIs and clomipramine to be effective.

Excoriation (Skin-picking) Disorder

It is characterised by repetitive picking of skin which results in skin lesions. Prior to skin picking, patients have an urge to pick their skin and often try to resist it. However, there is an increasing feeling of tension, which drives the patient to do the act of skin picking. The act of skin picking is associated with a sense of relief and, at times, even pleasure. However, later most patients feel guilty or embarrassed about their behaviour. Many patients try to hide the skin lesions caused by picking using bandages or make-up.

The mean age of onset is usually between 12 to 16 years of age, and the disorder is more common in females than males.

The treatment involves the use of behavioural therapy using habit reversal techniques and cognitive behavioural therapy. SSRIs and Naltrexone have also shown effectiveness in small trials.

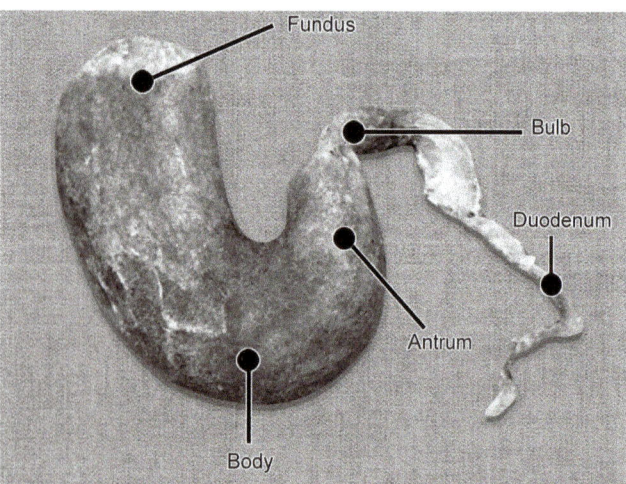

Fig. 6.2: Trichobezoar in trichotillomania.

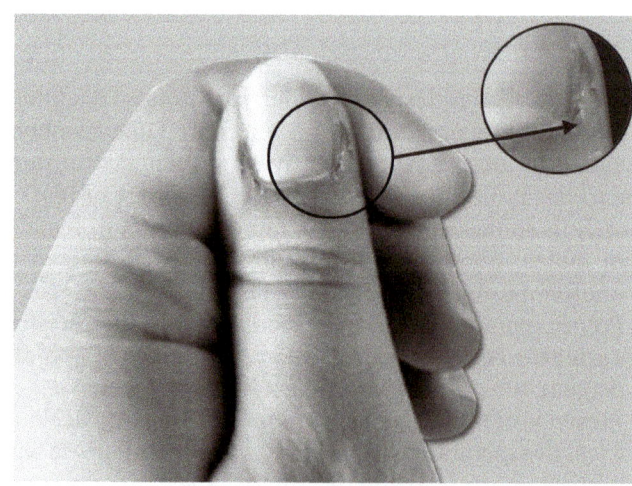

Fig. 6.3: Excoriation disorder.

OLFACTORY REFERENCE DISORDER

Olfactory reference syndrome is characterised by preoccupation with the belief that one is emitting a foul body odour. The others do not perceive any such foul odour; however, the patient persists with the belief. They may indulge in repetitive behaviours like repeatedly taking showers or changing clothes and may even start avoiding others. The insight may vary from good insight to absent insight. The treatment is on similar lines to other obsessive-compulsive and related disorders.

HYPOCHONDRIASIS

Hypochondriasis is characterised by a preoccupation with (or fear of) the possibility of having a serious, life-threatening illness. The preoccupation is usually secondary to a misinterpretation of normal or common sensations. For example, a patient may misinterpret the gurgling sounds from the abdomen as evidence of stomach cancer. The preoccupation is followed by excessive and repetitive health-related behaviours such as repetitive investigations and medical consultations. In ICD-11, hypochondriasis has been included in the section obsessive-compulsive or related disorders, whereas in DSM-5, the corresponding diagnosis of Illness anxiety disorder has been included in the section of somatic symptoms and related disorders. This topic has been explained in more detail in the Chapter 9 'Somatic Symptoms and Related Disorders'.

CASE BASED MCQ

An 18-year-old girl was quite distressed as she repeatedly thought she was 'not clean'. She would take hours to wash after defecation as she had the thought that 'the fecal matter is sticking to her body'. And she would also take a bath every time she went to urinate. The patient said, 'I know my thoughts are incorrect, but I feel so overwhelmed that I have to wash myself till I feel satisfied'. What is the likely diagnosis?
a. Delusional disorder
b. Major depressive disorder
c. Body dysmorphic disorder
d. Obsessive-compulsive disorder

Ans. d. The history is suggestive of the obsession of contamination followed by the compulsion of washing; the likely diagnosis is obsessive-compulsive disorder.

SUGGESTED READINGS

1. American Psychiatric Association. Diagnostic and Statistical Manual of Mental Disorders. Arlington, VA: American Psychiatric Publishing, 2013.
2. Sadock B, Sadock V, Ruiz P. Kaplan & Sadock's comprehensive textbook of psychiatry. 10th ed. Philadelphia: Wolters Kluwer; 2017.
3. Tasman A, Kay J, Lieberman J, First M, Riba M. Psychiatry. 4th ed. Chichester, West Sussex: Wiley Blackwell; 2015.
4. Boland R, Verdiun M, Ruiz P. Kaplan & Sadock's Synopsis of Psychiatry. Lippincott Williams & Wilkins; 2021.
5. Murthy RS. National mental health survey of India 2015–2016. Indian journal of psychiatry. 2017;59(1):21.
6. World Health Organization. International classification of diseases for mortality and morbidity statistics (11th Revision).

7 Impulse Control Disorders

Praveen Tripathi, Priyanka Goyal

Impulse control disorders are characterised by repeated failure to resist an **impulse or drive** to perform an act that is clearly harmful to the individual or others or both. Typically, every act is associated with three events:
a. First, there is an impulse to do a particular act; this impulse is associated with **increasing tension and arousal**, and in some cases, with anticipation of pleasure.
b. The impulse leads to action; the completion of the action brings **relief** from the mounting tension and often a feeling of **gratification.**
c. After some time, the individual feels **remorse or guilt.**

INTERMITTENT EXPLOSIVE DISORDER

Intermittent explosive disorder is characterised by repeated episodes of significant **aggression**, in which the individual may assault others or cause destruction of property. The aggressive episode is clearly out of proportion to the provocation, with a rapid onset and usually lasts for less than 30 minutes. After the episode, the individual expresses genuine regret or guilt, and there is no generalised aggressiveness in between the episodes (this helps in differentiation from antisocial personality disorder, in which aggression is in a regular pattern).

The intermittent explosive disorder is more common in men than in women and, in many cases, results in the individual being sent to correctional settings.

The cause appears to be multifactorial and is not completely known. There is an association between intermittent explosive disorder and an aversive childhood environment, including exposure to violence, neglect and physical abuse. Also, evidence suggests that serotonergic transmission is associated with impulsivity, and low levels of CSF, 5-HIAA (5-Hydroxyindoleacetic acid, the metabolite of serotonin) have been found to be correlated with increased impulsivity.

The treatment is usually a combination of pharmacotherapy and psychotherapy. Anticonvulsants (carbamazepine, valproate, phenytoin), lithium, antipsychotics, SSRIs, TCAs, and beta blockers like propranolol, have all been found to be effective in some cases.

Cognitive behavioural therapy and group psychotherapies have been found to be useful.

KLEPTOMANIA

Kleptomania is characterised by repetitive episodes of **stealing**. The individual is not able to resist the impulse to steal; the items stolen are usually of no value to the individual. The individuals experience mounting tension, which gets relieved with stealing and may be replaced by gratification. There may or may not be a feeling of guilt and remorse afterwards. The item stolen is often of low value and given away or returned back later. The goal of the individual is not to get any particular item but to indulge in the act of stealing.

Kleptomania is more common in females. Not much is known about the aetiology. Like other impulse control disorders, serotonin dysregulation appears to be involved. The treatment includes both pharmacological and non-pharmacological approaches. SSRIs and naltrexone have been found to be effective in some cases. Cognitive behavioural therapy and behavioural therapy have been used with variable success.

PYROMANIA

Pyromania is characterised by repetitive episodes of **deliberate fire setting**. The individuals feel a mounting urge before the episodes, and after setting the fire, there is a feeling of relief and gratification. These individuals are often fascinated by fires and things related to fire, and sometimes they become firefighters. Pyromania is more common in males than in females. The aetiology of pyromania is not clearly understood. The treatment includes both pharmacological and non-pharmacological approaches. Cognitive behavioural therapy is effective. In pharmacotherapy, SSRIs, anticonvulsants, lithium, naltrexone and antipsychotics have been used with variable success.

COMPULSIVE SEXUAL BEHAVIOUR DISORDER

It is characterised by a persistent pattern of inability to control **sexual impulses**, resulting in repetitive sexual behaviour. The repetitive sexual activities may become the main focus of life, often resulting in neglecting other aspects of life. The individual often makes attempts to stop repetitive sexual behaviour but is unsuccessful, and the repetitive sexual activities are continued despite adverse consequences. The individual may derive little or no satisfaction from the repetitive sexual acts and often feels guilt and remorse after the act.

Sometimes, the term 'sex addiction' is used for this condition. The term **'satyriasis'** and **'nymphomania'** have been used to describe excessive sexual desire in males and females, respectively.

SSRIs have been used to decrease libido. Medroxyprogesterone, too, can decrease the libido in men; antiandrogens like cyproterone have been used in women with variable success. 12 step self-help groups (such as sexaholics anonymous and sex addicts anonymous) have been beneficial in many cases. Cognitive behavioural therapy and insight-oriented psychotherapy have been successful in some cases.

CASE BASED MCQ

A 23-year-old female from an affluent family was caught stealing a pen from a mall. When confronted by the security about why she would steal something so inexpensive that she could have very easily bought, she replied, 'I am sorry, I couldn't stop myself, it's a problem for me, there are times when I have such a strong urge to steal that I just can't control myself, please forgive me, I am extremely embarrassed. What is the likely diagnosis?
a. Obsessive compulsive disorder
b. Pyromania
c. Kleptomania
d. Antisocial personality disorder

Ans. c. Kleptomania. A history of repetitive stealing items of no value, as the individual cannot control the impulse to steal, suggests kleptomania.

SUGGESTED READINGS

1. Boland R, Verdiun M, Ruiz P. Kaplan & Sadock's Synopsis of Psychiatry. Lippincott Williams & Wilkins; 2021.
2. Sadock B, Sadock V, Ruiz P. Kaplan & Sadock's Comprehensive Textbook of Psychiatry. 10th edition. Philadelphia: Wolters Kluwer; 2017.
3. American Psychiatric Association. Diagnostic and Statistical Manual of Mental Disorders. Arlington, VA: American Psychiatric Publishing, 2013.
4. Tasman A, Kay J, Lieberman J, First M, Riba M. Psychiatry. 4th edition. Chichester, West Sussex: Wiley Blackwell; 2015.

8 > Disorders Specifically Associated with Stress

Sujita Kumar Kar, Praveen Tripathi

PS9.1	Enumerate and describe the magnitude and aetiology of stress related disorders
PS9.2	Enumerate, elicit, describe and document clinical features in patients with stress related disorders
PS9.3	Enumerate and describe the indications and interpret laboratory and other tests used in stress related disorders
PS9.4	Describe the treatment of stress related disorders including behavioural and psychosocial therapy
PS9.5	Demonstrate family education in a patient with stress related disorders in a simulated environment
PS9.6	Enumerate and describe the pharmacologic basis and side effects of drugs used in stress related disorders
PS9.7	Enumerate the appropriate conditions for specialist referral in stress disorders

Stress is an inevitable part of human life. The response to stressful events has three components:
1. *An emotional response*: Emotional responses to stress include (a) anxiety symptoms such as palpitations, sweating, increased muscle tension, irritability and (b) depressive symptoms such as negative thinking, decreased activity levels and sadness of mood.
2. *A coping strategy*: Coping strategies are activities an individual does to deal with stressful events and reduce their impact. These may include activities such as problem-solving (e.g., when faced with financial stress, an individual reaches out to his parents for financial help) and emotion-reducing strategies (e.g., after losing a parent to a chronic illness, an individual talks to a family member and shares how he is feeling, and also tries to understand that it is for good that the parent no longer has to suffer the pain). Sometimes coping strategies can be maladaptive (e.g., use of alcohol and drugs) and may reduce the stress in the short term but create more problems in the longer term.
3. *A defense mechanism*: Unlike coping strategies, defense mechanisms are unconscious (i.e., the individual is not aware that he is using them). For example, when informed about it, a person refused to accept the diagnosis of cancer and any treatment for the same (this is the use of a defense mechanism called denial. This person is not aware that he is unconsciously using denial to deal with the stress of the diagnosis of cancer). Defence mechanisms are discussed in detail in the Chapter 18 'Psychoanalysis'.

Stress can impact the presentation of almost all the psychiatric disorders that have been discussed in this book. Stress can be a predisposing factor (increasing the vulnerability for the development of a particular disorder, e.g., a person working in a stressful situation is likely to develop substance use disorders), precipitating factor (resulting in the onset of an illness, e.g., A person with a strong family history of schizophrenia, had an onset of schizophrenia after failing in exams) or perpetuating factor (maintaining or altering the course of illness, e.g., a patient with a poor relationship with spouse, continued to have depressive symptoms for long duration) in development of a psychiatric disorder. However, in most of these disorders, the role of stress is not always clear, and these disorders can occur even in the absence of any stressful event.

In contrast, there are certain psychiatric disorders in which **stressful events directly affect causation**. In other words, **these disorders would not have occurred without the stressful event**. These disorders have been considered in this chapter. Kindly note that stressful events do not always result in the development of psychiatric disorders, and an individual's vulnerability and coping capacity play a significant role. In fact, most individuals who experience a stressful event do not develop any psychiatric illness.

POST-TRAUMATIC STRESS DISORDER

Post-traumatic stress disorder (PTSD) is an intense, long-term and at times delayed response to a traumatic experience and the traumatic event.

According to DSM-5, the traumas that can cause PTSD involve exposure to actual or threatened death, serious injury, or sexual violence.

The traumatic events that cause PTSD are so severe that they can **overwhelm** almost everybody. During the event, the patient usually feels fear and helplessness. The traumatic event can be an exposure to a life-threatening situation like war, natural disasters (e.g., earthquake), threatened or actual physical or sexual assault (e.g., severe physical attack, bomb blast, severe physical abuse, sexual abuse, robbery), being kidnapped, terrorist attack, severe road traffic accident or severe life-threatening medical illnesses (e.g., cancer, HIV infection). It is not necessary that a person should get injured in the trauma; exposure to the trauma faced by others can also cause PTSD. E.g., A police personnel who gets exposed to a horrible and violent crime as a part of his profession may also develop PTSD.

Epidemiology

Studies on soldiers who fought during world wars and, more recently, in American soldiers who were a part of the Gulf War, Afghanistan and Iraq wars have furthered the understanding of PTSD. According to DSM-5, the lifetime risk of developing PTSD in the USA is 8.7%. In high-risk groups (e.g., soldiers), the prevalence is much higher. PTSD is more common in females than males. In females, the trauma is usually assault or rape, whereas the trauma is usually combat-related in males.

PTSD is more common in young adults because of a higher likelihood of experiencing significant trauma; it is less prevalent in adolescents and children.

The most important risk factor for PTSD is the duration, severity and closeness to the traumatic event.

Aetiology

Stressor: PTSD is caused by an exceptional stressor, but not every individual exposed to an exceptional stressor develops PTSD. Different people have different vulnerabilities. The following factors increase the predisposition to the development of PTSD:
1. Female sex
2. Young adults
3. History of childhood trauma
4. Personal history of mood and anxiety disorders
5. Lower intelligence
6. Poor social support

Genetic factors: Twin studies have suggested a genetic component in predisposition to the development of PTSD.

Neurobiological factors: The following neurobiological changes have been found in patients with PTSD:
a. Increased sympathetic tone and an overactive noradrenergic system
b. A hyperactive endogenous opiate system, along with low levels of plasma beta-endorphins
c. Hyper regulation of hypothalamic-pituitary-adrenal axis, with low plasma and urinary free cortisol concentrations
d. Imaging studies have shown a lower hippocampal volume (the hippocampus is involved in memory formation) and an **overactive amygdala** (remember, the amygdala is involved in emotional processing). These findings suggest that in PTSD, emotionally charged memories are not processed correctly, resulting in symptoms.

Psychological Theories

Cognitive model: According to the cognitive model, PTSD results when the brain cannot properly process the emotionally charged information of the trauma. That is why unprocessed memory keeps on intruding into the awareness of the patient.

Behavioural model: According to the behavioural model of PTSD, trauma (unconditioned stimulus) results in a fear response (unconditioned response). In the second step, things associated with the trauma (e.g., For a person who survived a car accident, the sight of the same car model, the road where he met the accident, the song that he was listening to at the time of trauma) also start producing the fear response, because of pairing between unconditioned stimulus and conditioned stimulus.

Trauma (unconditioned stimulus) ⟶ Fear (unconditioned response)

Conditioned stimulus (thoughts and memories of trauma, things associated with trauma) become paired with the unconditioned stimulus.

Conditioned stimulus ⟶ Fear (conditioned response)

Clinical Features and Diagnosis

The major clinical features of PTSD include the following:
A. **Intrusion symptoms:** Intrusion symptoms involve the recollection and re-experiencing of the trauma. The following are the types of intrusion symptoms:
   1. **Flashbacks:** In 'flashbacks', the patient may feel as if the traumatic event is happening again and may also act as if he is in the middle of the traumatic event
   2. Recurrent, unwanted and distressing memories of the traumatic event
   3. Recurrent dreams (**nightmares**) about the traumatic event
B. **Avoidance symptoms:** Patients with PTSD avoid the memories, thoughts and feelings related to the traumatic event. Also, there is avoidance of events and situations that remind about the traumatic event and cause distress.
C. **Arousal symptoms:** Patients with PTSD are in a state of hyperarousal and may have the following symptoms:
   1. Insomnia and poor concentration
   2. Irritability and aggression
   3. Hypervigilance (it is a state of excessive alertness, in which the person keeps on looking for possible dangers in the surrounding) and exaggerated startle response (extreme physical and psychological response when startled)

Apart from these three major domains, patients often have negative thoughts and moods associated with traumatic events and may express negative beliefs about themselves (I am bad) and others and may even blame themselves for the trauma.

Patients may also present with emotional numbing, anhedonia, feeling of detachment, depersonalisation or derealisation.

The onset of symptoms may be delayed; if symptoms appear **6 months** after the trauma, it is diagnosed as PTSD with **delayed onset**.

For a diagnosis of post-traumatic stress disorder, the symptoms should be present for more than 1 month (several weeks according to ICD-11).

Comorbidity

Most patients with PTSD show at least one other mental disorder such as depressive disorder, substance use disorder, anxiety disorder or bipolar disorder.

Management

The management of PTSD involves the use of both pharmacotherapy and psychotherapy.

Psychotherapy

1. **Cognitive behavioural therapy:** Trauma-based cognitive behavioural therapy is considered the **treatment of choice.** It involves the use of exposure to trauma-related stimuli; the exposure may initially be imaginal and later in vivo (e.g., if a patient had developed PTSD after a car accident and is avoiding the street on which she had the accident, the patient is made to visit that street—which will initially increase the anxiety and stay there till the anxiety starts to decrease).

   Apart from exposure, cognitive restructuring (changing the dysfunctional beliefs, such as 'the world is an unsafe place') is also done.

2. **Eye movement desensitisation and reprocessing (EMDR):** This technique was designed to treat PTSD. In this technique, the therapist sits in front of the patient and keeps moving his finger from side to side. A saccadic eye movement is induced in the patient as he is asked to follow the side-to-side movement of the therapist's finger. Simultaneously, the patient is asked to imagine the traumatic events and an attempt is made to replace and reformulate the negative thoughts associated with images of the traumatic event. EMDR attempts to reprocess the memory of a traumatic event in a healthier manner.

3. Psychodynamic psychotherapy, group therapy and family therapy can also be used.

Pharmacotherapy

Selective serotonin reuptake inhibitors (**SSRIs**) are considered the first-choice medications in the management of PTSD.

Tricyclic antidepressants (amitriptyline, imipramine) are also useful in treating symptoms of PTSD. However, side effects limit the use of tricyclic antidepressants. Other drugs like—serotonin-norepinephrine reuptake inhibitors (SNRIs), monoamine oxidase inhibitors, carbamazepine, valproate, trazodone, prazosin and propranolol may be helpful in the treatment of PTSD.

Benzodiazepines may provide symptomatic relief but should not be used for long because of their dependence potential.

Recent evidence suggests the role of repetitive transcranial magnetic stimulation (rTMS) in PTSD. rTMS targeting the right dorsolateral prefrontal cortex has a promising role in reducing the symptoms of PTSD, as per the initial results.

Similarly, early evidence suggests that deep brain stimulation (DBS) targeting the basolateral amygdala might help reduce the symptoms of PTSD. The evidence regarding the effectiveness of these newer neuromodulation techniques in trauma and stress-related disorders is preliminary, and extensive research is needed to understand their therapeutic role in these disorders.

> **COMPLEX PTSD**
>
> It is a new diagnostic category in ICD-11. Complex PTSD may develop following exposure to an event or series of events of extremely threatening nature (usually in cases where the trauma is repetitive, e.g., in cases of slavery, repeated childhood sexual or physical abuse, or prolonged domestic violence). In complex PTSD, in addition to the symptoms of PTSD, the following are seen:
> - Severe abnormalities of affect regulation (i.e., severe emotional regulation disturbances)
> - Belief about oneself as being a defeated and worthless person and feelings of shame and guilt for the event
> - Inability to feel close to others and sustain a relationship

ACUTE STRESS REACTION AND ACUTE STRESS DISORDER

Acute stress reaction and acute stress disorder describe different phases of the stress response. Acute stress reaction describes the short-lasting response, whereas acute stress disorder describes the more prolonged response.

Acute Stress Reaction

ICD-10 used the diagnosis of 'Acute stress reaction' and described it as a transient disorder that develops in response to exceptional physical/mental stressors and subsides within hours or days. The stressors may be an exceptionally traumatic event (e.g., a natural catastrophe like earthquake, accident, war, criminal assault, rape) or a sudden change in social position/or network of a person (e.g., due to multiple deaths).

The symptoms described included an initial state of 'daze' (restriction of consciousness and attention, the person may appear disoriented and not be able to comprehend happenings around him) which may be followed by anxiety, depression, despair or agitation. Also, there could be the presence of autonomic symptoms of anxiety such as palpitations, sweating, and tremors.

The symptoms usually start immediately or within minutes of the stressor and disappear within 2–3 days (often within hours).

In ICD-11, acute stress reaction has been removed from the list of mental disorders, and it has been reclassified as a reaction to trauma. The aim is to depathologise brief periods of emotional upset that occur in response to trauma.

Acute Stress Disorder

DSM-5 describes the diagnosis of acute stress disorder. DSM-5 diagnosis of acute stress disorder is of more clinical importance. Acute stress disorder develops in response to an exceptionally stressful event that involves exposure to actual or threatened death, serious injury or sexual violation (e.g., exposure to war, physical assault, sexual assault, disasters such as earthquakes, severe motor vehicle accidents). The person may have directly experienced the trauma or witnessed it happening to others. Learning about the trauma that happened to a close friend/relative or repeated exposure to traumatic events due to professional work (such as police officers) can also cause acute stress disorder.

The symptoms of acute stress disorder are the same as that of PTSD, although the duration criterion is different. The symptoms usually start immediately after the trauma and persist for at least 3 days and up to 1 month (duration criterion: 3 days-1 month). Acute stress disorder may progress to PTSD after 1 month or may remit within 1 month.

Management

Immediately after the trauma, the following can be done:

Psychological first aid: Immediately after the trauma, comfort and consolation should be provided. The victim should be provided safety and taken away from the stressful situation. Along with physical care, the person should be connected to a support system (families, friends and professional services).

Crisis intervention: It is an essential modality of psychological intervention that needs to be done following exposure to trauma. It helps an individual understand and accept the trauma, cope with the consequences of trauma, and restore equilibrium after the traumatic event.

Debriefing: After a major incident, debriefing (or critical incident stress debriefing, CISD) can be provided. In debriefing, the victim is encouraged to process the event and describe their thoughts and feelings about the event. The effectiveness of debriefing in preventing subsequent psychological distress is questionable, and a few studies have found that debriefing may actually increase the chances of future PTSD.

Treatment of acute stress disorder: If the symptoms of acute stress disorder persist, trauma-focused cognitive behavioural therapy can be used.

Medications may help in symptomatic relief in acute stress disorder. Antidepressants and anxiolytic agents may be helpful in the short-term management of symptoms. Antipsychotic drugs may be needed if there is evidence of impending psychosis. Benzodiazepines and antidepressants may be useful in the short-term control of symptoms of acute stress disorder in some patients; however, the level of evidence regarding the effectiveness of these medications in acute stress disorder is low.

ADJUSTMENT DISORDER

Adjustment disorder is also a **direct result of a stressor**. However, unlike PTSD and ASD, the traumatic events (stressors) responsible for adjustment disorder have not been clearly defined in diagnostic guidelines. Adjustment disorders usually follow events that are critical but not uncommon, and one can expect such events during the course of life. Common events associated with adjustment disorder are change of job, change of school/college, retirement, migration, relationship difficulties, medical illnesses, workplace stress and legal disputes, death of a loved one, etc. These stressful life events result in continuing unpleasant circumstances resulting in adjustment disorder.

Compared to adjustment disorders, the stressful events associated with PTSD and ASD are more serious, threatening and overwhelming.

Symptoms

Patients usually present with symptoms of anxiety and depression, irritability, somatic symptoms such as palpitations, etc. Patients may indulge in self-harm, and substance abuse. The symptoms are severe enough to cause psychological distress and/or significant impairment.

The symptoms usually start within 3 months of the stressful event and resolve within 6 months of termination of stress or its consequences.

Management

Evidence on the effectiveness of psychological interventions and pharmacological interventions in adjustment disorders is limited. **Psychotherapy** is the **treatment of choice** for adjustment disorder.

Psychological interventions such as—coping skill training, relaxation exercises, mindfulness-based interventions, supportive counselling and family therapy are useful in adjustment disorders.

In adjustment disorder, group therapy is beneficial when a group of people have a common problem (e.g., mass migration).

Individual psychotherapy explores the specific stressor(s) and addresses them. Crisis intervention is helpful in the short-term management of stressors. The individuals, who have developed such disorders often, have a maladaptive way of coping, which needs to be addressed in therapy. Installing adaptive ways of coping helps individuals to deal with their stressors effectively. Various relaxation exercises (deep breathing exercises, progressive muscular relaxation, meditation and yoga) help in stabilising autonomic symptoms of anxiety and have a calming effect.

Antidepressants and benzodiazepines have some role in alleviating the symptoms of adjustment disorder. Antidepressants and anxiolytic agents are commonly used in the short-term management of symptoms. However, there is a lack of robust evidence regarding the use of pharmacological intervention in adjustment disorders. Spontaneous resolution of the symptoms may occur once the stress resolves.

ADJUSTMENT DISORDER AND DEPRESSION

Since adjustment disorder also presents with depressive symptoms, it is sometimes difficult to differentiate between major depression and adjustment disorder. It must be remembered that if the criterion for depression gets fulfilled, the diagnosis of depression should be given precedence. An episode being triggered by a stressor does not preclude the diagnosis of depression. However, if the episode was triggered by a stressor and presents with depressive symptoms, which are not enough to fulfil the criterion of depression, adjustment disorder is the preferred diagnosis.

PROLONGED GRIEF DISORDER (PERSISTENT COMPLEX BEREAVEMENT DISORDER)

Prolonged grief disorder is characterised by a prolonged grief response following the death of a close relative. The response includes persistent preoccupation with the deceased, persistent longing for the deceased, and intense emotional pain. The duration of symptoms must be at least 6 months (according to ICD-11, which uses the diagnosis of prolonged grief disorder). According to DSM-5, the symptoms must be present for at least 12 months (DSM-5 uses the diagnosis of persistent complex bereavement disorder).

REACTIVE ATTACHMENT DISORDERS AND DISINHIBITED SOCIAL ENGAGEMENT DISORDER

DSM-5 and ICD-11 describe two disorders in children, which are a direct result of negligent parenting and maltreatment and result in an inability of the child to develop a normal attachment to the caregivers. The maltreatment may include emotional neglect or physical abuse, or both. Children raised in foster care centres with changing staff or who have been hospitalised for a long duration are also susceptible.

The possibility of pathological parenting is more if the caregiver (parent) has a psychiatric disorder, substance use disorder, intellectual disability, poor upbringing as a child, or in cases of premature parenthood (as in adolescent parents). Although the aetiology remains the same, the two disorders present differently:

a. **Reactive attachment disorder:** In this disorder, the child remains emotionally withdrawn from the caregivers. Even when distressed, the child does not seek comfort from the caregivers, and when caregivers try to comfort the child, he does not respond to it. The child shows minimal emotional response to others too and often looks sad, irritable or miserable without any reason. Before diagnosing reactive attachment disorder, it is important to rule out autism spectrum disorder (as children with autism spectrum disorder often have disturbances of social interaction too).
b. **Disinhibited social engagement disorder:** In this disorder, the child often shows an array of disinhibited behaviours such as over-familiarity with stranger adults (e.g., a child may go and sit in the lap of a stranger), absence of inhibition or fear in approaching stranger adults, lack of search for his/her caregiver in unfamiliar situations and willingness to go out with an unfamiliar adult without reluctance.

To make a diagnosis of both reactive attachment disorder and disinhibited social engagement disorder, the minimum age of the child should be 9 months.

The **management** involves first ensuring the child's safety and taking action (including legal) if child abuse is suspected. The treatment focuses on improving the relationship between the caregiver and the child.

DEATH AND DYING

The topic of 'Death and dying' is being discussed in this chapter to maintain the continuity of the related topics.

When an individual is informed about impending death, he usually goes through a series of responses called stages of death.

Elisabeth Kubler-Ross proposed **these stages of death and dying.** Although it is not necessary that every person goes through all these stages, they still provide a basic framework for understanding the responses of a dying person.

Stage 1: Denial and shock— It is characterised by the refusal to accept the diagnosis and a reaction of shock. A patient may even refuse treatment in this stage.

*Stage 2: Anger—*This stage is characterised by irritability and anger at family members, friends, doctors, and even God. The patient may displace his anger on the treating team, and the clinician must understand that this anger is actually displacement.

*Stage 3: Bargaining—*In this stage, the patient may try to bargain with family members and even God. For example, they may pledge to God that they will regularly go to temples/mosques/churches if God cures them.

Stage 4: Depression— In this stage, the patient starts showing signs and symptoms of depression such as sadness of mood, withdrawal and suicidal thoughts. If a clinical depressive episode develops, it must be treated with antidepressants and other modalities used to treat depression.

*Stage 5: Acceptance—*In the stage of acceptance, the patient finally accepts that death is inevitable, and their feelings may change to neutral or even happiness and peace.

GRIEF, BEREAVEMENT AND MOURNING

Although these terms have been used interchangeably, they have specific meanings.

Grief is the **emotional and behavioural response** precipitated by the death of a loved one.

Bereavement is the **state** of being deprived of someone due to death.

Mourning is the **process** through which grief is resolved. Mourning involves socially sanctioned practices like funerals, burial and memorial services.

Grief: Grief response is usually described as having the following three stages:

First stage: There is a denial of death in the first stage. The person may not entirely accept that a loved one has died and may appear emotionally numb. The person may show restlessness as if searching for the deceased. The first stage lasts from a few hours to several days.

Second stage: In this stage, there is sadness, crying, anxiety, sleep and appetite disturbances, feeling of guilt (that they did not do enough for the deceased loved one), and social withdrawal. The patient may have a **longing to join** the deceased person and may even experience **transient hallucinations**. The feeling of loneliness, especially after losing a spouse, is a lasting manifestation. The second stage usually lasts from a few weeks to 6 months. However, recent studies have shown that it may last much longer, for years.

Third stage: In this stage, there is a recognition that the lost person will not come back, the symptoms start to subside, and the bereaved individual gradually returns, to normal functioning, although few symptoms may persist for years.

Complicated Bereavement (Complicated Grief Reactions/Abnormal Grief Reactions)

Many different names have been given to abnormal grief responses, such as complicated bereavement or complicated grief reactions. These are not diagnostic categories in DSM-5 or ICD-11, and these complicated bereavements would be diagnosed as adjustment disorder or prolonged grief reaction (or persistent complicated bereavement disorder) according to DSM-5 and ICD-11.

Still, these terms have been used for a long time, and it's worth mentioning them briefly.

Complicated bereavement can present in the following three patterns:
a. **Chronic grief:** Here, there is a **prolonged grief reaction. The duration of normal grief varies in different** cultures; however, by convention, a grief reaction continuing for more than 6 months can be considered chronic grief.
b. **Hypertrophic grief:** If the grief response is too intense with excessive symptoms, it is called hypertrophic grief. In other words, if the symptoms are more than 'expected', it would be classified as hypertrophic grief. The definition of 'expected' symptoms varies across cultures, and clinical skills are used to make this subjective judgment.
c. **Delayed grief:** If the first stage of grief does' not start within two weeks of the death of a loved one, it is classified as delayed grief.
Traumatic bereavement refers to grief that is both chronic and hypertrophic.

The differentiation between normal grief and adjustment disorder (including complicated bereavement) rests on the analysis of whether the symptoms are in the range of 'expected response' or more than that. As can be seen, this is a subjective judgement and needs careful assessment, keeping in mind the cultural norms.

Anniversary reaction is a form of grief reaction on specific days (birthday, anniversary) related to the deceased one. Over time, the intensity of the anniversary reaction diminishes and becomes brief.

Bereavement (Grief) and Depression

Grief is a complex experience in which both positive emotions (happy memories of the deceased) and negative emotions (sadness) coexist and alternate. In depression, the negative emotions predominate and do not change. The symptoms such as excessive guilt, suicidal thoughts, ideas of worthlessness and psychomotor retardation are not seen in grief, and their presence suggests depression.

The functional impairment in grief is transient and mild. In comparison, in depression, symptoms are more severe, and there is a significant functional impairment.

CASE BASED MCQ

A 34-year-old man lost his job 1 month back, following which he became irritable and often looked sad. Whenever there was a discussion in the family regarding future plans, he would get angry and, on occasions, shouted at the family members. He also had difficulties in sleeping and on occasions, took the sleeping pill that was prescribed to his mother. His appetite was normal, and there was no history of any weight loss. He reported that his mood was quite bad for the entire month, except for 2 days when he went out with his friends to watch movies. What is the likely diagnosis?
a. Generalised anxiety disorder
b. Adjustment disorder
c. Mixed anxiety depression
d. Moderate depression

Ans. b. Loss of job followed by mild depressive symptoms suggest adjustment disorder. The history of a significant negative life event followed by non-syndromal depressive symptoms goes in favour of the diagnosis of adjustment disorder.

SUGGESTED READINGS

1. American Psychiatric Association. Diagnostic and statistical manual of mental disorders (DSM-5®). American Psychiatric Pub; 2013.
2. Sadock BJ, Sadock VA, Ruiz P (Eds). Kaplan & Sadock's Comprehensive Textbook of Psychiatry, 9th edition, Lippincott Williams & Wilkins; 2009.
3. Sadock BJ, Sadock VA. Kaplan & Sadock's synopsis of psychiatry: Behavioral sciences/clinical psychiatry. Lippincott Williams & Wilkins; 2011.
4. Kar SK, Sarkar S. Neuro-stimulation Techniques for the Management of Anxiety Disorders: An Update. Clinical Psychopharmacology and Neuroscience. 2016;14(4):330.
5. World Health Organization. Guidelines for the management of conditions that are specifically related to stress. World Health Organization; 2013.

9 Somatic Symptoms and Related Disorders

Vijay Niranjan, Swayam Prava Baral, Praveen Tripathi

PS10.1	Enumerate and describe the magnitude and aetiology of somatoform, dissociative and conversion disorders
PS10.2	Enumerate, elicit, describe and document clinical features in patients with somatoform, dissociative and conversion disorders
PS10.3	Enumerate and describe the indications and interpret laboratory and other tests used in somatoform, dissociative and conversion disorders
PS10.4	Describe the treatment of somatoform disorders including behavioural, psychosocial and pharmacologic therapy
PS10.5	Demonstrate family education in a patient with somatoform, dissociative and conversion disorders in a simulated environment
PS10.6	Enumerate and describe the pharmacologic basis and side effects of drugs used in somatoform, dissociative and conversion disorders
PS10.7	Enumerate the appropriate conditions for specialist referral in patients with somatoform dissociative and conversion disorders

Somatic symptom and related disorders are characterised by **prominent somatic symptoms associated with significant distress and impairment**. The somatic symptoms may be multiple, vague and involve single or multiple body systems. These symptoms often have a significant adverse effect on the well-being and functioning of the individual and lead to excessive and inappropriate use of healthcare resources due to multiple doctor visits, unnecessary investigations and treatment. These somatic symptoms are believed to have a 'psychogenic origin'; however, unfortunately, the term' psychogenic origin' is often confused with 'imaginary symptoms'. It cannot be emphasised more that the symptoms and sufferings of the patient are 'real', and so is the associated distress.

Medicine has found these conditions difficult to classify. A variety of terms such as hysteria, **medically unexplained symptoms**, functional symptoms, somatisation, Briquet's syndrome, conversion, etc., have been used to describe these symptoms. Of particular interest is the diagnosis of 'hysteria', which was in use for a long-time. The term 'hysteria' is derived from the Greek word "hystera" (uterus) and dates back to the era of Hippocrates, when it was thought that the wandering uterus throughout the body creates symptoms in the various parts of the body.

In DSM-IV, the diagnosis of 'somatoform disorders' was used for these symptoms, and the DSM-IV criterion for somatoform disorder stressed upon the presence of 'medically unexplained symptoms (MUS) to make the diagnosis. However, it was rightly pointed out that just the absence of 'medical explanation' cannot be the basis for diagnosing a psychiatric disorder. In DSM-5, the core criteria have been modified as discussed below. However, even in DSM-5, some categories of 'somatic symptoms and related disorders' have 'medically unexplained symptoms' as a key feature.

Somatic symptoms and related disorders (SSD) include:
- Somatic symptom disorder
- Illness anxiety disorder
- Conversion disorder
- Psychological factors affecting other medical conditions
- Factitious disorder

SOMATIC SYMPTOM DISORDER (BODILY DISTRESS DISORDER)

Somatic symptom disorder is characterised by the following:
- One or more **somatic symptoms** (usually patients have multiple symptoms) that are distressing or result in significant disruption of daily life. The somatic symptoms may be specific, (e.g., pain, indigestion, bloating, and paraesthesia) or nonspecific, (e.g., fatigue and weakness)
- Presence of **excessive thoughts, feelings, or behaviours** related to the somatic symptoms or associated health concerns in one of the following ways:
  - Excessive thoughts about the symptoms (patient worries excessively about the symptoms and may consider them very serious despite reassurances by doctors)
  - Excessive feelings about the symptoms (patient has a high level of anxiety about the symptoms)

- Excessive behaviours related to symptoms (patient spends excessive time and energy visiting multiple doctors and getting unnecessary tests done)

According to DSM-5, the symptoms should last for at least 6 months to make a diagnosis. DSM-5 also adds a specifier of 'With predominant pain' in patients who have prominent pain symptoms. ICD-11 uses the diagnosis of **'Bodily distress disorder'** instead of somatic symptoms disorder.

The disorder usually begins by the third decade, and males and females are equally affected. According to DSM-5, the prevalence of somatic symptom disorder is around 5–7%.

Patients with somatic symptoms disorder most commonly present with pain, fatigue, gastrointestinal symptoms, cardiovascular symptoms, sexual symptoms and neurological symptoms (sensation changes, weakness, swallowing difficulty, etc.). The course of this disorder is usually chronic, with exacerbations and remissions in between.

People with somatic symptom disorder usually consult physicians initially. When the diagnosis is discussed, there is often a reluctance to accept that the symptoms have a psychological cause rather than a physical cause. It is important that before the diagnosis of somatic symptom disorder is made, a detailed medical and psychiatric evaluation is done. This is to rule out medical illnesses that may have a similar presentation, such as neurological disorders, endocrine disorders, occult malignancies etc., and psychiatric conditions like major depressive disorder, OCD or delusional disorder.

Aetiology

Biological theories: It has been hypothesised that individuals with somatic symptom disorder have a biological predisposition that makes them oversensitive to certain stimuli (e.g., a lower threshold to pain). This is probably due to differential activation of pain and other sensory pathways compared to healthy individuals. Thus, what may be a normal pressure sensation in the abdomen for a healthy individual, may be processed and perceived as abdominal pain in a patient with somatic symptom disorder. Neurotransmitters like serotonin, norepinephrine, and glutamate have been proposed to play a role in such biological predisposition.

Behavioural theories: According to behavioural theory, the disorder develops due to the reinforcing properties of the symptoms. To understand better, let's take an example of an 18-year-old boy who is forced to work in a family business against his wishes. This boy was allowed to take leave, whenever he had headaches. Since the headaches allowed him to avoid something unpleasant, they got reinforced. And the boy started having frequent unexplained headaches, which were distressing but at the same time helped him to avoid something he disliked.

Psychodynamic theory: The Psychodynamic theory uses the concept of "somatisation" to explain the somatic symptom disorder. Somatisation is a process whereby mental distress manifests as somatic symptoms. Freud and Breuer proposed that mental distress gets "converted" into physical dysfunction and leads to the development of somatic symptoms.

Management

Once the diagnosis of somatic symptom disorder is confirmed, unnecessary investigations and speciality referrals should be avoided. The symptoms should be duly acknowledged, and the patient should be provided education about the illness. At the same time, the patient should not be made to feel that the treating team is doubting the patient's symptoms or intentions. Patient education should be done using empathy, and a nonconfrontational attitude should be maintained. When necessary, regularly scheduled consultations and physical examinations reassure the patients that their complaints are being taken seriously.

Pharmacotherapy: Depressive disorder, anxiety disorder, and substance abuse disorders often coexist with somatic symptom disorders and should be treated with appropriate pharmacotherapy. However, studies supporting the effectiveness of pharmacological interventions targeting specific somatic symptom disorders are limited.

Cognitive behaviour therapy: Cognitive behaviour therapy (CBT) is an effective treatment of somatic symptom disorders. It focuses on the cognitive distortions (faulty patterns of thinking) and behaviours that underlie somatic symptoms and anxiety about the symptoms. Behavioural interventions also focus on improving self-esteem and increasing the capacity to express emotions effectively.

BODY INTEGRITY DYSPHORIA

It is a rare and less understood condition characterised by a mismatch between the physical body and mental body image. The patients do not identify with a particular body part and have a desire to get rid of it. The patient presents with an intense and persistent desire to become physically disabled in a significant way, such as by amputation of a limb or severing the spinal cord to become paralysed. The patient may pretend to be disabled or may attempt to actually get disabled, causing severe harm to the health.

ILLNESS ANXIETY DISORDER

Illness anxiety disorder is characterised by the following:
- The patient has a **preoccupation with having or acquiring a serious illness.** The preoccupation continues despite negative laboratory results and reassurances from the doctor.
- There is significant anxiety about the health.
- The patient indulges in **excessive health-related behaviours,** (e.g., searching on the internet about the illness, checking the body for signs of illness).
- Somatic symptoms, if present, are mild. The patient may misinterpret normal sensations and consider them to be arising due to an underlying 'serious illness'.

The illness preoccupation should be for at least 6 months to make a diagnosis. There are two types of Illness anxiety disorder:
1. **Care seeking type:** In this type, frequent visits to doctors and frequent investigations are sought.
2. **Care-avoidant type:** In this type, medical care is avoided.

SOMATIC SYMPTOM DISORDERS VERSUS ILLNESS ANXIETY DISORDER

A patient with somatic symptom disorder is mainly concerned with the 'symptoms'. In contrast, in illness anxiety disorder, the primary concern is with the 'illness/diagnosis' and not with symptoms. For example, a patient with somatic symptom disorder will complain of bloating, indigestion etc., whereas a patient with an illness anxiety disorder will complain that he probably has 'stomach cancer'.

DSM-IV used the diagnosis of 'hypochondriasis' for patients who had a preoccupation with the fear of having a serious physical illness or the idea that they already have a serious physical illness based on the misinterpretation of bodily symptoms. According to DSM-5, most of the patients with hypochondriasis would be diagnosed with 'somatic symptom disorder', and a minority will be diagnosed with 'illness anxiety disorder'. ICD-11 still uses the diagnosis of hypochondriasis and groups it is in the section' obsessive-compulsive and related disorders as described earlier.

ILLNESS ANXIETY DISORDER VERSUS DELUSIONAL DISORDER

Patients with an illness anxiety disorder are usually convinced that they have a serious illness; however, the conviction is not at the level of delusion. In delusion, the belief is 'fixed' and 'unshakeable'. In contrast, in illness anxiety disorder, the belief though strong, is not 'fixed' and even if only for a short-time, the patient may be amenable to reassurances and reasoning by the doctor.

The aetiology of this disorder is not clearly understood, but postulated theories are similar to that of somatic symptom disorder.

Psychodynamic theories propose that distressing unconscious wishes are converted into 'fear of physical illness'.

Behaviour theory explains the continuation of symptoms as a learned behaviour due to the reinforcement of symptoms. The patient takes a 'sick role' that offers escape and avoidance from tense and stressful situations.

A familial predisposition to this disorder is also reported.

Management

After diagnosis, it is necessary to avoid repetitive and unnecessary diagnostic tests and interventions. Treatment involves cognitive behaviour therapy and pharmacotherapy. The use of selective serotonin reuptake inhibitors (SSRIs) has some empirical support. SSRIs also help by reducing the coexisting depressive and anxiety symptoms. Cognitive behaviour therapy modifies the patient's dysfunctional thoughts and behaviours. It also includes psychoeducation (educating the person about the illness) and techniques for distraction and relaxation.

PSEUDOCYESIS

In pseudocyesis (or false pregnancy), the patient has a false belief of being pregnant along with the development of objective signs of pregnancy such as abdominal enlargement (although the umbilicus does not get everted), reduced menstrual flow or amenorrhoea, subjective sensations of fetal movements, nausea, breast engorgement and labour pains at the expected date of delivery. Some endocrine changes may also be present. When detailed history is taken, it often reveals that the patient had a powerful desire for pregnancy. The disorder shows how the body can get impacted by psychological factors. Usually, a negative pregnancy test leads to the resolution of symptoms; however, in some cases, the patient may develop a delusional belief of being pregnant. Treatment is on the lines of other somatic symptom disorders and primarily focuses on psychotherapy.

Chronic fatigue syndrome (myalgic encephalomyelitis): This syndrome is frequently diagnosed in Western countries. For diagnosis, the symptoms should be present for at least 6 months and include severe, debilitating fatigue, malaise, headaches, pharyngitis, low-grade fever, cognitive complaints, gastrointestinal symptoms and tender lymph nodes. There are no pathognomonic features, and symptoms are often **nonspecific**. **Epstein–Barr virus** has been implicated as the causative agent in a few studies, but most other studies have been inconclusive. There are no reliable patterns of laboratory abnormalities, although in some cases, immunological abnormalities have been found in patients with chronic fatigue syndrome. Comorbid psychiatric symptoms are common. Depression is the most common comorbidity. The diagnosis of chronic fatigue syndrome is not included in either ICD-11 or DSM-5. Treatment is primarily supportive and symptomatic, such as the use of analgesics for pain. In many cases, psychotherapy, particularly **cognitive behavioural therapy**, is useful.

CONVERSION DISORDER (FUNCTIONAL NEUROLOGICAL SYMPTOM DISORDER)

Conversion disorder is characterised by the following:
1. The symptoms include loss of voluntary motor or sensory functions, (i.e., neurological symptoms)
2. The symptoms cannot be explained by any recognised neurological or medical condition, (i.e., the clinical findings are incompatible with any recognised neurological or medical condition)
3. The symptoms are judged to have been caused by a psychological stressor, and usually, there is a temporal relationship between the stressor and the onset of symptoms.
4. The symptoms of conversion disorders are not produced intentionally.

Common conversion symptoms include the following:
1. **Motor symptoms:** The common motor symptoms include paralysis, weakness, abnormal movements, and gait disturbances.
2. **Sensory symptoms:** The common sensory symptoms include anaesthesia, paraesthesia, blindness, tunnel vision and deafness.

3. **Seizure symptoms:** The patient may have a seizure-like episode called pseudoseizures.

The most common symptoms of conversion disorder are paralysis, blindness and mutism. The term 'functional' is often used to convey that these symptoms have a psychogenic origin. In comparison, the term 'organic' is used for symptoms caused by neurological causes.

The diagnosis of conversion disorder is challenging as it is difficult to rule out a medical disorder with complete certainty. The fact that patients with conversion disorders often have comorbid neurological and medical conditions makes the task even tougher.

La belle indifference: Patients with conversion disorder often show a lack of concern towards their serious symptoms. This lack of concern is called 'la belle indifference'. Though usually described in relation to conversion disorders, la belle indifference is not specific to the conversion disorder and can be seen in other disorders too. Also, it must be remembered that a patient with conversion disorder may show great concern towards his symptoms, and la belle indifference is not always present in these patients.

When present, certain signs can help diagnose conversion disorder, as they suggest a psychogenic origin of symptoms rather than a neurogenic origin. These include:

1. **Hoover's sign:** Hoover's sign is based on the fact that in normal subjects, in the supine position, involuntary hip extension occurs on attempting flexion of the contralateral hip against resistance.

   Suppose a patient presents with weakness of hip extension, and differentiation between neurological weakness and conversion disorder needs to be made. The patient is asked to lie down in the supine position, and the examiner places his hand under the heel of the weak leg. Now, the patient is asked to press the heel down forcefully. No downward pressure would be felt on the hand of the examiner in both neurological weakness or conversion disorder.

   In the second step, while keeping the hand under the weak leg, the patient is asked to flex the contralateral hip against resistance. In patients with conversion disorder, the examiner will now feel the patient pressing the heel of the 'weak leg' downwards, due to involuntary hip extension. This is a **positive Hoover's sign**. No downward pressing would be present in the neurological disorder, even in the second step.

2. **Tremor entrainment test:** This test helps differentiate a functional tremor (as seen in conversion disorder) from an organic tremor (as seen in a neurological disorder). In this test, a unilateral tremor can be identified as 'functional' if the tremor changes when the patient is distracted. In the test, the examiner makes a rhythmic hand movements, and the patient is asked to copy this movement with their unaffected hand. When patient copies the examiner's movement with the unaffected hand, it results in a change in the 'functional tremor' too, as it tends to copy the rhythm (gets entrained) of the unaffected hand. Else, the 'functional tremor' may simply get suppressed. A 'real' tremor would not get affected by the movements of the other hand.

3. Seizures can be differentiated from 'pseudoseizures' (also called 'psychogenic nonepileptic seizures') on the basis of the following points (refer to **Table 9.1**).

Table 9.1: Clinical manifestations in seizure versus pseudoseizure.

	Seizure	Pseudoseizure
Precipitating factor	Uncommon	Usually, a psychological stressor is present before the onset of pseudoseizures
During sleep	Common	Pseudoseizures are very rarely seen in sleep
Audience presence	True seizures occur irrespective of the presence or absence of an audience	Usually occurs only when others are around
Duration	Few minutes	Minutes to hours
Semiology	Mostly fixed	Variable
Reflexes	Babinski reflex and pupillary constriction usually present after the seizure episode	No pathological reflexes
Convulsive movement	Rhythmic and synchronous, characteristic tonic–clonic movements often present	Asynchronous and irregular movement of limbs, characteristic tonic–clonic movement is usually absent
Injury	• Accidental injuries are fairly common • May include lateral tongue bites, posterior dislocation of the shoulder	• Injuries are rare • Occasional tongue bite (tip) may be present
Consciousness	Complete or partial loss	Usually present, may fluctuate, but some response to pain is present
Incontinence during the episode	Common	Uncommon
Eyes	Usually open during the episode, the pupillary reflex is absent	Usually closed, the patient may forcefully close the eyes if an attempt is made to open them. Pupillary reflex is present
Electroencephalogram (EEG) findings during the episode	Epileptiform changes usually present	Normal EEG even during the episode
Postictal confusion	Usually present	Usually absent
Prolactin levels after episode	Increased	No changes

The usual age of onset for conversion disorders is between 10–35 years. Onset is usually acute, and symptoms are usually of short duration but may persist in certain cases. It is two to three times more common in females than males. The disorder is more common in rural populations, lower socioeconomic status, and in those with minimal medical or psychological knowledge.

Aetiology of Conversion Disorder

Following are the theories on the aetiology of conversion disorder. Psychoanalytic theories were very famous in the early 20th century; however, as research is progressing, more emphasis is now given to biological and behavioural theories.

A. **Psychoanalytic view:** According to psychoanalytic theory, the defence mechanisms involved in the development of conversion disorder are repression, conversion, symbolisation and identification. To understand it better, let us take an example of a person who had unconscious, unacceptable sexual impulses towards his mother. Usually, the mind uses 'repression' (a defence mechanism by which unacceptable impulses and wishes are kept away from the conscious mind to prevent the development of anxiety) and prevents these urges from entering the conscious mind. However, in the presence of a stressor (e.g., marriage against wishes), repression fails to keep the anxiety-provoking urges hidden inside the unconscious mind. In this scenario, the mind has to use another defense mechanism to prevent the unacceptable urges from entering the conscious mind. This second defence mechanism is 'conversion', and it converts intrapsychic anxiety into a physical symptom. The physical symptoms produced, (e.g., paralysis of the body below the waist), symbolises the original unacceptable impulse (defense mechanism of 'symbolisation'). Also, in many cases, patients have witnessed the symptom in some important person in the past (identification) (e.g., in his childhood, the patient had witnessed his uncle developing paraplegia after a stroke)

When a physical symptom is produced, it results in a decrease in intrapsychic anxiety. This is called 'primary gain', (i.e., the primary benefit of symptom production). Since the development of symptoms results in anxiety relief, patients often show a 'la belle indifference' towards the symptoms.

Once the physical symptoms are produced (e.g., paralysis), the patient gets sympathy and attention and can avoid certain duties. This is called 'secondary gain' (i.e., attention and decreased workload is the secondary benefit of symptom production)

The presence of primary and secondary gain results in the continuation of symptoms.

B. **Learning theory (Behavioural theory):** According to learning theory, classical conditioning can explain conversion symptoms. Symptoms of illness learned in childhood are called forth to deal with a stressful situation. Once the symptoms develop, there is a psychological relief as the stressor can be avoided. Hence, the symptoms get reinforced according to the principles of operant conditioning. Further, reinforcement occurs due to the secondary gains (in the form of attention and reduced responsibility)

C. **Biological theory:** Recent evidence suggests that in conversion disorder, there are disturbances in the neural circuits that connect the brain areas involved in volition (volition refers to the will), with brain areas controlling perception and movement. The areas in the prefrontal cortex have been studied primarily. It has been found that when an action is to be initiated, there is an activation of the dorsolateral prefrontal cortex and supplementary motor area, and when an action needs to be stopped, there is the activation of the orbitofrontal cortex.

It was demonstrated in a patient who had a conversion symptom of paralysis of the leg that whenever she attempted to move her paralysed leg, there was activation of the orbitofrontal cortex (which has an inhibitory role) and no activation of the motor cortex. These findings have increased interest in the biological underpinnings of conversion disorder.

Treatment of Conversion Disorder

The doctor must establish a good therapeutic relationship while treating a patient with conversion disorder. Patients should never be told that their symptoms are 'imaginary' or 'all in their mind'. Patients must be made to feel that the doctor trusts them and is genuinely interested in helping them. The treatment is primarily psychological.

A. **Symptom resolution:** An attempt should be made for as quick a resolution of symptoms as possible. The symptoms become resistant to treatment if they are chronic. It should be conveyed to the patient and family members that the symptoms are not serious and should resolve soon. Family members should be instructed to cut the secondary gains, and the patient should not be given extra attention or care.
   1. Benzodiazepines can be used in the short-term to provide an anxiolytic effect.
   2. Relaxation exercises can be used to decrease anxiety symptoms.
   3. If symptoms do not resolve, sodium amobarbital or pentothal interviews can be conducted in certain cases. In these interviews, the patient is given an injection of barbiturates (sodium amobarbital or pentothal), and the dose is titrated to lower the level of consciousness. In this state, the patient is interviewed, and an attempt is made to identify the stressor that is likely to have precipitated the episode. During the interview, suggestions can also be given to the patient that may be helpful in the resolution of symptoms.
   4. Aversion techniques that used painful stimuli (e.g., pressure over the eyeballs or sternum) to resolve the symptoms were used commonly in the past. But the use of such techniques is unethical and should be avoided.

B. **Dealing with the stressor:** Once the symptom resolution has been achieved, the aim is to find out the stressor and resolve it. Detailed interviewing is required for the same. Psychoanalytic techniques such as insight-oriented psychotherapy too can be used. All attempts should be

made to cut the secondary gains and encourage self-sufficiency in the patient.
C. **Abreaction:** Abreaction is the process by which unconscious thoughts, impulses and memories are brought to conscious awareness, along with the release of associated emotions. Abreaction can be achieved by the use of hypnosis, free association (described in detail in the Chapter 18 'Psychoanalysis') or the use of drugs like amobarbital or pentothal.
D. In case comorbid anxiety disorder or depression is present, it should be treated with appropriate pharmacotherapy and psychotherapy.

> In ICD-11, conversion disorder is considered a type of dissociative disorder. The corresponding diagnosis for conversion disorder in ICD-11 is 'Dissociative neurological symptom disorder'.

PSYCHOLOGICAL FACTORS AFFECTING OTHER MEDICAL CONDITIONS

The concept of psychosomatic disorders (physical disorders caused by or aggravated by psychological factors) has been there for a long time. It is a known fact that stress can cause many somatic symptoms. Stress is described as any circumstance that disturbs or is likely to disturb an individual's normal physiological or psychological functioning.

Hans Selye described a model of stress called **general adaptation syndrome**. According to this model, the body reacts to stress in three stages.

Stage 1, the alarm reaction: It is the immediate response characterised by a fight or flight response.

Stage 2, the stage of resistance: It is also known as the stage of adaptation. In this stage, the body adapts to stress. For example, when faced with starvation, the body reduces energy consumption and decreases physical activity.

Stage 3, the stage of exhaustion: If the stress continues, the body's resistance gradually decreases and finally body collapses.

Almost all organ systems can get affected by psychosomatic disorders. The important examples include:
A. *Gastrointestinal system*: Many gastrointestinal disorders such as peptic ulcers, Crohn's disease, and ulcerative colitis are affected by psychological factors. Irritable bowel syndrome, which is characterised by symptoms such as abdominal pain, cramps, and alteration of bowel habits (diarrhoea or constipation), is a well-known example of a psychosomatic disorder.
B. *Respiratory system*: Psychological factors play a role in asthma, chronic obstructive pulmonary disease (COPD) and hyperventilation syndrome. Hyperventilation syndrome is characterised by rapid and deep breathing for several minutes and accompanying symptoms of suffocation, giddiness, paraesthesia and syncope due to falling PCO_2 levels in the blood.
C. *Cardiovascular system*: Cardiovascular disorders such as hypertension, coronary artery diseases, and cardiac arrhythmias are known to be affected by psychological factors.
D. *Musculoskeletal system*: Disorders like rheumatoid arthritis and systemic lupus erythematosus are known to be impacted by psychological factors. Of particular importance is fibromyalgia, a disease characterised by pain and stiffness of soft tissues such as muscle and ligaments. The patient often reports local areas of tenderness, also known as "trigger points". There might be associated symptoms such as anxiety, fatigue and inability to sleep.
E. Other disorders such as endocrinological disorders, skin disorders and headaches too get impacted by psychological factors.

Treatment: The treatment is usually focused on helping the patient understand the effect of psychological factors in the development of somatic symptoms while acknowledging that the symptoms are 'real' and distressing to the patient. Psychotherapeutic techniques such as group psychotherapy, insight-oriented psychotherapy, behaviour therapy, cognitive therapy and hypnosis may be useful. Relaxation techniques and stress management training may also be required.

According to the DSM-5, "**psychological factors affecting other medical conditions**" is diagnosed when there is a "medical symptom or condition" and psychological or behavioural factors are adversely affecting that symptom or condition, such as by causing exacerbations or poor adherence to the treatment and thereby leading to changes in the course of the medical condition.

FACTITIOUS DISORDER (MÜNCHHAUSEN SYNDROME)

Richard Asher, in 1951 coined the term 'Münchhausen's syndrome'. The disorder is named after Baron Hieronymus Friedrich Freiherr von Münchhausen, a German cavalry officer who served in the Russian army. Von Münchhausen was known to entertain people by telling exaggerated and false stories about his war heroics.

Factitious disorder is characterised by the production of false symptoms (physical or psychological) or exaggeration of actual symptoms to get medical attention. For example, a patient may inject himself with insulin to produce hypoglycaemia or inflict injuries (occasionally life-threatening) on himself to get into medical care.

Factitious disorder is also called '**hospital addiction**'/'**polysurgical addiction**', and patients are sometimes referred to as 'professional patients'. These patients distort the history and make stories (called pseudologia fantastica) to convince the doctor and get admitted. They can also use fake identities and claim to be important figures like war heroes (i.e., impostorship) to get medical attention. The patients are often from medical and related fields and have a basic understanding of the signs/symptoms of various disorders.

Examination often reveals signs suggestive of previous interventions, such as surgical scars. In case multiple surgeries were done in the past, the patient may have a **gridiron abdomen** (mass of scars on the abdomen is called gridiron abdomen or washboard abdomen).

These patients are usually quite eager for investigations and medical procedures, including invasive investigations and procedures.

When the investigations do not show any abnormalities, these patients may get angry and accuse the doctors of incompetency. They may suddenly leave the hospital, only to go to some other hospital and repeat the cycle.

Sick role: Patients with factitious disorders try to assume a sick role (i.e., they want to be treated as if they are quite sick or ill) and demand attention from doctors and medical staff.

FACTITIOUS DISORDER BY PROXY/ MÜNCHHAUSEN SYNDROME BY PROXY

It is characterised by the production of false symptoms (physical or psychological) or exaggeration of actual symptoms, in another person under the individual's care. For example, a mother may give her child an oral Hypoglycaemic drug, induce signs of Hypoglycaemia and then take the child to the emergency department for admission. The purpose could be to take the sick role indirectly or be relieved of caretaking by getting the child admitted.

The age of onset of factitious disorder is generally before 30 years. Factitious disorder is more common in females and workers from the healthcare sector.

> DSM-5 describes two categories of Factitious disorders, factitious disorder imposed on self and factitious disorder imposed on another (described here as factitious disorder by proxy).

Treatment

Patients with factitious disorders are usually reluctant to see a psychiatrist. To initiate the treatment, it is essential to establish a therapeutic relationship with the patient. The patient must be helped to identify the motivations behind the desire to assume a sick role. Unnecessary investigations and procedures should be avoided to prevent iatrogenic complications. The treatment is primarily by psychotherapy. Pharmacotherapy is used for comorbidities like depression, anxiety disorders etc.

As Münchhausen syndrome by proxy is commonly associated with child abuse, proper precautions must be taken. Appropriate government child welfare agencies should be involved in case of suspicion of Münchhausen syndrome by proxy. In severe cases, it may be necessary to remove the child from the care of the offending guardian.

Conversion Disorder and Factitious Disorder

In conversion disorder, symptoms are not produced voluntarily; the symptoms are produced unconsciously.

In factitious disorder, false symptoms are wilfully created by the patient; the symptoms are produced consciously.

MALINGERING

Malingering is not a psychiatric disorder. It is discussed here as it is an important differential diagnosis of conversion disorder and factitious disorder. Malingering involves the intentional production of false physical or psychological symptoms, with a motivation of getting some external incentives such as financial incentives, avoiding military or other tough duty, or avoiding legal cases.

Malingering should be suspected if:
- There is a medicolegal case involved, including referrals by **courts of law**
- There is a marked **discrepancy** in complaints by patients and objective findings on examination
- Lack of co-operation by the patient during diagnostic evaluation and treatment
- The person has antisocial personality disorder **factitious disorders and malingering**

Both factitious disorder and malingering involve the production of fake symptoms. The difference lies in the reasons for symptom production. Patients with factitious disorders want to get medical attention and assume a 'sick role'. In contrast, those who indulge in malingering do so to get external incentives such as financial gains or to run away from duties/law.

Culture bound syndromes: These syndromes are limited to a particular culture and are not seen worldwide. It is believed that local cultural beliefs and patterns of behaviour strongly influence the presentation of these syndromes. A few important common culture-bound syndromes include:
- **Dhat syndrome:** It is prevalent in the Indian subcontinent. The characteristic features are anxiety and distress about the loss of semen or 'dhat', and the attribution of various physical and psychological symptoms to the loss of semen. The patient complains of a white discharge in the urine or stool and believes that it is semen. Loss of semen is considered equivalent to the loss of vitality. Patients present with anxiety, depressive symptoms, and physical complaints such as weakness, fatigue and sexual symptoms. The urine analysis in most of these patients does not show any abnormality. This syndrome is most widely seen in India and Pakistan
- **Koro:** The patient presents with a sudden episode of anxiety that the penis (or vulva in females) will retract into the abdomen and would result in death
- **Latah:** It is usually seen in Malaysia and Indonesia. Patients present with an exaggerated startle to minimal stimuli. This is followed by automatic obedience, echolalia and echopraxia

CASE BASED MCQ

A 35-year-old male keeps changing his doctor as no one is able to help him with his primary complaint of 'feeling of abdominal fullness'. Despite multiple consultations and repeated investigations, no cause could be found for his symptom. The patient spends a significant amount of time reading about the possible causes on the internet and has been irregular at work as the 'abdominal fullness interferes with his thinking capacity'. What is the likely diagnosis?

a. Somatic symptom disorder
b. Illness anxiety disorder
c. Conversion disorder
d. Factitious disorder

Ans. a. Preoccupation with a somatic symptom along with the presence of excessive behaviours, thoughts or feelings related to the somatic symptoms is suggestive of somatic symptom disorder.

SUGGESTED READINGS

1. American Psychiatric Association. Diagnostic and statistical manual of mental disorders (4th Edition, text rev.). Washington, DC 2000.
2. American Psychiatric Association. Diagnostic and statistical manual of mental disorders (5th Edition.). 2013 Washington, DC 2013.
3. Barsky A, Ahern D. Cognitive Behavior Therapy for Hypochondriasis. JAMA. 2004;291(12):1464-70.
4. Mayou R, Kirmayer LJ, Simon G, Kroenke K, Sharpe M. Somatoform disorders: time for a new approach in DSM-V. Am J Psychiatry 2005;162(5):847-55.
5. Boland R, Verdiun M, Ruiz P. Kaplan & Sadock's Synopsis of Psychiatry. Lippincott Williams & Wilkins; 2021 Feb 9.
6. World Health Organization. International classification of diseases for mortality and morbidity statistics (11th Revision).
7. Blom RM, Hennekam RC, Denys D. Body integrity identity disorder. PLoS One. 2012;7(4):e34702.

10 > Dissociative Disorders

Vijay Niranjan, Swayam Prava Baral, Praveen Tripathi

PS10.1	Enumerate and describe the magnitude and aetiology of somatoform, dissociative and conversion disorders
PS10.2	Enumerate, elicit, describe and document clinical features in patients with somatoform, dissociative and conversion disorders
PS10.3	Enumerate and describe the indications and interpret laboratory and other tests used in somatoform, dissociative and conversion disorders
PS10.4	Describe the treatment of **somatoform** disorders including behavioural, psychosocial and pharmacologic therapy
PS10.5	Demonstrate family education in a patient with somatoform, dissociative and conversion disorders in a simulated environment
PS10.6	Enumerate and describe the pharmacologic basis and side effects of drugs used in somatoform, dissociative and conversion disorders
PS10.7	Enumerate the appropriate conditions for specialist referral in patients with somatoform dissociative and conversion disorders

These disorders were previously classified as "hysteria", but that term is no longer used. French psychiatrist Pierre Janet first coined the term 'dissociation'.

Dissociative disorders are characterised by an involuntary disruption in the normally integrated mental functions of consciousness, identity, memory, perception and motor behaviour. It means that usually the above-mentioned mental functions are integrated; however, in dissociative disorders, the defense mechanism of '**dissociation**' results in the segregation of one/or a group of these mental functions from the rest. Dissociative disorders usually have a sudden onset and are often precipitated by psychological trauma. For better understanding, let us take an example.

A 21-year-old man was travelling with his parents in a car, when the car met with an accident. In the accident, both parents died, whereas the man escaped with minor injuries. While being treated, it was found that the man had no recollection of the accident and death of his parents, and there was no memory of the entire episode. He insisted that there was no accident and parents must be at home. After ruling out any brain injury, he was diagnosed with dissociative disorder (dissociative amnesia).

In this patient, the sudden death of his parents was an excruciating memory. If allowed to remain in consciousness, it would have caused unbearable anxiety to the man. To protect him from this unbearable anxiety, the patient's mind used an unconscious defence mechanism of dissociation and segregated this painful memory from the rest of memories and other mental functions. It can be said that the painful memory was buried inside the unconscious mind to ensure that it does not cause unbearable anxiety. This is 'dissociation' at work.

The development of dissociative disorders is often explained in terms of primary, secondary and tertiary gains. All these gains function unconsciously.

Primary gain: It refers to the internal psychological motivation or benefit of symptom production. For example, in the example mentioned above, the primary gain is 'keeping an extremely painful and unbearable memory out of consciousness'.

Secondary gain: It refers to external psychological motivation. For example, this patient who developed sudden memory loss got a lot of attention from the extended family. He was not expected to work or make money for the family and was relieved of his duties.

Tertiary gain: It refers to the gain that a third person derives because of the patient's symptoms. For example, this patient's wife started getting money regularly from her parents, as they felt sympathetic towards her.

All these gains function unconsciously, which means that patient is not aware of any of these.

The following are the types of dissociative disorders.

DISSOCIATIVE IDENTITY DISORDER (MULTIPLE PERSONALITY DISORDER)

☐ Dissociative identity disorder is characterised by the presence of two or more distinct identities (or "personality states" or '**alters**') in an individual, which recurrently take control of the individual. These identities usually have their own thinking, behaviour, and memory patterns. The identities develop involuntarily and cause distress and impairment in the individual's functioning.

- In some cases, the different identities are aware of each other's existence. Usually, the different personalities are completely unaware of each other. Sometimes two personalities struggle for control of the person.
- The disorder appears to be culture-bound because it is primarily restricted to North America. Relatively few cases have been reported elsewhere. Women constitute the majority of cases of multiple personality disorder. Dissociative identity disorder is commonly associated with traumatic events and/or abuse in childhood.

> **PARTIAL DISSOCIATIVE IDENTITY DISORDER**
>
> Like dissociative identity disorder, there are two or more distinct identities. However, only one personality state is dominant and controls daily life. There are occasional and transient intrusions by the nondominant personality states. During these intrusions, the individual's consciousness is controlled by the nondominant personality states, leading to significant socio-occupational impairment.

DISSOCIATIVE AMNESIA

In dissociative amnesia, the characteristic feature is an inability to recall important personal information, usually involving a traumatic or stressful event. The memory loss cannot be attributed to any medical cause, such as head injury or any particular medical condition, or due to the direct effects of substance abuse. An acute psychological trauma usually precipitates it.

Dissociative amnesia can be of multiple types:

a. **Localised amnesia:** Amnesia (inability to recall) is for a particular period of time
b. **Generalised amnesia:** Amnesia is for the entire lifetime
c. **Selective amnesia:** Amnesia is about a particular event/events
d. **Continuous amnesia:** In this type, the patient is unable to form memories of new events as they occur, and it results in amnesia for successive events
e. **Systematised amnesia:** In this type, amnesia (inability to recall) is about a specific category, such as for a particular person.

The memory loss in dissociative amnesia is usually reversible. The onset is usually sudden, but in some cases, the symptoms may develop gradually over the years.

> **DISSOCIATIVE FUGUE**
>
> - Dissociative fugue has features of dissociative amnesia, plus a history of a sudden, unexpected travel from one's usual place of stay or work. The travel is purposeful, and the person usually goes to a place with some emotional significance. During the journey, the person appears normal to the others, maintains basic self-care (e.g., hygiene etc.) and indulges in regular social interactions (e.g., taking directions)
> - There is amnesia for the period of travel, and the patient may find it difficult to recall most of the past.
> - There may be confusion about the personal identity, and in some cases, the individual may take a completely new identity and live with the new identity for a period of time.
>
> *Cont'd...*

Cont'd...

> (For example, a young 15-year-old boy, who lived with his abusive father and was repeatedly beaten by him, left the house one day after getting beaten up badly. He travelled for an entire day using public transport. He reached the neighbouring city where the family lived before the mother's death. When the police found him, he could not tell his name and could not remember anything about how he reached there).
>
> Traumatic circumstances usually trigger episodes of dissociative fugue. Usually, the person experiences strong emotions (such as anger, fear) and a strong wish to flee before the episode.
>
> In the earlier classification, the dissociative fugue was a separate diagnosis. However, both DSM-5 and ICD-11 have removed it. In DSM-5, dissociative fugue has been made a subtype of dissociative amnesia. So, if the patient presents with the symptoms mentioned above, the diagnosis according to DSM-5 would be dissociative amnesia with dissociative fugue.

TRANCE DISORDER (DISSOCIATIVE TRANCE)

This disorder is characterised by trance states. In trance states, there is a significant change in the state of consciousness, (i.e., the patient is not fully alert and awake and may feel confused) and narrowing of awareness of surroundings, (i.e., the patient can focus on only limited things in his surroundings). There may be a loss of ordinary sense of personal identity, (i.e., the patient may not feel and behave like his usual self) and the patient's movements and speech may become restricted. He may repeat certain movements and words and may experience as if he is not in control of his speech and movements. There is no assumption of a distinct identity.

For example, a young girl whose marriage was fixed against her wishes had episodes of abnormal behaviour which lasted for around 20 minutes. During the episodes, she would stare blankly and mumble, not respond to family members, and suddenly cry. After the episode, her mental state would be normal, although she would not be able to recall the episodes completely.

POSSESSION TRANCE DISORDER

This disorder is characterised by trance states, in which there is a significant change in the state of consciousness, and the patient's identity gets replaced by a "possessing external identity" (it appears that the patient's identity has been taken over by another identity, e.g., that of a god, or an ancestor etc.). The patient's behaviour appears to be totally in control of the 'possessing identity'.

For example, a 23-year-old female whose marriage was fixed against her wishes had episodes of abnormal behaviour which lasted for around 20 minutes. During the episode, the patient would rotate her head several times. Her voice would become heavy, and her eyes would be wide open. She would claim that she is an 'angry goddess' and that if the girls of the house are not respected well, the entire family will die. After the episode, the patient would collapse, and when she regained her senses, there would be no recollection of the episode.

It must be remembered that a diagnosis of dissociative trance disorder or possession trance disorder can only be made if the trance state or possession trance state is considered both involuntary and unwanted by the patient and is not socially and culturally acceptable. For example, if someone is voluntarily entering a trance state as a part of acceptable religious practice, it would not be considered a trance disorder.

DEPERSONALISATION/DEREALISATION DISORDER

Depersonalisation is characterised by feelings of unreality or detachment from oneself or one's body. The patient feels "as if" he has changed, although he finds it difficult to describe what exactly has changed. The patients frequently report that they feel as if they were detached from their bodies and were watching themselves, like in a movie. Depersonalisation is often accompanied by derealisation, in which the patient experiences as if the world is unreal.

These experiences are not very rare in the general population. According to the DSM-5, about half of all adults may experience single brief episodes of depersonalisation, usually during times of extreme stress.

> *ICD-11 describes another type of dissociative disorder, dissociative neurological symptoms disorder. The DSM-5 instead calls it conversion disorder and classifies it separately from dissociative disorders.*

OTHER DISSOCIATIVE DISORDERS

Ganser's Syndrome

The characteristic symptom of Ganser's syndrome is **approximate answers (also called Vorbeigehen)**. Approximate answers are the answers which are not correct but bear an obvious relation to the question, indicating that the question was understood. For example, when asked about the colour of the sky, a patient answered, red. Although the answer is not correct, it is obvious that the patient understood that the question was about colour. Other symptoms of Ganser's syndrome include **clouding of consciousness, auditory and visual hallucinations** and other dissociative symptoms. Ganser's syndrome is most commonly seen in **prisoners** but is **not exclusive to** that population group.

AETIOLOGY OF DISSOCIATIVE DISORDERS

The aetiology of dissociative disorder has been described using different models.

1. **Psychodynamic theory:** According to psychodynamic theory, dissociative disorders are caused by the use of the defence mechanism of repression (in repression, a painful and anxiety-provoking thought or wish is hidden inside the unconscious mind), e.g., in dissociative amnesia, anxiety-provoking memory is repressed. Another defence mechanism involved is dissociation.
2. **Learning theory or behavioural theory: According to learning theory, the development of symptoms can be explained on the basis of classical conditioning and operant conditioning. This theory has already been discussed in the last chapter in the aetiology of conversion disorders.**
3. **Diathesis–Stress model:** According to this model, certain personality traits, such as proneness to fantasies, high susceptibility to hypnotism, and openness to altered states of consciousness, may predispose individuals to develop dissociative experiences in the face of extreme stress.
4. **Neurobiological theories:** Neurobiological studies are still in infancy, but a few studies have shown that areas of the brain involved in emotional processing, memory, attention regulation, arousal and cognitive control may be dysfunctional in patients with dissociative disorders.

TREATMENT OF DISSOCIATIVE DISORDERS

It is exactly similar to the treatment of conversion disorders. (kindly refer to the last Chapter for details)

CASE BASED MCQ

A 16-year-old boy complained of a strange feeling of having changed from inside. He reported feeling as if he is different from his usual self and 'unreal'. He was quite tensed and anxious yet could not point out the precise change in him. This phenomenon is best called:
a. Delusional mood
b. Depersonalisation
c. Autochthonous delusion
d. Overvalued idea

Ans. b. Depersonalisation is characterised by feelings of unreality or detachment from oneself or one's body.

SUGGESTED READINGS

1. American Psychiatric Association. Diagnostic and statistical manual of mental disorders (4th edition, text rev.). Washington, DC, 2000.
2. American Psychiatric Association. Diagnostic and statistical manual of mental disorders (5th edition). Washington, DC, 2013.
3. Barsky A, Ahern D. Cognitive Behavior Therapy for Hypochondriasis. JAMA. 2004;291(12):1464.
4. Cutler J. Psychiatry. 3rd ed. Oxford India Press.
5. Dorahy M. Dissociative identity disorder and memory dysfunction: the current state of experimental research and its future directions. Clinical Psychology Review. 2001;21(5):771-95.
6. Spanos N. Multiple identity enactments and multiple personality disorder: A sociocognitive perspective. Psychological Bulletin. 1994;116(1):143-65.
7. Maldonado JR, Butler LD, Spiegel D. Treatments for dissociative disorders. In: Nathan PE, Gordon JM (Editors). A Guide to treatments that work. New York: Oxford University Press.; 1998. pp. 423-46.
8. Sadock B, Sadock V, Ruiz P, Kaplan H. Kaplan & Sadock's synopsis of psychiatry, 11th edition. Philadelphia, Pa: Wolters Kluwer, 2015.

11 Substance Related and Addictive Disorders

Praveen Tripathi, Anweshan Ghosh

PS4.1	Describe the magnitude and aetiology of alcohol and substance use disorders
PS4.2	Elicit, describe and document clinical features of alcohol and substance use disorders
PS4.3	Enumerate and describe the indications and interpret laboratory and other tests used in alcohol and substance abuse disorders
PS4.4	Describe the treatment of alcohol and substance abuse disorders including behavioural and pharmacologic therapy
PS4.5	Demonstrate family education in a patient with alcohol and substance abuse in a simulated environment
PS4.6	Enumerate and describe the pharmacologic basis and side effects of drugs used in alcohol and substance abuse
PS4.7	Enumerate the appropriate conditions for specialist referral in patients with alcohol and substance abuse disorders

In this chapter, we will discuss the mental and behavioural disorders caused by psychoactive substances and certain specific repetitive, rewarding and reinforcing behaviours.

DISORDERS DUE TO SUBSTANCE USE

In this section, we will discuss the disorders caused by the use of alcohol, caffeine, cannabis, hallucinogens, inhalants, opioids, sedatives and hypnotics, stimulants, tobacco, and other substances. But before discussing specific substances, it is essential to understand the terms relevant to the discussion.

Terminology

1. **Intoxication:** A transient condition that develops following the use of a substance, in which mental functions such as consciousness, thinking, perception or behaviour are altered.
2. **Tolerance:** Tolerance is the phenomenon in which increasing amounts of a substance are required to get the desired effect (e.g., a person who would felt the 'high' with two pegs of alcohol in the past now requires five pegs to get the same 'high').
3. **Withdrawal symptoms:** Withdrawal symptoms are the typical physiological or psychological symptoms that develop when substance intake is reduced or stopped (e.g., a person who used alcohol daily for many years developed tremors and nausea on suddenly quitting alcohol)
4. **Dependence:** It is a disorder in which an individual is unable to regulate the use of a substance after repetitive or continuous use. Dependence on a **substance is characterised by a strong drive to use it, as manifested by:**
   a. Difficulty in controlling substance taking behaviour in terms of its onset, termination or levels of use. The patient finds it difficult to control, when to use the substance (e.g., a patient starts consuming alcohol immediately after getting up in the morning), when to stop (e.g., a patient may not be able to stop himself from drinking until he **passes** out), or amount to be used (e.g., a patient continues drinking till the last drop is left in the bottle)
   b. Increasing priority is given to substance use over other activities and there is progressive neglect of other interests because of substance use.
   c. Persistence with substance in terms of its onset, termination or levels of use despite harmful or negative consequences (e.g., a patient realised that alcohol is responsible for his liver disease but still continued to consume alcohol regularly)

Along with these, the other features include:
   d. Strong desire or urge to use the substance **(craving)**
   e. **Tolerance**
   f. **Withdrawal symptoms** if the substance use is stopped or reduced. Dependence encompasses behavioural dependence (reflected as substance seeking behaviours), physical dependence (physiological effects of substance use as reflected in the development of tolerance and withdrawal symptoms) and psychological dependence (reflected by continuous or intermittent craving).

These features usually become evident over a period of at least 12 months; however, if the substance use is continuous (daily or almost daily), the diagnosis can be made in 1 month.

5. **Harmful pattern of use:** It is a state where substance use is causing harm, but the criterion of dependence is not met. According to ICD-11, harmful use is defined as a pattern of substance use that causes damage to a person's **physical health** (e.g., hepatitis due to alcohol use) or **mental health** (e.g., an episode of depression secondary to heavy alcohol consumption) or has resulted in behaviour leading to harm to the health of others.
6. **Single episode of harmful use:** A single episode of substance use that has caused damage to a person's physical or mental health or has resulted in behaviour leading to harm to the health of others.
7. **Use disorder:** While ICD-11 uses the diagnosis of 'dependence' and 'harmful use', DSM-5 uses a diagnosis of 'substance use disorder'. DSM-5 further provides for the diagnosis of mild, moderate and severe substance use disorders, depending on the number of criteria met.

Criteria

According to DSM-5, the following are the criterion for substance use disorders:

1. Substance intake is often in larger amounts or for a longer period than intended
2. There is a persistent desire or unsuccessful efforts to cut down on substance use
3. Excessive time is spent on substance-related activities (in its procurement, use or recovery after use)
4. Recurrent substance use results in failure to fulfil personal and professional obligations
5. Continued use despite it causing social or interpersonal problems
6. Progressive neglect of other recreational activities
7. Recurrent use in situations in which it is physically hazardous (e.g., drinking alcohol while driving)
8. Persistent use despite clear evidence that it is causing physical or psychological problems
9. Craving or a strong urge to take the substance
10. Tolerance
11. Withdrawal symptoms

DSM-5 requires the presence of at least two of the above, in the last 1 year to make a diagnosis of '**substance use disorder**'.

Further, DSM-5 says that substance use disorder can be mild (2–3 symptoms are present), moderate (4–5 symptoms are present) or severe (6 or more symptoms are present).

As one can see, the criteria of ICD-11 and DSM-5 are not much different; however, ICD-11 allows two levels of diagnosis (dependence and harmful use), whereas DSM-5 allows a single diagnosis (use disorder) but allows for severity to take care of various levels of pathological use.

EPIDEMIOLOGY

Epidemiological studies in substance use disorders are inherently difficult to conduct. One of the most important reasons is that people try to hide their substance use pattern, which is more true for illicit substance users. Further, substance users (more so, illicit substance users) tend to make their own closely connected and often underground groups, and it is difficult to find a representative sample. Due to these difficulties, certain special survey techniques are used to estimate the prevalence of substance use disorders. These include:

1. **Key informant technique:** In this technique, certain key informants (such as head of household, teachers in schools or colleges, village heads, etc.) are interviewed, and data is collected.
2. **Snowball technique:** In this technique, initially, few substance users are identified, and then these users help in identifying more users, and this process is repeated to identify all the users in a particular area. This technique is especially useful for illicit substance users as they tend to remain underground.

Apart from these, certain indirect indicators also help identify the prevalence of substance use disorders in a population. For example, morbidity and mortality rates due to hepatic cirrhosis indicate the prevalence of alcohol use disorders in the population.

The data from de-addiction centres and outpatient-based substance use treatment centres also helps identify the prevalence of drug use and the types of drugs being used in the community.

Worldwide, alcohol is the **most commonly** used substance, followed by tobacco, and cannabis is the most commonly used illicit substance. Substance use disorders are more common in males than females, although this distinction is more pronounced in the developing world than the developed world.

In India, the **National Mental Health Survey (NMHS)-2016** was conducted on a nationally representative sample from 12 states across the country. The following were the findings:

1. The prevalence of tobacco use disorder (including moderate and high dependence on tobacco) was 20.9%, and it was the **most common** substance use disorder in the country.
2. The prevalence of alcohol use disorder (including harmful use of alcohol and alcohol dependence) was 4.6%
3. The prevalence of illicit substance use disorders (including abuse and dependence) was 0.6%. The illicit substances included cannabis products, opioid drugs, stimulant drugs, inhalant substances and prescription drugs. Cannabis is the most commonly used illicit drug in the country (remember, tobacco and alcohol consumption is legal as long as certain regulations are followed).

The prevalence of all substance use disorders (including tobacco, alcohol and illicit substances) was much higher in males than females.

AETIOLOGY

The development of substance use disorders is best explained by a **biopsychosocial model**. It means that there is an interaction of biological factors, psychological factors, and social factors, resulting in substance use disorders.

Neurobiology

The pathway in the brain that mediates the feeling of pleasure and reward is called the '**brain reward pathway**'. It primarily consists of dopaminergic neurons connecting the ventral tegmental area to the nucleus accumbens. Whenever we do something that we enjoy or find pleasurable (e.g., playing a game or finishing a task that gives us a sense of achievement), it is due to the release of dopamine in the brain reward pathway.

In some individuals, there is a deficiency of dopamine receptors (primarily D2) in this pathway. Hence, these individuals cannot get a feeling of reward or pleasure in usually rewarding activities (called **reward deficiency syndrome**). However, using a substance may release enough dopamine and provide the much-needed feeling of 'reward or pleasure' and hence may be repeated again and again. So, reward deficiency syndrome may increase the vulnerability to the development of substance use disorder.

The release of dopamine in the nucleus accumbens is regulated by other neurotransmitters such as serotonin, opioids, glutamate and GABA. As the understanding of the role of these neurotransmitters becomes better, it would help develop newer pharmacological modalities in the treatment of substance use disorders.

Genetic Factors

Most of the studies on genetics have been conducted in relation to alcohol use disorders. The family studies have shown that the prevalence of alcohol use disorders is much higher in relatives of patients with alcohol use disorders than in control groups. Further, the monozygotic concordance rate is much higher than the dizygotic concordance rate for alcohol use disorder, providing a clear indication of the role of genetics in the development of the disorder. Similarly, adoption studies have shown that the children of parents with alcohol use disorders, who were raised by parents without any alcohol use disorders (due to adoption), still showed a much higher rate of alcohol use disorders than the control group, thus showing the clear role of genetics.

Although fewer studies are available for other substances, the findings are quite similar, suggesting a role of genetics in the development of substance use disorders.

Behavioural Factors

Apart from biological factors, learning and conditioning are also known to contribute to the development of substance use disorder. The use of a substance can cause an intense sense of euphoria. Hence, to experience that state, a person is likely to use the drug repeatedly (**positive reinforcement**, wherein the frequency of a behaviour increases if it results in a positive consequence). Substance use also frequently alleviates negative emotions (such as sadness and anxiety) and withdrawal symptoms. Again, this is likely to increase substance taking behaviour (**negative reinforcement**, wherein the frequency of a behaviour increases as it helps avoid a negative state).

With time, the drug itself and the paraphernalia (such as needles, cigarette packs, bottles) and other cues (such as liquor shop, seeing a friend smoking) can cause a craving and an intense desire to consume the substance.

Other factors like peer pressure, social acceptance, legal controls, easy availability, and the individual's personality type also contribute to the development of substance use disorders. For example, the social permissiveness towards alcohol consumption has been associated with a higher prevalence of alcohol use disorder in the states of Punjab and Goa.

COMORBIDITY

Antisocial personality disorder, depression and anxiety disorders are the most common psychiatric disorders comorbid with substance use disorders. Substance use disorder is a major risk factor for suicide (studies have shown that around 15% of patients with alcohol use disorder die by suicide).

ALCOHOL

Ethyl alcohol (CH_3-CH_2-OH) is the active ingredient of alcoholic drinks. The concentration of ethyl alcohol (ethanol) varies across the preparations. The standard drink or a unit of alcohol corresponds to 10 mL of absolute alcohol or 7.8 g of absolute alcohol (specific gravity of alcohol is 0.78). The concentration of alcohol in commonly used preparations has been summarised in **Table 11.1**.

Table 11.1: Absolute alcohol concentration in various preparations.	
Preparation	Concentration of alcohol by volume (% ABV)
Spirits (whiskey, rum, gin, vodka, brandy, etc.)	40
Arrack	33
Fortified wines	14–20
Wines	5–13
Beer (strong)	8–11
Beer (standard)	3–4

Note: One standard drink = 1 peg (30 mL) of spirits = 1 glass (125 mL) of wine = 1 glass (60 mL) of fortified wine = 1/2 packet of arrack = 1/2 bottle of standard beer = 1/4 bottle of strong beer.

Arrack is the country-made liquor. Fortified wines are prepared by adding brandy to wine.

Absorption

About 10% of alcohol is absorbed from the stomach and the remainder from the **small intestine (80% from the duodenum and jejunum)**. However, when alcohol is consumed with food, the absorption gets delayed due to the slowing down of gastric emptying. The peak blood alcohol concentration is reached in 30–90 minutes (usually 45–60 min), depending on whether the alcohol was ingested empty stomach (absorption is faster) or with food (absorption is slower). Further, if alcohol is consumed rapidly, the peak blood concentration is reached in lesser time.

However, if alcohol is consumed in excessive amounts, the concentration of alcohol in the stomach gets too high, leading to the closure of the pyloric valve. In this case, absorption gets reduced as alcohol cannot pass into the small intestine. Also, pylorospasm results in nausea and vomiting.

Mellanby Effect

Studies have shown that intoxicating effects of alcohol are greater at a given blood alcohol level when blood alcohol concentration (BAC) is increasing than when it is falling. So, an individual would appear more intoxicated at a particular BAC while consuming the alcohol than when the levels are falling after stopping the alcohol consumption.

Reverse Tolerance

This refers to the phenomenon where the intoxicating effects of alcohol are seen progressively with **lower dosages**. The individual reports of getting intoxicated with much smaller amounts of alcohol in comparison to the past. It is believed to be secondary to decreasing levels of alcohol metabolising enzymes due to progressive liver dysfunction (A similar concept of **sensitisation** is seen with cocaine, amphetamines, opioids and cannabis, wherein augmented stimulant response is observed with repeated, intermittent exposure to a specific drug. It is believed to be due to changes in the brain's reward pathways).

Metabolism

About 90% of absorbed alcohol is metabolised through oxidation in the liver; the remaining 10% is excreted unchanged by the kidneys and the lungs. The alcohol in alveolar air is in equilibrium with alcohol in blood passing through pulmonary capillaries; hence determining the alcohol levels in breath by breath analyser gives a good estimation of blood alcohol levels.

The rate of oxidation of alcohol by the liver is constant and is around 7–10 g an hour (which is the amount of alcohol in one standard drink). Alcohol is converted into acetaldehyde (CH_3CHO) by the enzyme alcohol dehydrogenase, which is further oxidised into acetate by the enzyme aldehyde dehydrogenase. Acetate is converted into carbon dioxide and water.

Women may experience more intoxication symptoms than men after drinking a similar amount of alcohol. The reason for the same appears to be lower alcohol dehydrogenase levels in females than males.

Acute Intoxication

Alcohol is a central nervous system depressant. The excitement that follows alcohol use is due to decreased conscious self-control.

Mechanism

The acute effects of alcohol are hypothesised to be mediated by changes in the fluidity of the neuronal membranes. Short-term use of alcohol increases the membrane's fluidity (long-term use makes the membrane rigid), which in turn impacts the release of various neurotransmitters leading to the intoxicating actions of alcohol. For example, the release of dopamine and opioids in the 'reward pathway' leads to the feeling of pleasure, and the facilitation of GABA activity decreases anxiety.

The symptoms and signs of alcohol intoxication depend on the blood alcohol concentration. The **Table 11.2** below describes the intoxication symptoms at different blood alcohol concentrations:

Table 11.2: Symptoms of alcohol intoxication.	
Blood alcohol concentration (mg/dL)	**Symptoms**
20–30	Slowness of motor performance and decreased thinking ability. **30 mg/dL** is the legal limit for driving in India
30–80	Worsening of motor performance and a further decrease in thinking ability
80–200	Incoordination, judgment errors, mood lability
200–300	Nystagmus, slurring of speech, **alcoholic blackouts**
>300	Impaired vital signs and possible death

At higher levels, death occurs secondary to respiratory depression or the inhalation of vomitus.

> Idiosyncratic alcohol intoxication (or **mania a potu**): It refers to the marked changes in behaviour (such as extreme aggression) that occur within minutes of taking small amounts of alcohol.

> **Alcoholic blackout**: It refers to the **anterograde amnesia** that may develop during intoxication. The individual cannot recall the events that happened when his blood alcohol levels were between 200–300 mg/dL, although while consuming alcohol, his behaviour appeared to be goal-directed, and the individual didn't appear confused. For example, a person (while his BAC was around 250 mg/dL) made elaborate plans about a new business with his friend and appeared to be coherent; however, he could not recall that discussion the next day.

Alcohol Withdrawal

It refers to the symptoms that develop after cessation of alcohol intake. Withdrawal symptoms are usually seen in individuals who have been consuming alcohol heavily for years. They typically manifest on waking up the next day after blood alcohol concentration has dropped during sleep. Many individuals start drinking alcohol immediately after waking up to relieve the withdrawal symptoms **(early morning drinking is highly suggestive of alcohol dependence)**.

Comorbid physical illnesses, malnutrition, or fatigue can act as predisposing (or aggravating) factors for precipitating alcohol withdrawal symptoms.

The following sequence is seen in most patients, though all symptoms do not necessarily manifest in all the patients.

- **After 6–8 hours:** The earliest and the most common feature of alcohol withdrawal is **tremulousness (coarse tremors)** that affects the hands, legs, and trunk. Other symptoms include gastrointestinal symptoms (like nausea and vomiting), sympathetic autonomic hyperactivity including arousal, anxiety, sweating, hypertension, mydriasis and tachycardia.
- **After 12–24 hours: Perceptual disturbances and psychotic symptoms**. It refers to the illusions or hallucinations that develop in the absence of any disturbances of consciousness. Rarely, delusions may also be present.
- **After 24–48 hours: Alcohol withdrawal seizures**. The seizures are usually generalised and tonic-clonic. Usually, patients have >1 seizure in a span of 3–6 hours; hence often, the term **cluster seizures** is used for alcohol withdrawal seizures.
- **After 48–72 hours: Delirium tremens**. Alcohol withdrawal delirium is a medical emergency, and if left untreated, the mortality rate is around 20%. The symptoms and signs include disturbances of consciousness, disorientation to time, place and person, hallucinations (**most commonly visual**, but sometimes also auditory and tactile hallucinations), coarse tremors, autonomic hyperactivity and gross tremulousness of hands. Other signs and symptoms seen in delirium can also be present (please remember delirium tremens is nothing but delirium precipitated by alcohol withdrawal). Medical comorbidities such as hepatitis and pancreatitis increase the predisposition to delirium tremens.

Protracted Withdrawal

After acute withdrawal symptoms resolve, symptoms like anxiety, insomnia, and autonomic hyperactivity may continue for 2–6 months. The persistence of these symptoms may increase the risk of relapse, as the patient may go back to drinking to relieve these symptoms. Although the evidence is limited, anti-craving drugs like acamprosate may help relieve some of these symptoms. Psychoeducation and cognitive behavioural therapy is also helpful in some patients.

Alcohol Dependence, Harmful Pattern of Use of Alcohol and Alcohol Use Disorders

These diagnoses are made if alcohol use fulfils the DSM-5 or ICD-11 criterion as mentioned in the terminology section.

ALCOHOL-INDUCED DISORDERS

Physical Disorders

Excessive consumption of alcohol can cause physical disorders by different mechanisms that include:
a. Direct toxic effect on tissues like brain and liver
b. Poor dietary intake and poor absorption resulting in a deficiency of vitamin B and protein
c. Increased risk of accidents

One can refer to any standard textbook of medicine for the details. Here, we would focus primarily on psychiatric disorders.

Psychiatric Disorders

Many psychiatric disorders can develop during or soon after intoxication with alcohol or during withdrawal from alcohol. These disorders usually resolve within 1 month of cessation of alcohol intake. If the symptoms of the mental disorder persist beyond that, the possibility of an independent mental disorder should be entertained. Alcohol-induced psychiatric disorders include:

1. Alcohol-induced psychotic disorders.
2. Alcohol-induced bipolar disorders
3. Alcohol-induced depressive disorders.
4. Alcohol-induced anxiety disorders, alcohol-induced sleep disorder.
5. Alcohol-induced sexual dysfunction.

A detailed discussion is warranted about alcohol-induced neurocognitive disorders.

These include:
A. *Alcohol-induced dementia*: Long term alcohol use can result in the development of cognitive disturbances that meet the criteria of dementia. The symptoms tend to improve with abstinence, but in many, despite abstinence, long term deficits may continue.
B. *Alcohol-induced persistent amnestic disorder* (**Wernicke-Korsakoff syndrome**): Long term alcohol use can cause amnestic syndrome (amnestic syndromes are characterised by primary abnormality of short-term memory), which has been classically called as Wernicke-Korsakoff syndrome and includes:
   a. **Wernicke's encephalopathy:** It is the acute neurological complication characterised by the following symptoms (mnemonic GOA):
      - G: **G**lobal **confusion**
      - O: **Ophthalmoplegia,** usually due to 6th nerve palsy (second most common is 3rd nerve palsy) leading to horizontal nystagmus and gaze palsy)
      - A: **Ataxia**

   Although Wernicke's encephalopathy can be **reversed** with treatment, **residual ataxia** and horizontal nystagmus

often persist. Ophthalmoplegia responds rapidly to thiamine treatment and may get reversed within hours. The patients, when treated adequately, have the following course: (1) Ophthalmoplegia starts to resolve within hours, though horizontal nystagmus often persists. (2) Ataxia begins to improve within the first week; however, around 50% of patients are left with some residual abnormalities. (3) Global confusion begins to clear within 2–3 weeks and resolves completely in 1–2 months.

Despite treatment, some patients can progress to Korsakoff's syndrome.

If untreated, Wernicke's encephalopathy may clear spontaneously in days to weeks or may progress to Korsakoff's syndrome.

b. **Korsakoff's syndrome:** It is the **chronic** neurological complication of long-term alcohol use. It is characterised by impaired recent memory, **anterograde amnesia** (inability to form new memories), **retrograde amnesia** (inability to recall old memories) and **confabulations** (making of false stories to fill memory gaps, which is unintentional). Anterograde amnesia is much more prominent than retrograde amnesia.

The cause for both Wernicke's syndrome and Korsakoff's syndrome is **thiamine deficiency**.

In Wernicke's korsakoff syndrome, the neuropathological lesions are usually symmetrical and involve **mammillary bodies**. Other lesion sites include the thalamus, hypothalamus, midbrain, pons, medulla, fornix and cerebellum.

Treatment: Wernicke's encephalopathy is treated with a high dose of parenteral thiamine. Korsakoff syndrome is treated with oral thiamine for around 3–12 months. Only about 20% of patients with Korsakoff syndrome recover completely.

> **Marchiafava–Bignami disease:** It is a rare neurological complication of long-term alcohol use. It is characterised by epilepsy, ataxia, dysarthria, hallucinations and intellectual deterioration. The pathophysiology is the demyelination of **corpus callosum**, optic tracts and cerebellar peduncles.

> **Fetal alcohol syndrome:** Consumption of alcohol during pregnancy can damage the fetus as alcohol inhibits intrauterine growth. The term 'fetal alcohol syndrome, is used for the constellation of symptoms that develop due to the use of alcohol during pregnancy. Fetal alcohol syndrome presents with:
> ❖ Facial abnormality
> ❖ Small stature
> ❖ Low birth weight
> ❖ Low intelligence
> ❖ Overactivity

Evaluation

A. **Screening test:** One of the most commonly used screening tests for alcohol use disorder is **CAGE questionnaire**, which includes the following four questions:

C: Have you ever felt that you should **C**ut down on your drinking?

A: Have people **A**nnoyed you by criticising your drinking?

G: Have you ever felt bad or **G**uilty about your drinking?

E: Have you ever had a drink first thing in the morning to steady your nerves or to get rid of hangovers (**E**ye-opener)?

A positive response to **two or more** of these questions suggests alcohol use disorder. Another commonly used screening test is **AUDIT** (**alcohol use disorders identification test**). Others tests such as **SADQ** (**severity of alcohol dependence questionnaire**) are used to determine the severity of dependence.

B. **Diagnostic markers:** Apart from the screening tests, the blood tests may also help identify heavy drinkers who are susceptible to alcohol use disorders.

- **Blood alcohol concentration:** It can be used to judge tolerance to alcohol. For example, if a person has high blood alcohol concentration without any signs of intoxication, it indicates the presence of tolerance and a high likelihood of alcohol use disorders.

  Blood alcohol concentration is usually measured using breath analysers. It can also be estimated using **the Widmark formula** if the amount of alcohol consumed and body weight is known.

- **Carbohydrate deficit transferrin (CDT):** The **most sensitive** and **specific** laboratory test to identify heavy drinking is elevated blood levels of carbohydrate deficit transferrin.

- **Gamma-glutamyl transferase (GGT):** Elevated levels of GGT are again suggestive of heavy drinking. However, GGT has poor sensitivity and specificity (50–60%). The levels of both CDT and GGT return to normal within days to weeks of stopping drinking.

- **Alanine aminotransferase (ALT) and aspartate aminotransferase (AST):** These liver enzymes are even less sensitive than GGT, however, they have higher specificity. **ALT has higher specificity** out of the two, as it is found mostly in the liver. A ratio of AST:ALT is a good marker for heavy alcohol consumption.

- **Mean corpuscular volume:** MCV is frequently elevated in individuals who indulge in heavy drinking.

- Other tests include elevated levels of alkaline phosphatase, which indicate liver injury secondary to heavy drinking.

Treatment

Detoxification

The first step in the treatment of alcohol use disorders (or dependence/harmful use) is detoxification, which focuses primarily on managing the withdrawal symptoms. In regular users, the brain adapts to the constant presence of alcohol (which is a CNS depressant). When there is a sudden cessation of alcohol, the brain remains in a hyper-excited state resulting in withdrawal symptoms. It is vital to manage the withdrawal symptoms, as they are a common cause of relapse.

The aim is to make the withdrawal symptoms tolerable rather than completely suppress them, as the medicines used for such purposes themselves carry a moderate to high abuse liability.

Benzodiazepines are considered the **drug of choice** for the management of alcohol withdrawal. Benzodiazepines have cross-tolerance with alcohol and hence reduce the alcohol withdrawal symptoms. The commonly used benzodiazepines include chlordiazepoxide (considered to have low dependence potential), diazepam or lorazepam. Short-acting benzodiazepines, such as oxazepam or lorazepam, are preferred in patients with impaired liver function. The dose of benzodiazepines is gradually tapered off, and they are stopped in 5–7 days.

Carbamazepine can also be used to manage alcohol withdrawal, though other anticonvulsants have no role.

Oral thiamine must be given to prevent the development of Wernicke-Korsakoff syndrome. In cases of severe withdrawal symptoms or when medical comorbidities are present, and inpatient detoxification is being done, parenteral thiamine is recommended as a prophylaxis for Wernicke-Korsakoff syndrome.

Thiamine is required for the metabolism of glucose. Alcohol-dependent patients are often deficient in thiamine due to poor intake and absorption. Hence, in a patient with alcohol withdrawal symptoms, if IV.

Glucose is administered; it may precipitate acute deficiency of thiamine and lead to Wernicke's encephalopathy. Thus, thiamine must always be given before glucose in this patient group.

Apart from medical treatment, brief counselling sessions are also taken during the detoxification stage.

> **Alcohol withdrawal seizures:** The drugs of choice for alcohol withdrawal seizures are benzodiazepines. Carbamazepine can be used, other anticonvulsants have no role.

> **Delirium tremens:** Treatment of delirium tremens must be done in an inpatient setting as it is a medical emergency. The following points must be remembered:
> - Intravenous benzodiazepines are the drugs of choice
> - Parenteral thiamine (and other B vitamins) must be administered
> - Supportive measures include administration of IV fluids and maintaining electrolyte balance
> - Antipsychotics can be used to manage hallucinations and agitation, although they must be used carefully as they can reduce seizure threshold and may cause other side effects
> - The environment should be protective, and sensory stimuli should be minimal

Relapse Prevention (Maintenance of Abstinence)

This stage follows detoxification. In this stage, the goal is to prevent the patient from relapsing to alcohol use. Both pharmacological and psychosocial approaches are used.

1. **Pharmacotherapy:** The medications that have shown effectiveness in relapse prevention include:
   a. **Naltrexone:** Naltrexone is an opioid antagonist. Endogenous opioids play a role in increasing the dopaminergic activity after consumption of alcohol, which leads to the feeling of 'pleasure'. Opioid receptor block prevents this dopaminergic activity, and hence alcohol consumption cannot produce the 'high'. This prevents the rewarding effects (positive reinforcement) of alcohol and also reduces the craving. Naltrexone can be started when patients are still drinking or during detoxification. Naltrexone is metabolised by the liver and must be used carefully in patients with hepatic insufficiency.
   Common side effects: Nausea, vomiting, headache, dizziness, weight loss, abdominal pain.
   b. **Acamprosate:** It acts by decreasing the excitatory effects of glutamate (NMDA antagonism) and increasing inhibitory GABAergic function. It reduces the craving for alcohol. Acamprosate can be started during detoxification as it has a potential neuro-protective effect. It is not metabolised by the liver and is excreted by the kidneys.
   Common side effects: Diarrhoea, abdominal pain, nausea, vomiting, fluctuations in libido and pruritus.
   c. **Disulfiram:** Disulfiram acts by inhibiting the enzyme aldehyde dehydrogenase leading to the accumulation of acetaldehyde after alcohol consumption. This results in an unpleasant reaction called as 'disulfiram ethanol reaction'. It is characterised by the following symptoms:
      - Facial flushing
      - Throbbing headache
      - Hypotension, tachycardia
      - Nausea, vomiting
      - In some cases, cardiac arrhythmias and collapse may occur (hence avoided in patients with a history of congestive heart failure, coronary artery disease, and hypertension)

   Disulfiram acts as a deterrent agent (aversive agent) as the patient avoids using alcohol to avoid this unpleasant reaction. However, the efficacy of unsupervised disulfiram use is limited as patients often stop the medicine. The evidence about the effectiveness of disulfiram is weaker than naltrexone and acamprosate, and it is considered a 'second-line' drug now.
   Common side effects: Drowsiness, nausea, constipation, dermatitis, metallic taste. Rarely psychosis, peripheral neuropathy, hepatitis, and optic neuritis.

   Other drugs that are sometimes used for relapse prevention in alcohol include nalmefene, topiramate, and baclofen.

2. **Psychosocial treatment:** Along with medications, psychosocial techniques too play an important role in relapse prevention. Before talking about the different types of useful techniques, it is important to understand how behavioural change develops in a patient with alcohol use disorder (or any substance use disorder). The **transtheoretical model of change**, which was proposed by Prochaska and DiClemente, is considered the most

influential model of change. According to this model, the following are the stages of change:
  a. **Precontemplation:** In this stage, the substance user does not see any problem in his behaviour and does not think about quitting.
  b. **Contemplation:** In this stage, the substance user realises that he has a problem and is taking the substance excessively. He considers the **pros and cons** of stopping substance use. However, he is yet to make any decision.
  c. **Preparation:** In this stage, the substance user decides to quit the substance and starts making a plan to quit.
  d. **Action:** In this stage, the substance user stops taking the substance and changes his behaviours to ensure the same. (e.g., he stops meeting the friends with whom he used to consume the drugs or seeks medical help to quit the substance use).
  e. **Maintenance:** In this stage, the patient continues to stay away from substances (drugs) and continues with the treatment and other behaviours to prevent relapse.

A patient may remain in the maintenance stage or may relapse if he starts using the substance again. Usually, a patient has few relapses before attaining complete abstinence (freedom) from substance use.

Psychological treatment methods that are useful in the treatment of substance use disorders include:
1. **Motivational interviewing:** This clinical method is used to increase a substance user's motivation for a transition from the stage of precontemplation/contemplation to the stage of action (technique can be used in all the stages of change). The technique involves encouraging the person to decide on change while the therapist facilitates this process by providing clarifications, advice if needed, and accurate feedback while avoiding confrontation all along.
2. **Motivational enhancement therapy (MET):** In MET, the clinical style of motivational interviewing is used, and also specific emphasis is given to personalised assessment, providing feedback and making change plans.
3. **Relapse prevention:** 'Relapse prevention' is a general term used for multiple approaches that are used to prevent relapse. Many relapse prevention approaches use cognitive and behavioural techniques to decrease the possibility of relapses.
4. **Family and marital therapy:** Involvement of family members and spouses often help in the treatment process.
5. **Brief intervention:** As the name suggests, it is a brief and initial approach that can be used by general physicians and involves giving education and advice about safe levels of alcohol drinking.
6. **Alcoholics anonymous (12-step self-help group):** Alcoholics Anonymous is a self-help group where people with a similar problem (i.e., alcohol use disorder) help each other out. The treatment rationale is not medical and instead based on 'faith' and religion. It is known to work as an effective adjunct to medical treatment.

OPIOIDS

There are three broad classes of opioids:
1. Naturally occurring opium alkaloids (called **opiates**), such as morphine and codeine.
2. Semi-synthetic that are produced by modifying natural opium alkaloids. For example: Heroin, oxycodone and hydrocodone.
3. Pure synthetic compounds that are not produced from opium and may have chemical structures different from opium alkaloids. For example: Fentanyl and methadone.

The term **opioids** is a broader term used for all compounds with effects like opiates and includes all the above three classes.

The primary impact of opioid drugs is mediated by µ-opioid receptors (mu), κ-opioid receptors (kappa) and Δ-opioid receptors (delta). Out of these, µ receptors are responsible for the development of dependence.

Heroin (diacetylmorphine) is the **most commonly** abused opioid. Since it is more lipid-soluble than morphine, it crosses the blood-brain barrier faster and has a more rapid onset of action. Heroin was initially used to treat morphine addiction; however, it was later realised that the dependence potential of heroin is higher than morphine. The street names of heroin include "smack" and "brown sugar", amongst others. The street forms are often impure and have adulterants like starch (fructose and sucrose), quinine, chalk powder, paracetamol and talcum powder.

Opioids can be taken orally (In India, orally used forms include '*affim*' and '*doda*', mostly used in the country's Northern States), snorted intranasally, smoke can be inhaled through a straw (also called chasing the dragon), and injected intravenously or subcutaneously. The intravenous use (called mainlining) tends to gradually shift from peripheral veins to larger veins (as more and more veins collapse). The intravenous route is particularly dangerous as it can lead to potential transmission of HIV and Hepatitis B and C due to sharing of contaminated needles.

As more and more veins collapse, the user may progress to subcutaneous administration of heroin (known as "**skin popping**").

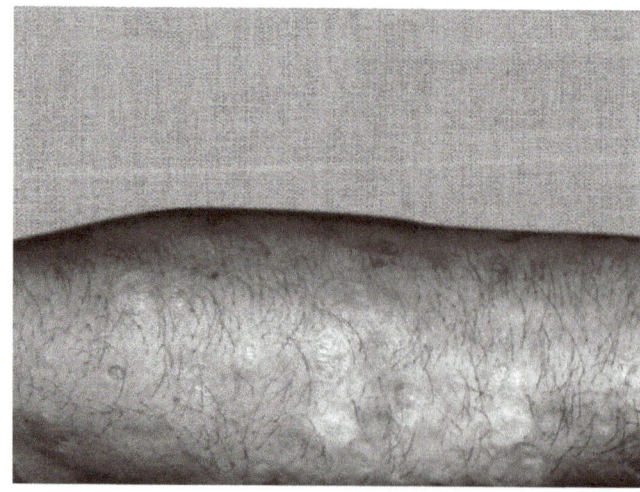

Fig. 11.1: Skin popping.

> The close proximity of India to two major opium-producing regions, the so-called **golden crescent** (which includes Pakistan, Afghanistan and Iran) and the **golden triangle** (Thailand, Laos and Myanmar), makes the trafficking of drugs from these regions into India easier and poses a big challenge for country's law enforcement agencies.

Intoxication

Opioid use (especially intravenous) leads to a feeling of intense euphoria (known as "rush"). The other symptoms include a feeling of warmth, heaviness of extremities and facial flushing. There is also relief from pain and anxiety and a dream-like state, with decreased responsiveness to the environment.

This initial euphoria is followed by a period of sedation (known as "nodding off").

In people who are not dependent, the use of morphine or heroin may lead to an unpleasant feeling.

Overdose

Opioid overdose can be lethal due to **respiratory depression**. The overdose symptoms include slow respiration rate, hypothermia, **hypotension**, bradycardia, pinpoint pupils, cyanosis, and coma.

Withdrawal Symptoms

The sudden cessation of opioids after prolonged use or intake of opioid antagonists like naltrexone can precipitate withdrawal symptoms. The short-term use of opioids decreases the activity of noradrenergic neurons, and long-term use results in compensatory hyperactivity. When opioids are suddenly stopped, there are symptoms due to rebound noradrenergic hyperactivity. This hypothesis also explains the effectiveness of clonidine (alpha-2 adrenergic receptor agonist, which decreases norepinephrine release) in managing opioid withdrawal.

The withdrawal symptoms usually appear around **6–8 hours** after the last intake, peak during the second or third day and subside during the next 7–10 days. The withdrawal from opioids results in a **flu-like syndrome** with the following symptoms:
- **Lacrimation**, **rhinorrhea**, sweating, **diarrhoea**
- **Yawning** and **piloerection**
- Pupillary dilation
- Muscle cramps and generalised body ache
- **Insomnia**, anxiety, hypertension and tachycardia
- Nausea, vomiting and anorexia.

Opioid dependence, harmful pattern of use of opioids and opioid use disorders.

These diagnoses are made if opioid use fulfils the DSM-5 or ICD-11 criterion, as mentioned in the terminology section.

Treatment

A. **Detoxification:** In this stage, the main focus is on managing withdrawal symptoms. The medications usually used are long-acting opioids like **methadone** or **buprenorphine**. Due to agonist action at opioid receptors, both medications suppress the withdrawal symptoms. Dextro-propoxyphene can also be used. Levo-alpha-acetylmethadol was also used in the past but was found to increase the QTc interval and hence is no longer recommended.

Usually, the detoxification phase continues for 2–3 weeks.

Clonidine can also be used for the detoxification of opioids. However, clonidine provides considerably less symptom relief than buprenorphine or methadone. Clonidine is thus mostly used as an adjunct to methadone or buprenorphine during detoxification.

Accelerated detoxification: In this method, patients with opioid use disorders are initially given low doses of naltrexone to precipitate the withdrawal symptoms. The withdrawal symptoms are then managed using clonidine. This method reduces the detoxification period to 4–5 days.

B. **Maintenance treatment:** It follows detoxification, and the goal is to prevent relapse. There are two different pharmacological approaches for the maintenance phase.
  1. **Opioid substitution therapy:** In this method, the illicit, parenterally administered and short-acting opioids (like heroin) are replaced with medically safe, orally taken and long-acting opioids. The long-acting opioids such as **methadone** and buprenorphine are primarily used. Levo-alpha-acetylmethadol was also used in the past; however, it has since been stopped as it can cause torsades de pointes.

     These orally used opioids are given at government-approved centres. Though the patient continues to remain opioid-dependent, however, he is protected from the medical consequence of parenteral opioids (such as HBV, HCV, and HIV infection) and does not need to indulge in criminal activities to fund illicit opioid use. This is also referred to as the harm reduction approach.

     Methadone is considered the **gold standard** for the treatment of opioid dependence. Once the patient is stable, methadone can be gradually tapered and stopped. Methadone withdrawal symptoms are less severe than the withdrawal symptoms of heroin and can be managed using clonidine.

  2. **Opioid antagonist treatment: Naltrexone** can be given to the patient after detoxification is complete. The rationale is that naltrexone will block the opioid receptors, and any opioid use would fail to produce the euphoric response and hence would not be repeated.

C. **Psychosocial treatment:** All the psychosocial treatment approaches that are used to treat alcohol dependence can be used in the treatment of opioid use disorders, including the self-help groups (called narcotics anonymous) approach.

D. **Overdose treatment:** The opioids are lethal in overdose. The drug of choice for treatment of opioid overdose is IV **naloxone** (short-acting opioid antagonist). The signs of overdose reversal with naloxone include increased respiratory rate and pupillary dilatation. In case overdosage is with a long-acting opioid such as methadone, or LAAM, repeated administration of IV naloxone might be required as naloxone has a short half-life. Recently, the FDA has approved the **nasal spray of naloxone** to treat opioid overdose.

CANNABIS

Cannabis preparations are derived from the hemp plant, *Cannabis sativa*. The plant has several varieties named after the regions where it is found (e.g., *Cannabis sativa* indica in India, *Cannabis sativa* americana in the USA).

The active ingredient responsible for the psychoactive effects of cannabis is **Δ-9 tetrahydrocannabinol (THC), although there are about 60 more chemicals similar to Δ-9 THC in the plant (known as cannabinoids).**

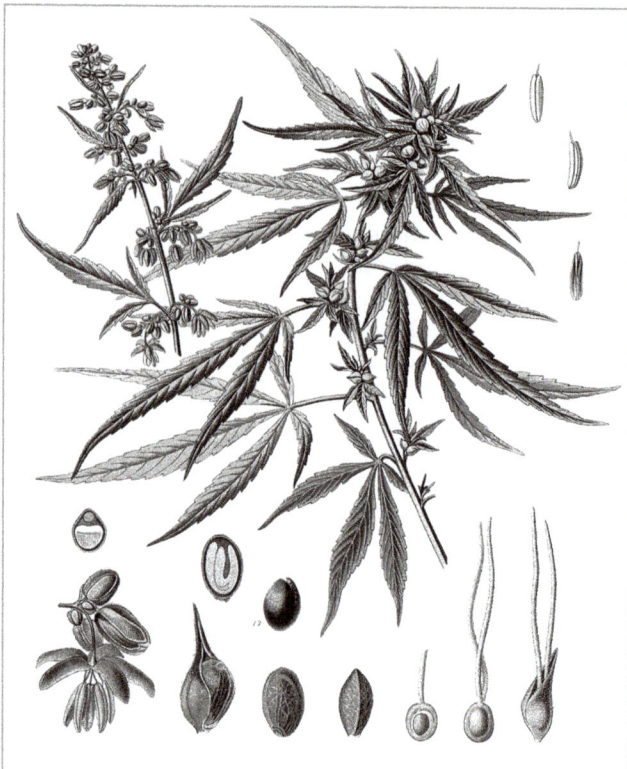

Fig. 11.2: *Cannabis* plant and seeds.

Cannabis is the **most commonly used illegal drug** in the world and India.

The street names include joints, marijuana, grass, pot, weed, etc.

The various preparations of *Cannabis* are given in the **Table 11.3** below.

Table 11.3: THC concentration in various *Cannabis* preparations.

Cannabis preparations	THC content (%)
Bhaang (paste of leaves of the plant or dried leaves)	1
Ganja (derived from the dried flowering stem of the plan)	1–2
Hashish/*Charas* (derived from resinous exudates)	8–14
Hash oil (made by extracting cannabinoids from the resin using organic solvents)	15–40

Cannabis can be ingested orally or can be smoked. In North India, some people use *Cannabis* orally in a milk-based drink called *Thandai* during the festivals of *Holi* and *Shivratri*. More commonly, *Cannabis* is smoked by mixing the preparations of *Cannabis* with tobacco in cigarettes. *Cannabis* is unsuitable for intravenous use because of poor solubility in water. Also, if taken intravenously, there is a risk of anaphylaxis due to undissolved particulate matter.

The pharmacological actions of cannabinoids are mediated through specific cannabinoid receptors in the central nervous system. These receptors are found in various brain parts but not in the brainstem (hence *Cannabis* causes a minimal effect on respiratory and cardiac functions).

The cannabinoids do not stimulate the 'reward pathway', and although tolerance and psychological dependence develops to *Cannabis*, the physiological dependence is weak.

Intoxication

It is characterised by euphoria, a subjective sense of slowing of time, a sense of floating in the air, **reddening of the conjunctiva** (due to dilatation of conjunctival blood vessels), **increased appetite** and dryness of the mouth. Other symptoms include impairment of motor skills, depersonalisation, derealisation, **and synesthesia** (cross over of sensory perceptions. For example, the patient may report that he is "seeing" music and "hearing" lights).

In some cases, after consuming *Cannabis*, the person might feel restless, fearful, paranoid, extremely anxious (similar to a panic attack) and may think that he will go crazy. This unpleasant experience is known as a **"bad trip"**.

Withdrawal Symptoms

Earlier it was believed that *Cannabis* does not cause physical dependence, and there are no withdrawal symptoms associated with *Cannabis* use. However, recent studies have shown mild withdrawal symptoms do develop within 1–2 weeks of cessation of cannabis use. These include **irritability**, anxiety, decreased appetite, depressed mood and sleep difficulties (including insomnia and strange dreams). Physical complaints such as abdominal pain, tremors, headache, sweating, fever or chills can also be present.

Cannabis Dependence, Harmful Pattern of Use of *Cannabis* and *Cannabis* Use Disorders

These diagnoses are made if cannabis use fulfils the DSM-5 or ICD-11 criterion as mentioned in the terminology section.

Cannabis-related Disorders

Some of the important psychiatric disorders associated with cannabis use include:

1. ***Cannabis* induced psychotic disorder (hemp insanity):** The patient develops psychotic symptoms such as delusions and hallucinations. The psychotic symptoms usually resolve within a month of cessation of *Cannabis* use. On occasions, the 'bad trips' may present with psychotic symptoms; in such cases, too, a diagnosis of *Cannabis*-induced psychotic disorder is made.

2. **Flashbacks:** *Cannabis* flashbacks are not as common as flashbacks associated with hallucinogens use. The flashbacks are characterised by re-experiencing, when the individual is sober, of one or more perceptual symptoms that were experienced while intoxicated with *Cannabis*.
3. ***Cognitive impairment:*** Long term *Cannabis* use can impair cognitive functions like memory, attention and the ability to work effectively with complex information.
4. **Amotivational syndrome:** In individuals who use *Cannabis* frequently, there may be a decrease in the desire to work or compete with others. The individual shows an unwillingness to persist in any task, whether at school or at work. The individual appears uninterested, lethargic and apathetic.

> **Run amok:** It is the development of rage following *Cannabis* use, in which the person may hurt or even indiscriminately kill others.

Treatment

As withdrawal symptoms are mild, no medications are usually required. If needed, the benzodiazepines can be used in the short term.

Long-term treatment usually involves the psychotherapeutic approach. The psychosocial treatment methods described in the management of alcohol dependence are also used for *Cannabis* dependence treatment.

HALLUCINOGENS

As the name suggests, hallucinogens use primarily results in perceptual disturbances like hallucinations and illusions. Hallucinogens are natural and synthetic substances, also called psychedelics or psychotomimetics. The most common naturally occurring hallucinogens are psilocybin and mescaline. Other naturally occurring hallucinogens include ayahuasca, cathinone (present naturally in the khat plant and synthetically made and known as bath salts), ibogaine, and *Salvia divinorum*.

The classic synthetic hallucinogen is **LSD (lysergic acid diethylamide)**. Nowadays, LSD is mostly sold as "blotter acid" as stamps soaked in LSD (paper sheets soaked with LSD are dried and perforated in small squares and stamped with designs). Other synthetic drugs include 3, 4 methylenedioxyamphetamine (MDMA, also called ecstasy), phencyclidine (PCP, **angel dust**) and ketamine.

Phencyclidine (PCP) and Ketamine are closely related compounds and are called "dissociative anaesthetics", as when consumed, they produce a condition where the patient appears dissociated or cut off from the environment despite being awake. Both act by blocking NMDA receptors.

Intoxication

Hallucinogen intoxication manifests with heightened perceptions (colours look richer, there is a heightened response to smell and taste), illusions, hallucinations (usually visual, often of geometric figures), **synesthesia** (also called reflex hallucinations wherein the patient may report cross over of sensory perceptions), depersonalisation, derealisation, and autonomic hyperactivity features such as pupillary dilatation, tachycardia, sweating, palpitations, tremors, etc.

Phencyclidine intoxication may result in severe symptoms, including the development of delusions and hallucinations. Phencyclidine intoxication also produces a few characteristic symptoms such as vertical or horizontal nystagmus, ataxia, dysarthria and extreme agitation and assaultiveness.

Similar to *Cannabis*, hallucinogen intoxication may also result in an unpleasant experience characterised by restlessness, paranoia and a state of panic (bad trip).

Usually, no withdrawal symptoms are seen with hallucinogens use. The tolerance is associated with the use of any of the hallucinogens.

Hallucinogen-persisting perception disorder (flashbacks): These are characterised by re-experiencing, when the individual is sober, of one or more of perceptual symptoms that were experienced while intoxicated with hallucinogens. During the flashback, insight is retained, and the person remains aware that the disturbances are linked to the effect of drugs. Stress, sensory deprivation, or use of another substance like alcohol or *Cannabis* may trigger flashback episodes.

Treatment

The treatment of hallucinogens intoxication usually involves reassuring the patient that symptoms are due to drugs and would improve with time. In the presence of severe symptoms, benzodiazepines are used. If agitation is significant or psychotic symptoms are present, antipsychotics may be required. For hallucinogen-persisting perception disorders, benzodiazepines can be used. Antipsychotics are used when psychotic symptoms are present.

Mostly psychotherapeutic techniques are used to prevent relapses.

STIMULANTS

The two major classes of stimulants include cocaine and amphetamines.

Cocaine

Cocaine is derived from the plant *Erythroxylum coca*. Sigmund Freud had studied its pharmacological effects and is also believed to be addicted to cocaine for a long time. Coca-cola used to contain cocaine till 1903, after which it ceased to be an ingredient.

Cocaine was initially used as a local anaesthetic (action mediated by blockade of fast sodium channels), especially for eye, nose and throat surgery, for its vasoconstrictive and analgesic effects.

The most common method of using cocaine is the inhalation of finely powdered form into the nose (known as **snorting** or tooting). Due to its vasoconstrictive properties, nasal inhalation of cocaine leads to nasal congestion and long term use can result in nasal septal perforation.

Other intake methods are intravenous or subcutaneous injection and smoking (known as **freebasing**) and subcutaneous or intravenous injections. Freebasing involves mixing street cocaine (which usually has procaine or sugar as adulterants) with freebase (chemically extracted pure cocaine). A particularly potent way of consumption is taking cocaine and heroin (called speedball) together.

Crack is a freebase form of cocaine that is smoked. It is highly potent, and even a single use can cause intense cravings. Crack users can do extremes of violence to obtain more crack.

Cocaine acts primarily by inhibiting the reuptake of dopamine by blocking D1 and D2 receptors. It also inhibits the reuptake of norepinephrine and hence has a significant sympathomimetic effect. When consumed, cocaine causes marked vasoconstriction of peripheral arteries resulting in hypertension. In some cases, vasoconstriction of the epicardial coronary arteries can lead to ischemic myocardial injury. Cocaine use can also cause seizures. Cocaine (**most common**) and amphetamines (second most common) are the drugs that are commonly associated with seizures.

Amphetamines

The most commonly used amphetamines include dextroamphetamine, methamphetamine and a mixed dextroamphetamine-amphetamine salt. The street names for these include ice, crystal, speed and crystal meths. Some amphetamine-like compounds include methylphenidate, ephedrine, pseudoephedrine, and phenylpropanolamine. MDMA (methylenedioxymethamphetamine) is a substituted amphetamine (MDMA has been classified as a hallucinogen too).

Amphetamines are FDA approved for the treatment of attention deficit hyperactivity disorder (ADHD) and narcolepsy.

Amphetamines are abused to increase performance and for their euphoric effects. Students preparing for exams and professionals who want to improve their performance are known to abuse amphetamines.

Apart from amphetamines and cocaine, another class of stimulants are derived from *Catha edulis* or 'Khat', a plant that is indigenous to Africa. The plant contains the stimulants cathinone and cathine. Khat is chewed like tobacco for its stimulant action. Synthetic cathinones have been prepared, and are packaged in various types of disguise, most famously as 'bath salts'.

Stimulant Intoxication

Stimulant ingestion results in a feeling of euphoria, improved physical and mental efficiency, and improved concentration. Higher dosages may result in irritability, agitation, aggression and psychotic symptoms.

Stimulant Withdrawal

After intoxication, a 'crash' follows, characterised by feeling depressed, lethargy, fatigue, tremulousness and insatiable hunger. There may be suicidal ideations or behaviour too. There may be a strong craving to use cocaine to relieve these unpleasant withdrawal symptoms.

Stimulant Induced Psychotic Disorders

Stimulant induced psychotic disorders are characterised by the presence of paranoid delusions (delusion of persecution) and hallucinations (most commonly auditory hallucinations). The presentation of substance-induced psychotic disorder is quite similar to paranoid schizophrenia. Cocaine use can also cause tactile hallucinations (sensation of insects crawling under the skin), also known as **cocaine bugs** or **formication** or **magnan phenomenon.** For the treatment of psychotic symptoms, antipsychotics are used.

Treatment

The withdrawal symptoms are usually mild, and no specific pharmacological agents reduce the intensity of withdrawal. Treatment primarily relies on psychotherapeutic interventions like cognitive behavioural therapy, group therapy, and support groups such as narcotics anonymous. Network therapy is a specialised combination of individual (using psychodynamic and cognitive-behavioural approaches) and group therapy (engaging in a group support network composed of the patient's family and peers) that yields better results in the outpatient-based treatment of addicted patients.

CLUB DRUGS

Partygoers use a group of drugs (called club drugs) to enhance their experience, especially in raves (all-night parties), dance clubs and bars. These include LSD (lysergic acid diethylamide), γ-hydroxybutyrate (GHB), ketamine, methamphetamine, MDMA (ecstasy), and Rohypnol or "roofies" (flunitrazepam). GHB, ketamine, and Rohypnol are sometimes called date rape drugs because they produce disorienting and sedating effects and often amnesia. These drugs may be given surreptitiously, such as slipped into a drink, or a person might be coerced to take the drug.

■ TOBACCO

It is the **most commonly** used substance in India (caffeine, not considered). Tobacco is consumed in various ways, including smoking, chewing, applying, sucking and gargling. In India, *beedi* smoking is the most common form of use, followed by cigarette smoking. The active ingredient of tobacco, which causes addiction, is nicotine, and the constituents responsible for cardiovascular disorders are nicotine and carbon monoxide.

Nicotine has a stimulant action and improves attention, learning, reaction time and problem-solving ability. Tobacco users also report that cigarette smoking lifts their mood, decreases tension, and lessens depressive feelings.

The withdrawal symptoms can develop within 2 hours of smoking the last cigarette and peak in 24–48 hours. These include:
- Craving for nicotine
- Irritability

- Anxiety
- Poor concentration
- Bradycardia
- Drowsiness and paradoxical trouble sleeping
- Increased appetite and weight gain

Treatment

Pharmacotherapy

1. **Nicotine replacement therapy:** It is used to relieve the withdrawal symptoms by substituting nicotine in tobacco with nicotine in safer forms (as they do not contain the other harmful constituents present in tobacco). The various preparations include nicotine gums, nicotine lozenges, nicotine patches, nicotine inhalers and nicotine spray. Nicotine replacement therapy doubles the cessation rate as they reduce the withdrawal symptoms. They are used for a maintenance period of 6–12 weeks and then gradually tapered over another 6–12 weeks.
2. Non-nicotine medications that are useful include varenicline, bupropion, clonidine and nortriptyline (second line).

Varenicline: Varenicline is a new first-line treatment for smoking cessation. The clinical effectiveness is due to partial agonism at **α4β2 nicotinic acetylcholine receptors**. When a person smokes a cigarette, the absorbed nicotine binds to α4β2 nicotinic acetylcholine receptors, leading to the release of dopamine in the nucleus accumbens. This is responsible for the 'high' as well as reinforcement of smoking behaviour. When a person stops smoking, the nicotinic acetylcholine receptors are left unstimulated, and dopaminergic activity falls, resulting in craving and withdrawal symptoms.

As varenicline is a partial agonist, it's binding to α4β2 nicotinic acetylcholine receptors results in much lesser dopamine release and lesser reinforcement. At the same time, as receptors are occupied, the craving and withdrawal symptoms get controlled. Further, it competitively inhibits the nicotine from binding to α4β2 nicotinic acetylcholine receptors, and hence even if a person smokes, the reinforcement of smoking behaviour is prevented.

Before starting varenicline, the patient is advised to set a quit date (the day smoking will be stopped). Varenicline is started a week before the quit date. Varenicline is started at dosages of 0.5 mg/day for the first 3 days; from the fourth day, the dose is increased to 0.5 mg twice a day, and finally, from the 8th day, it is increased to 1 mg, twice a day. The treatment is continued for 3 months. For those who have successfully stopped smoking at the end of 12 weeks, an additional course of 12 weeks of treatment with varenicline is recommended to increase the likelihood of long-term abstinence further.

The most common adverse effects include nausea, headache and insomnia. Initially, the FDA issued a black box warning for potential neuropsychiatric adverse effects such as depressed mood, agitation, suicidal ideations, and suicide. Later, the research showed that varenicline doesn't worsen the psychiatric symptoms and is not associated with any increased risk for suicide. FDA warning about the neuropsychiatric adverse effects was hence withdrawn.

Other Treatment Approaches

Apart from medications, **behavioural therapy** is considered beneficial. To prevent relapse, high-risk situations (situations in which the patient is likely to smoke) are identified, and the patient is suggested to avoid these situations. Cognitive and behavioural skills that can be used to avoid smoking in high-risk situations are taught, and the patient is asked to practice them. Stimulus control involves eliminating cues (cues that intensify the craving, e.g., seeing the ashtray) for smoking in the environment. Some patients benefit from a series of hypnotic sessions (hypnotherapy).

OTHER DRUGS

1. **Inhalants or volatile solvents:** These include gasoline (petrol), glues, thinners, and industrial solvents. These solvents are soaked in a cloth and sniffed (vapours are inhaled). Inhalant abuse is more commonly seen in children and adolescents. Long-term use may cause irreversible damage to livers and kidneys, peripheral neuropathy and brain damage.
2. **Benzodiazepines and other sedative-hypnotics:** Benzodiazepines can produce physical and psychological dependence. The withdrawal symptoms usually include anxiety, irritability, insomnia, and in some cases, seizures. The treatment usually involves slow tapering and then stopping benzodiazepines and supportive measures.
3. **Caffeine:** Caffeine is the most widely used psychoactive substance worldwide. Caffeine use is associated with a feeling of improved efficiency, increased energy levels and concentration. Excessive use can cause anxiety, restlessness and irritability. Caffeine can also cause physiological dependence, and withdrawal symptoms include anxiety, irritability, mild depressive symptoms, nausea and vomiting.
4. **Synthetic cannabinoids:** These are synthesised chemical compounds that are potent agonists of endogenous cannabinoid receptors. The synthetic compound is typically sprayed into a vehicle, such as *Cannabis* or tea leaves and then smoked. Ingestion of these compounds can result in psychotic symptoms like paranoia or hallucinations, along with the euphoric effects.

DISORDERS DUE TO ADDICTIVE BEHAVIOURS

The ICD-11 has added a new block called "disorders due to addictive behaviours," which includes gambling disorder and gaming disorder. Disorders due to addictive behaviours are recognisable and clinically significant syndromes that cause distress or impairment of functioning due to a person engaging in repetitive rewarding behaviours other than the use of dependence-producing substances. They have the following features:

- Difficulty in controlling the behaviour (e.g., onset, frequency, intensity, duration, termination, context);
- Increasing priority is given to the behaviour, and it takes precedence over other life interests and daily activities

(e.g., a college student stops going out with friends and playing cricket and spends long hours playing online games)
- The behaviour is continued or escalated despite the occurrence of negative consequences (e.g., despite losing large sums of money, gambling is still continued)

The following are the types:
- **Gambling disorder:** In gambling disorder, the individual indulges in persistent or recurrent gambling behaviour, which may be online (i.e., over the internet) or offline.
- **Gaming disorder:** In gaming disorder, the individual is involved in persistent or repeated gaming behaviour ('digital gaming' or 'video-gaming'), which may be online (i.e., over the internet) or offline.

Treatment

Pharmacotherapy

Pharmacological treatment was once considered ineffective in managing gambling and other behavioural addiction disorders; however, recent data proves otherwise. Drugs used in the management of pathological gambling include antidepressants, particularly SSRIs and bupropion; mood stabilisers, including lithium sustained-release formulations and lamotrigine; atypical antipsychotics; and opioid agents such as naltrexone. It is still not clear whether the antidepressants or mood stabilisers have a direct effect on gambling cravings or the effect is mediated by symptom reduction in comorbid depressive or bipolar disorders.

Pharmacotherapy for gaming disorder has not been well evaluated, but the use of the antidepressant bupropion holds some promise.

Apart from pharmacotherapy, psychosocial techniques are used in the treatment.

Gamblers anonymous (GA), modelled on alcoholic anonymous, may be useful for some patients with gambling disorders. Cognitive behavioural therapy, insight-oriented psychotherapy and family therapy can also be used.

Cognitive behavioural therapy and motivational interventions have been used in treating adolescents and adults with gaming disorder.

CASE BASED MCQ

A 43-year-old male who has been consuming around 180 mL of whisky daily for the last five years suddenly quit taking alcohol. Two days later, he appeared confused, could not identify where he was, and claimed he was being taken to jail. He also said that small insects were attacking him and looked terrified. What is the likely diagnosis?
a. Alcoholic hallucinosis
b. Schizophrenia
c. Delirium tremens
d. Dementia

Ans. c. History of quitting alcohol two days back followed by symptoms suggestive of disturbance of consciousness (appeared confused), disorientation (couldn't identify where he was) and hallucinations (small insects are attacking him) are suggestive of delirium tremens.

SUGGESTED READINGS

1. Lal R. Substance use disorder: manual for physicians. New Delhi: AIIMS. 2005:8.
2. David A, Fleminger S, Kopelman M, Mellers J, Lovestone S. Lishman's organic psychiatry: a textbook of neuropsychiatry.
3. American Psychiatric Association. Diagnostic and Statistical Manual of Mental Disorders. Arlington, VA: American Psychiatric Publishing, 2013.
4. Boland R, Verduin M. Kaplan & Sadock's Concise Textbook of Clinical Psychiatry. Lippincott Williams & Wilkins; 2021.
5. Harrison P, Cowen P, Burns T, Fazel M. Shorter Oxford textbook of psychiatry. Oxford university press; 2017.
6. Taylor DM, Barnes TR, Young AH. The Maudsley prescribing guidelines in psychiatry. John Wiley & Sons; 2021.
7. Neeraj A, Vyas JN. Text book of postgraduate psychiatry. New Delhi: Jaypee Brothers Medical Publishers (P) LTD. 2003.
8. Sadock BJ, Sadock VA, Ruiz P. Comprehensive textbook of psychiatry 10th edition.
9. https://main.mohfw.gov.in/sites/default/files/boolbehavioural.pdf retrieved on 25/10/2021
10. King DL, Delfabbro PH, Wu AM, Doh YY, Kuss DJ, Pallesen S, Mentzoni R, Carragher N, Sakuma H. Treatment of Internet gaming disorder: An international systematic review and CONSORT evaluation. Clinical Psychology Review. 2017 Jun 1;54:123-33.
11. Reddy KN, Murty OP. The essentials of forensic medicine and toxicology. New Delhi, India: Jaypee Brothers Medical Publishers; 2014.

12. Neurocognitive Disorders

Sujita Kumar Kar, Praveen Tripathi

CONSCIOUSNESS AND COGNITION (COGNITIVE FUNCTIONS)

It is essential to understand the meaning of consciousness and cognition before talking about neurocognitive disorders.

Consciousness has two components:
a. **Basic arousal**: It refers to the 'activation of cortex' by the ascending activating system (reticular activating system arouses and activates the cortex).
b. **Content of consciousness**: It refers to the higher cognitive and emotional functions, which can be carried out optimally only after the basic arousal of the cortex.

Cognition (cognitive functions): The term 'cognition' is used to describe the mental processes that are utilised to gain knowledge. These include memory, language, attention, orientation, judgment, performing actions (praxis) and problem-solving.

Levels of Consciousness

There are five levels of consciousness:
1. **Alertness**: The individual is awake, aware of internal and external stimuli, and can respond to them.
2. **Lethargy (or somnolence)**: The individual is not fully alert, awareness is limited, and if not actively stimulated, drifts into sleep. Even when aroused, the person is not able to give close attention.
3. **Obtundation**: The individual is difficult to arouse and appears confused when aroused. Constant stimulation is needed to get even minimal cooperation from the individual.
4. **Stupor (or semicoma)**: The individual does not show any spontaneous response in the stupor and remains akinetic (lack of movement) and mute. The individual may respond only to persistent and vigorous stimulation by groaning or mumbling and moving restlessly in bed.
5. **Coma**: Coma is a state of complete unawareness. The individual cannot be aroused by external stimulation and does not respond to internal stimuli either. Eyes are closed.

Few other terms have been used to describe the abnormalities of consciousness. These include:
1. **Torpor**: Torpor is a state of lowering of consciousness, short of stupor.
2. **Twilight state**: It is a dream-like state (also known as the **oneroid state**) in which awareness is restricted, and the individual may feel as if he is in a dream. The twilight state corresponds to the 'obtundation' stage.

NEUROCOGNITIVE DISORDERS

Neurocognitive disorders are characterised by a primary abnormality in cognitive functioning, which is acquired and is not developmental. This definition emphasises two points:
1. The core feature of neurocognitive disorders is an abnormality of one or more **cognitive functions**. Hence, psychiatric disorders, such as schizophrenia, in which cognitive deficits may be present but are not the core feature (in schizophrenia, the thought disorder, delusions and hallucinations are the core clinical features), would not be classified as neurocognitive disorders.
2. The deficits of cognitive function develop later in life, i.e., from previously attained levels of cognitive functioning, there is a decline. Hence, disorders such as intellectual impairment (or mental retardation), in which cognitive deficits are present from birth or develop during the developmental period, are not neurocognitive disorders.

The older name for neurocognitive disorders was 'organic mental disorders'. The term 'organic' referred to the fact that these disorders were caused by a demonstrable disturbance (such as infarcts, infections, etc.) of cerebral functioning.

In contrast, the disorders in which no disturbance of the brain could be found were called 'functional disorders'. Disorders such as schizophrenia and mood disorders were classified as 'functional disorders'. The functional disorders were considered as 'disorders of mind', compared to the 'organic mental disorders', which were considered 'disorders of brain'.

With the advancement in the understanding of psychiatric disorders, it became clear that the so-called functional disorders like schizophrenia, too are caused by demonstrable disturbances of the brain (elicited using advanced structural and functional neuroimaging). Hence, this classification of 'organic vs functional' has been discarded.

DELIRIUM

The hallmark of delirium is **an acute decline in the level of consciousness** along with impairment of cognitive functions, particularly attention. In the past, terms like ICU psychosis and acute confusion state were used for patients in delirium, but these terms have added to the confusion and should be avoided.

Delirium is more common in elder lies and in the presence of medical comorbidities. It has been estimated that delirium is present in 10–15% of general surgical patients, with the prevalence being higher in patients with open heart surgery (30%) and hip fractures (50%). The prevalence is even higher in patients admitted to intensive care units (70–85%) and terminally ill patients (80%). Delirium is a poor prognostic factor. The one-year mortality rate for patients with an episode of delirium is around 50%, with the underlying pathology that caused delirium often being the cause of death.

Clinical Features

Along with the disturbance of consciousness, the following are the clinical features of delirium:

1. **Disturbance in attention and reduced awareness of the environment:** Patients may have difficulty directing attention to a particular stimulus, sustaining the attention, or shifting attention from one stimulus to another. Along with attention deficits, patients also have reduced awareness of the environment (also called disorientation to the environment) and may struggle to understand what's going on around them. At times, terms like 'clouding of consciousness' and '**altered sensorium**' are used for attention and awareness disturbances.
2. **Presence of other cognitive deficits:** Apart from attention deficit, patients often have the following cognitive deficits:
   A. **Disorientation to time, place and person:** There may be a loss of orientation to time (not able to tell the day, date, month), place (not able to name the city, locality, building, etc.) and person (not able to identify the familiar persons). Orientation to person usually gets disturbed in the last.
   B. **Memory deficits:** Typically, disturbances of immediate and recent memory are seen in patients with delirium. The remote memory is usually preserved.
   C. **Language disturbances:** The patient may have disturbances of organisation of thought, manifesting as language disturbances, ranging from mild tangentiality to incoherence.
   D. **Visuospatial ability disturbances:** Visuospatial ability is the capacity to relate visual information to the space around. For example, when a person crosses the road, he can look at and judge the speed of incoming vehicles using his visuospatial ability. Patients may show visuospatial deficits in delirium.
   E. **Perceptual abnormalities:** Classically, hallucinations are present, and visual hallucinations (followed by auditory hallucinations) are the most common. The hallucinations may vary from elementary hallucinations (e.g., seeing a shape on the wall) to elaborate and vivid scenes. In some cases, instead of hallucinations, illusions may be present.
   F. **Delusions:** Patients with delirium may have transient delusions, with the delusion of persecution (e.g., belief that nurses and doctors are giving poison) being the most common type.

Associated disturbances include:
A. **Disturbances of psychomotor activity:** The patient may have agitation (**hyperactive delirium**), and aggression or may be sluggish and lethargic (**hypoactive delirium**, hypoactive delirium may sometimes be mistaken as depression).
B. **Emotional disturbances:** It includes irritability, anger, depression, emotional lability, etc.
C. **Sleep-wake cycle changes:** These may range from insomnia, mild excessive daytime sleepiness to complete reversal of the sleep-wake cycle.
D. **Floccillations (or carphologia):** Aimless picking behaviour in which the patient appears to be picking at his clothes/bed.
E. **Occupational delirium:** The patient behaves as if he is still at work, e.g., a tailor kept on asking for scissors and clothes while lying on the hospital bed.

Delirium classically has a sudden onset (within hours to days), a brief and fluctuating course, and improves rapidly once the causative factor is identified and removed. The symptoms of delirium tend to worsen during the night; this phenomenon is called '**sundowning**'.

Pathophysiology

A decrease in **acetylcholine** levels has been hypothesised to cause delirium. This hypothesis is supported by the observation that many drugs with anticholinergic activity can cause delirium.

The neuroanatomical area involved in the development of delirium is reticular formation. The reticular formation consists of a set of interconnected nuclei in the brain stem. The **ascending reticular activating system (ARAS)** comprises many neuronal circuits that originate in reticular formation and project via the thalamus to the cortex. The ARAS is responsible for maintaining arousal of the cortex and achievement of consciousness.

Aetiology

Certain factors, such as old age, male sex, pre-existing dementia or depression, and sensory impairment (hearing or vision loss) predispose an individual to delirium by decreasing the threshold of insult required to precipitate it.

In general hospital patients, delirium is usually caused by the toxicity of certain medications (most commonly opioids and anticholinergics) or metabolic derangements. The following are the **major causes** of delirium:

A. **Medication-induced:**
   1. Opioid analgesics (morphine, meperidine)
   2. Anticholinergic agents
   3. Serotonin syndrome
   4. Neuroleptic malignant syndrome
      (it must be remembered that any medication can cause delirium)
B. **Metabolic causes:**
   1. Uremic encephalopathy
   2. Hepatic encephalopathy
   3. Electrolyte disturbances (hyponatraemia, hypernatraemia, hypocalcaemia, hypercalcaemia, hypomagnesaemia, hypermagnesaemia)
   4. Hypoglycaemia, hyperglycaemia
   5. Wernicke's encephalopathy, pellagra
C. **Substance intoxication** (alcohol, opioids, cannabis, hallucinogens, sedatives, amphetamines, cocaine, inhalants)
D. **Substance withdrawal** (alcohol, sedatives and hypnotics)
E. **Central nervous system disorders:** Seizures, migraine, head trauma, subarachnoid haemorrhage, brain tumour, abscess, subdural or epidural haematoma, stroke, meningitis, encephalitis
F. **Systemic effects of infection:** Sepsis, pneumonia, urinary tract infection
G. **Post-operative delirium**
H. **Others:** Autoimmune disorders, endocrine disorders (adrenal insufficiency, Cushing's syndrome, hyperthyroidism), pulmonary disorders (chronic obstructive pulmonary disease, obstructive sleep apnoea, respiratory failure), cardiac causes (cardiac failure, arrhythmias, myocardial infarction, cardiac surgery), heavy metals and aluminium toxicity. Delirium can develop in older patients wearing eye patches after cataract surgery (due to sensory deprivation), also known as black-patch delirium.

The history of a medical disorder followed by a sudden development of disturbance of consciousness, cognitive and psychiatric symptoms such as hallucinations and delusions is strongly suggestive of delirium.

Management

Assessment

Delirium is a **clinical diagnosis**, and the presence of characteristic symptoms with a sudden onset helps make the diagnosis. Mental status examination and tools like **mini-mental status examination** (MMSE) are used to assess cognitive impairment and track the course of illness. Other tools such as **the confusion assessment method** have been developed to identify patients with delirium.

A detailed physical examination and investigations can give clues about the cause of delirium.

Electroencephalogram (EEG) in a patient with delirium typically shows **generalised slowing** (however, delirium caused by alcohol or sedative/hypnotic withdrawal shows low voltage fast activity).

Treatment

The main goal is to identify the cause and remove it. After removal of the causative factors, delirium tends to improve, and recovery usually occurs in 3–7 days. Symptomatic treatment involves environmental measures as well as pharmacological treatment.

Environmental measures: The environment should be neither understimulating nor overstimulating. The room in which the patient is kept should be quiet. At the same time, clocks on the wall, large calendars and windows in the room are important to ensure that patient is in touch with the environment. The presence of a familiar face like a family member or friend in the room also helps.

Pharmacotherapy: Symptomatic pharmacotherapy is used to manage psychotic symptoms (delusions, hallucinations, agitation) and insomnia. Most antipsychotics can be used, although haloperidol is often considered a good first choice. Benzodiazepines (short or intermediate-acting) can be used for insomnia and agitation, although they should be avoided as they may further worsen the confusional state.

Delirium versus Dementia

The following points help in differentiating delirium from dementia:

	Delirium	Dementia
Onset	Sudden onset	Insidious onset
Consciousness	Disturbance of consciousness (and attention) is present	Not present
Course	Fluctuating course	Stable and usually progressive course
Attention, alertness and orientation	Impaired	Usually intact in the early phase and may be affected in late dementia
Sleep cycle	Disrupted	Intact in the early phase
Sun-downing phenomenon	Present	Less common
Perceptual abnormalities (Hallucinations/illusions)	Present	Usually absent in the early phase

Sometimes patients with dementia develop superimposed delirium (called beclouded dementia).

Delirium versus Schizophrenia

Delirium (especially in patients with agitation, hallucinations and delusions) must be differentiated from schizophrenia. Patients with delirium have a disturbance of consciousness and disturbances of orientation, which are not seen in patients with schizophrenia. Further, the delusions and hallucinations in schizophrenia are more constant and well organised (elaborate), unlike those in delirium.

> ### MMSE
> Mini-mental status examination (MMSE) is a tool used to assess an individual's cognitive functioning. MMSE assesses the following five cognitive functions and gives them different weightage:
> 1. Orientation (10 points): Patient is asked, what is the (year) (season) (date) (day) (month) and where are we (state) (country) (town) (hospital) (floor). One point is given for each correct response.
> 2. Registration (3 points): Examiner names three objects, e.g., Home, Tree and Car. And the patient is asked to repeat them. For every correct repetition, one point is given.
> 3. Attention and concentration (5 points): The patient is asked to serially subtract 7 from 100 (for five times, i.e., 100..93..86..79..72) and gets 1 point for every correct subtraction. Alternatively, the patient can be asked to spell WORLD backwards (D-L-R-O-W)
> 4. Recall (3 points): The patient is asked to recall the three objects that were named while testing registration. One point is given for each correct recall.
> 5. Language (9 points):
>   - The patient is shown two objects (e.g., watch and pencil) and asked to name them (2 points)
>   - The patient is asked to repeat the phrase "No ifs, ands or buts" (1 point)
>   - The patient is asked to follow a 3 stage command "Take a paper in your hand, fold it in half and put it on the floor" (3 points)
>   - The patient is asked to follow a written command (1 point) (paper is given which says "Close your eyes", the patient is supposed to close the eyes after reading it)
>   - The patient is asked to write a sentence (1 point)
>   - The patient is shown a design and is asked to copy it (1 point)
>   - The maximum score for MMSE is 30. A score <24 is indicative of cognitive impairment

DEMENTIA (MAJOR NEUROCOGNITIVE DISORDER)

Dementia is defined as '**progressive impairment of cognitive functions in the absence of any disturbances of consciousness**'. Many times, the term dementia is considered equivalent to memory disturbances, which is incorrect. In dementia, multiple cognitive functions get progressively impaired, with memory disturbances being one of them. The general clinical picture of all types of dementia is characterised by a progressive deterioration of intellect, memory, personality, behavioural problems, and gradual loss of functioning abilities.

Epidemiology

The prevalence of dementia increases with age, with the prevalence of moderate to severe dementia being around 5% in the population older than 65 years and prevalence of 20–40% in the population older than 85 years. Alzheimer's disease, the **most common** type of dementia, is more common in females, whereas vascular dementia, the second most common type, is more common in males.

Symptoms

The symptoms of dementia include:
1. **Cognitive impairment**: Cognitive impairment is characterised by four A's: *a*mnesia, *a*phasia, *a*praxia and *a*gnosia.
   A. **Amnesia**: Amnesia refers to memory impairment. Typically, recent memory gets impaired first, the immediate memory (working memory) impairment follows and finally, at later stages of illness, remote memory is lost.

   Different kinds of memory deficits are observed in patients with dementia. These include:
   a. **Episodic memory deficits**: Episodic memory is the memory for events. For example, when you try to recall your first day in medical college, you are trying to remember an event; hence, it's an episodic memory. There is a gradient of impairment for episodic memory deficits, with memory for recent events getting impaired first than memory for remote events.
   b. **Semantic memory deficits**: Semantic memory is the knowledge of facts, rules, words and language. For example, when you try to recall the most common type of carcinoma in males, you are trying to retrieve semantic memory. Semantic memory is preserved in the early stages of dementia and gets disturbed later as the disease progresses.
   c. **Visuospatial skills deficits**: Visuospatial processes help in understanding the surroundings. These skills help interpret the visual signals and create a correct mental impression of objects in three-dimensional space. For example, when you try to pick a cup of tea from the table, you use visuospatial skills to identify the position of the cup in the 3D space and reach for it precisely. Visuospatial skills deficits manifest with the symptom of disorientation in a strange environment initially and getting lost even in a familiar environment later.
   B. **Aphasia (more precisely dysphasia)**: It refers to the disturbances of language function. In the early stages, the patient may have word-finding difficulties (e.g., a patient was shown a watch and asked to name it, he replied that this thing is used to tell time but could not say that it's a watch). As the disease progresses, symptoms such as inability to complete sentences, decreased fluency, echolalias (imitation of the speech), and perseveration (repetition of the same response) may develop.
   C. **Apraxia (more precisely dyspraxia)**: It refers to the inability to perform learned motor functions in the absence of any primary motor deficits. For example, a patient may have difficulty buttoning the shirt or combing their hair. Apraxia can lead to deterioration of self-care.

D. **Agnosia:** Agnosia is the inability to interpret a sensory stimulus and presents with difficulty in recognising objects. For example, a patient with visual agnosia could see a red spherical object that appeared leathery in consistency but could not interpret this information to understand that it was a 'ball'. One interesting type of agnosia, in which patients cannot identify faces, is called '**prosopagnosia**'. In some cases, the patients cannot identify their own faces, known as **autoprosopagnosia**. These patients may look at the mirror and not recognise their own reflection (mirror sign) and may even converse with their reflection.

E. **Executive function disturbances**: Apart from the 4 A's, disturbances of executive functioning (i.e., planning, organising, sequencing and abstracting) is another important cognitive impairment seen in patients with dementia. For example, if an individual wants to go to the bank, it needs planning, such as selecting the bank branch, deciding the time of visit, leaving from home accordingly, choosing the transport, carrying a pen to fill forms, etc. A patient with executive function disturbances will struggle to plan and execute these activities. Executive functioning is considered to be primarily a frontal lobe function. If a patient has executive function loss with speech deficits and relative memory sparing, it suggests that dementia predominantly involves the frontal lobe.

Patients with executive function disturbances gradually develop difficulties in performing everyday tasks (activities of daily living or ADLs).

2. **Behavioural and psychological symptoms:** Apart from the cognitive symptoms, patients with dementia often present with behavioural and psychological symptoms such as:
   A. **Psychotic symptoms**: Delusions are more common than hallucinations, with the delusion of persecution and delusion of theft being the common types. Visual hallucinations are the most common type of hallucinations, followed by auditory hallucinations.
   B. **Mood symptoms:** Patients may have mood disturbances such as depression and anxiety symptoms.
   C. **Activity related symptoms:** Patients may present with symptoms such as apathy, agitation and aggression.
   D. **Personality changes:** There might be significant changes in the patient's personality. The patient may become introverted and may appear to lack concern for others, or the patient may become hostile. Some patients may indulge in inappropriate behaviours, cracking silly jokes and passing inappropriate comments. The personality changes are more prominently present in patients with frontal and temporal lobe involvement.

   Complaints of personality changes in an individual older than 40 years of age should always be a reason to initiate a dementia assessment.
   E. **Catastrophic reaction:** Sometimes, patients may have an emotional outburst in a stressful situation when they are aware of their intellectual deficits. This is known as a "catastrophic reaction". For example, a surgeon got extremely angry at his residents on realising that he is not able to put sutures properly during the surgery.

3. **Other neurological signs and symptoms:** Patients can present with seizures, myoclonic jerks, exaggerated tendon reflexes, extensor plantar response or primitive reflexes. Focal neurological deficits are often present in patients with vascular dementia, with deficits corresponding to the location of vascular insult.

Sundowner syndrome: Patients with dementia may show worsening of symptoms in the evening and may appear confused, agitated or drowsy in the late afternoon and evening. This is called sundowner syndrome, and the trigger for it seems to be the fading light.

Reversible and Irreversible Dementia

Dementia can be divided into reversible and irreversible types. It is essential to do a detailed workup of a patient with dementia as around 15% of cases are reversible if identified early. The **reversible causes** of dementia include:

A. Neurosurgical conditions such as subdural haematoma, normal pressure hydrocephalus, intracranial tumours, and intracranial abscess.
B. Infectious causes such as meningitis, encephalitis, neurosyphilis, Lyme disease.
C. Metabolic causes such as vitamin B12 or folate deficiency, niacin deficiency, hypo and hyperthyroidism, hypo and hyperparathyroidism.
D. Others (drugs and toxins, alcohol abuse, autoimmune encephalitis).

Cortical and Subcortical Dementias

Depending on the brain area, which gets affected first by the dementia process, dementia can be divided into cortical and subcortical types.

Cortical Dementias

These disorders are characterised by early involvement of cortical structures and hence the **early appearance of cortical dysfunction.** Patients with cortical dementia have an **early and severe presentation of the A's**: *a*mnesia, *a*praxia, *a*phasia, *a*gnosia and acalculia (impaired mathematical skills), reflecting the cortical involvement. Alzheimer's disease is the prototype of cortical dementia. Other examples include Creutzfeldt-Jakob disease, Pick's disease and other frontotemporal dementias.

Subcortical Dementias

These disorders are characterised by early involvement of subcortical structures like basal ganglia, brain stem nuclei and cerebellum. These disorders are characterised by the **early presentation of motor symptoms** (abnormal movements like tics, chorea, dysarthria, etc.), significant disturbances of executive functioning and prominent behavioural and psychological symptoms like apathy, depression, bradyphrenia (slowness of thinking), etc. Examples of subcortical dementia include Parkinson's disease, Wilson's disease, Huntington's disease, multiple sclerosis, progressive supranuclear palsy, and normal pressure hydrocephalus.

Some types of dementia, such as vascular dementia, and dementia with lewy body, have a mixed presentation.

ALZHEIMER'S DISEASE (DEMENTIA OF THE ALZHEIMER TYPE)

The most common cause of dementia is Alzheimer's disease. The prevalence of Alzheimer's disease increases with age. It is more common in females than males at all ages, by a ratio of 2 or 3:1 except in early-onset familial forms (inherited as autosomal dominant disorder) in which the sex ratio is 1:1.

Based on age at onset, Alzheimer's disease can be classified as:
1. *Early-onset Alzheimer's disease*: Onset before 65 years of age
2. *Late-onset Alzheimer's disease*: Onset after 65 years of age

Early-onset is seen in 5–10% of cases, with late-onset being the more common presentation.

The onset is usually insidious, and progression is gradual. The insight (awareness of illness) is lost relatively early in the illness. Alzheimer's disease, being a cortical dementia, presents with memory disturbances early in the course of the illness; gradually, apraxia, agnosia, aphasia, and acalculia develop, and executive functioning gets disturbed. Along with the cognitive symptoms, behavioural and psychological symptoms are also commonly present. Neurological symptoms like tremors, rigidity, and spasticity may develop later.

Risk Factors

Age is the most important risk factor for Alzheimer's disease, and other risk factors include head injury, hypertension, insulin resistance, and depression. Few studies have claimed that smoking is a protective factor against Alzheimer's disease, but other studies have contradicted this finding. High education levels and remaining physically and mentally active till late in life are protective factors against Alzheimer's disease.

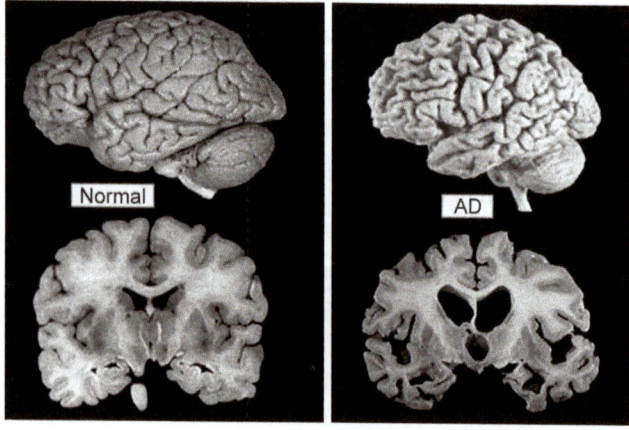

Fig. 12.1: Brain atrophy in advanced Alzheimer's disease.

Neuropathology

Amyloid deposits are the hallmark of Alzheimer's disease. The following are the neuropathological findings.

Gross Findings

The classical gross neuroanatomical finding in Alzheimer's disease is diffuse atrophy of the brain with flattened cortical sulci and enlarged cerebral ventricles. Alzheimer's disease predominantly affects parietal and temporal regions.

Typically, atrophy begins in medial temporal lobes before spreading to lateral and medial parietal and temporal lobes and lateral frontal cortex. At autopsy, the earliest and most severe degeneration is found in the medial temporal lobe (entorhinal/perirhinal cortex and hippocampus), lateral temporal cortex and nucleus basalis of meynert.

Microscopic Findings

The classical microscopic findings in Alzheimer's disease are neuritic (senile) plaques and neurofibrillary tangles:

a. **Neuritic plaques**: Neuritic plaques (senile plaques, amyloid plaques) are extracellular deposits of protein, **amyloid β-peptide (Aβ)**, Aβ (or β/A4) is derived from the breakdown of a precursor protein, amyloid precursor protein (APP). The neuritic plaque is made up of an amyloid core surrounded by neuritic changes. The neuritic plaques are found in all cortical areas, striatum and cerebellum. The number and density of neuritic plaques in the postmortem brain correlate with the severity of Alzheimer's disease.

Senile plaques are not exclusive to Alzheimer's disease; they are seen in Down's syndrome and, in some cases, in normal healthy elderlies.

In addition to the brain parenchyma, amyloid β-peptide also gets deposited in the vessel walls leading to cerebral amyloid angiopathy (CAA).

b. **Neurofibrillary tangles**: Neurofibrillary tangles are intraneuronal aggregates of **tau protein**. Initially, they appear as aggregates in the cell body, and as the cell body gets increasingly filled, they extend into the axon hillock. Neurofibrillary tangles can be readily visualised using silver staining techniques, such as the bielschowsky technique. When the bielschowsky technique is used, fine hair-like structures known as neuropil threads are also visualised. Neuropils, in all likelihood, are neurofibrillary tangles that have accumulated in the axons and dendrites of affected neurons.

Usually, tau protein is present in the axon, and its function is to bind and stabilise the microtubules (essential for axonal transport). The tau protein in the neurofibrillary tangle is highly phosphorylated and gets redistributed from axon to cell body. Highly phosphorylated tau protein gets aggregated in paired helical filaments, resulting in the development of tangles. The tangles first develop in the entorhinal cortex and later spread to the hippocampus and wider cortical structures. However, they are never found in the cerebellum. Tangles are insoluble and remain after the neuron dies when they are called 'ghost' or 'tombstone' tangles. Neurofibrillary tangles are not exclusive to Alzheimer's disease and are found in other disorders such as Down's syndrome and dementia pugilistica and in healthy older adults.

The levels of phosphorylated tau protein are increased in cerebrospinal fluid in patients with Alzheimer's disease, and the CSF levels of phosphorylated tau protein may be used in the future as a biomarker for Alzheimer's disease.

Synaptic losses and neuronal losses accompany the accumulation of neuritic plaques and neurofibrillary tangles.

Both senile plaques and neurofibrillary tangles can be present in older people without dementia. However, in patients with dementia, the senile plaques and neurofibrillary tangles are extensive and widespread. The neuropathological diagnosis of Alzheimer's disease requires the extensive presence of both **senile plaques (extracellular deposits) and neurofibrillary tangles (intracellular inclusions).**

Apart from plaques and tangles, other findings in Alzheimer's disease include **Granulovacuolar degeneration (GVD)** of neurons and Hirano bodies. Hirano bodies are eosinophilic inclusions present in the cytoplasm of hippocampal neurons in patients with Alzheimer's disease. Both granulovacuolar degeneration and Hirano bodies can be present in older healthy individuals; however, they are more severe and widely spread in Alzheimer's disease.

Amyloid Cascade Hypothesis

This hypothesis explains the formation of neuritic plaques and neurofibrillary tangles. Before understanding the hypothesis, it is essential to understand the metabolism of the amyloid precursor protein.

Amyloid precursor protein (APP) is metabolised by three secretase enzymes:

a. α secretase
b. β secretase or β amyloid cleaving enzyme (BACE)
c. γ secretase

Sequential cleavage of APP by β secretase and γ secretase, yields fragments of Aβ of 40–42 amino acids in length, whereas cleavage by α secretase does not yield Aβ.

According to the amyloid cascade hypothesis, mutations in the *APP* gene near the cleavage site favour the cleavage by β and γ-secretase, resulting in increased production of Aβ. Aβ (more so Aβ-42) combines to form oligomers and finally plaques. Aβ oligomers induce tau phosphorylation, possibly by inducing glycogen synthase kinase (GSK)-3 enzyme, which is a tau kinase.

Phosphorylated tau protein aggregates into tangles. Phosphorylated tau cannot function effectively as a microtubule-binding protein, which results in disturbed axonal transport, abnormal neuronal function and neuronal death.

Hence, the formation of plaques and tangles results in synaptic losses and neuronal losses.

Neurochemistry

Alzheimer's disease, at least partially, is a disorder of **cholinergic neurons.** Studies have found that cholinergic neurons are lost the earliest and maximally in Alzheimer's disease. Animal studies have also shown that cholinergic neurons are essential for memory.

Studies have demonstrated reductions in cholinergic neurons in the nucleus basalis of meynert in Alzheimer's disease.

Apart from cholinergic neurons, loss of noradrenergic neurones in locus ceruleus and serotonergic neurones in the dorsal raphe nucleus has been found too.

> **NINCDS-ADRDA**
>
> The diagnostic criterion for Alzheimer's disease proposed by the National Institute of Neurological and Communicative Disorders and Stroke and the Alzheimer's Disease and Related Disorders Association (NINCDS-ADRDA criteria) are often used for making the diagnosis.

Genetic Factors

Genetic factors play a significant role in the development of Alzheimer's disease, as suggested by positive family history in a significant number of cases and a much higher monozygotic concordance rate than dizygotic concordance rate. Different factors are involved in early-onset and late-onset Alzheimer's disease.

A. **Early-onset autosomal dominant familial Alzheimer's disease:** Early-onset Alzheimer's disease runs in several families in an autosomal dominant pattern. Linkage in these families has been mapped to chromosomes 21, 14 and 1.
   a. **Chromosome 21:** The gene in the candidate region is amyloid precursor protein (APP). Multiple mutations have been identified, and these mutations are at the site recognised by γ secretase and β secretase. These mutations favour cleavage of APP by γ secretase and β secretase, resulting in increased production of Aβ.
   b. **Chromosome 14:** The mutations were found in a gene called presenilin-1 on chromosome 14. These mutations result in a change in amyloid precursor protein processing.
   c. **Chromosome 1:** The mutations have been found in a gene called presenilin-2 on chromosome 1. Presenilin-2 mutations are much rarer than presenilin-1 mutations.
   Presenilin 1 and the closely related presenilin 2 constitute the catalytic component of the γ-secretase enzyme. The mutations in presenilins are believed to increase γ-secretase activity, resulting in increased production of Aβ.

B. **Late-onset Alzheimer's disease:** Previously, late-onset Alzheimer's disease was considered a sporadic condition. Later, it was found that a positive family history is present in up to one-third of the patients with late-onset Alzheimer's disease. Twin studies suggest that the heritability of late-onset Alzheimer's disease is 60–70%. Heritability describes how much of the variation in a given trait can be attributed to genetic variation. Heritability can range from zero to one. A heritability of 0 would mean that the trait is completely dependent on environmental factors, and there is no genetic component, e.g., Language spoken. The language spoken by a child is totally dependent on what is taught (environmental factor) to the child, and the genes do not contribute at all.

On the other hand, the heritability of 1 would mean that genetic differences are responsible entirely, with no contribution from environmental factors. For example, disorders that are caused by single-gene mutations, such as phenylketonuria (PKU), have high heritability.

A gene unequivocally linked to late-onset Alzheimer's disease is the *APOE* gene. There are three common alleles, APOE2, APOE3, and APOE4. The research suggests:

The APOE4 variant in the heterozygous state increases the risk for Alzheimer's disease by three to four times.

The APOE4 variant in the homozygous state increases the risk for Alzheimer's disease by ten times.

APOE gene does not cause the disease directly; instead, it modulates the risk by some yet unknown mechanism. It has been suggested that APOE4 alters risk by altering the age of onset of Alzheimer's disease. However, it must be remembered that the role of APOE4 is limited, and most patients with Alzheimer's disease do not carry APOE4. The testing for APOE genotype is not recommended as of now, as it does not improve diagnostic accuracy and cannot be used to predict Alzheimer's disease, either.

Patients with Down's syndrome have a significantly higher risk of developing Alzheimer's disease. In Down syndrome, there are three copies of the *APP* gene (amyloid precursor protein, *APP* gene is located on chromosome 21), and in the presence of a mutation at codon 717 in the *APP* gene, excessive deposition of Aβ occurs.

Difference between Alzheimer's Disease and Normal Ageing

In normal ageing, too, there may be the development of some memory disturbances. Early symptoms of Alzheimer's disease often go unnoticed as family members confuse those symptoms with changes seen in 'normal ageing'.

However, the evidence suggests a fundamental difference between the two conditions. The memory decline in late age is a secondary effect of poor information processing resulting in the poor encoding of information. Also, older individuals are less efficient in using strategies and instructions to retrieve information, and these factors combined result in memory decline in old age.

In comparison, in Alzheimer's disease, there is a primary loss of memory, language and spatial cognition that results in the symptoms.

Older individuals without any symptoms of dementia can also have senile plaques and neurofibrillary tangles (as documented by many post mortem studies); however, the number of plaques and severity of tangles is significantly more in the brain of patients with Alzheimer's disease than in older individuals without dementia. Also, the postmortem studies found that in patients with dementia, plaques were present in all layers of the cortex, whereas they were restricted to superficial layers in older people who had shown no intellectual decline. Similarly, tangles were found in the hippocampus of healthy aged subjects, but they were seldom found in the neocortex in the absence of dementia.

Management of Alzheimer's Disease

Early diagnosis and treatment are of utmost importance in patients with Alzheimer's disease. **MMSE (mini-mental status examination)** is often used as a screening test, and a score of less than 24 on MMSE suggests dementia. Neuroimaging (MRI) can help differentiate Alzheimer's disease from vascular dementia.

The treatment of Alzheimer's disease has several goals: controlling the symptoms, managing comorbidities, limiting the disability, improving the individual's functioning, treating the behavioural and psychological symptoms associated with dementia, and caregiver support. These goals are achieved through pharmacological and psychosocial interventions.

Pharmacological Interventions

Procognitive agents (cognitive enhancers): The commonly used procognitive agents are cholinesterase inhibitors (e.g., Donepezil, Rivastigmine, Galantamine). These drugs increase the levels of acetylcholine by inhibiting the enzyme acetylcholine esterase. Another commonly used drug is memantine, which increases the neurons' survivability by inhibiting the activity of the excitotoxic neurotransmitter, glutamate.

These drugs are well tolerated, and along with the procognitive role, they are also effective in reducing the behavioural and psychological symptoms associated with dementia.

Drugs for management of behavioural and psychological symptoms associated with dementia:

- *For insomnia*: Zolpidem and benzodiazepines are useful.
- *For depression*: Antidepressants, preferably those without anticholinergic properties, are used. SSRIs like escitalopram and sertraline are safe choices.
- *For anxiety symptoms*: SSRIs like escitalopram and sertraline are safe choices.
- *For psychotic symptoms or marked aggression*: Antipsychotic drugs in low doses may be used. Please note that antipsychotics can increase the mortality rate in patients with dementia by increasing the incidence of congestive heart failure, sudden death and infections such as pneumonia.

Aducanumab: In June 2021, the FDA granted accelerated approval to aducanumab, making it the first drug in the last 18 years to get approval for managing Alzheimer's disease. Aducanumab is a monoclonal antibody that binds soluble oligomers and insoluble fibrils of Aβ plaques and has been shown to reduce Aβ plaques in the brain. In a small subset of patients, a reduction in phosphorylated tau was also observed. However, the link between the reduction of Aβ plaques and clinical improvement is yet not clearly established, making this a controversial approval by FDA. The European agencies have refused to approve aducanumab for the same reason.

Psychosocial Interventions

The psychosocial interventions include:
a. Psychoeducation about the illness, its course and outcome to the patient and family members.
b. Supportive psychotherapy
c. Cognitive stimulation therapy (various cognitive exercises have been designed)

VASCULAR DEMENTIA

It is the **second most common type** of dementia after Alzheimer's disease and was formerly called "multi-infarct dementia". It is more common in men than women and often results from vasculopathies involving small to medium-sized cerebral blood vessels. The occlusion of vessels by thrombus or emboli results in the infarction of the brain parenchyma.

In vascular dementia, the onset of symptoms mostly correlates with a cerebrovascular event, and progressive decline in cognitive function in a stepwise manner may be observed (step ladder pattern of progression caused by a sequential decline in cognitive function with every cerebrovascular event), although it's not apparent in all cases.

Risk factors for vascular dementia include diabetes, hypertension, atherosclerosis, dyslipidaemia, and smoking.

Binswanger disease is a type of vascular dementia caused by multiple subcortical infarcts of the white matter while sparing the cortex.

Diagnosis of Vascular Dementia

In patients with vascular dementia, the general symptoms of dementia are present. In addition, there may be significant mood changes (depression), apathy, and irritability. Delusion and hallucination may be present.

General physical examination in patients with vascular dementia often reveals signs of atherosclerosis or hypertension. Neurological examination may show focal neurological deficits. Neuroimaging in patients with vascular dementia often reveals multiple infarcts.

NINDA-AIREN

NINDS-AIREN criterion is often used to make the diagnosis of vascular dementia National Institute of Neurological Disorders and Stroke (NINDS) and the Association Internationale pour la Recherche et l'Enseignement en Neurosciences (AIREN).

Many patients with dementia (around 10–15%) have coexisting vascular dementia and Alzheimer's disease.

Treatment of Vascular Dementia

In patients with vascular dementia, preventive measures are particularly important. These include appropriate treatment of diabetes, dyslipidaemia, hypertension, and obesity. Quitting smoking and regular exercise too is important.

The pharmacological and non-pharmacological treatment is similar to Alzheimer's disease.

FRONTOTEMPORAL DEMENTIA (PICK DISEASE)

The term 'frontotemporal dementia' (FTD) is used for the dementias characterised by the predominant degeneration of the frontal and temporal lobes. There is some confusion between the terms frontotemporal dementia and Pick disease. It must be remembered that frontotemporal dementia is a clinical diagnosis used for all dementias characterised principally by the degeneration of frontal and temporal lobes, as detected by the clinical presentation, neuroimaging or postmortem examination.

A variety of neuropathological substrates can cause frontotemporal dementia, with **Pick's disease** being one of them. Pick's disease is a neuropathological diagnosis; it is characterised by the presence of a neuronal inclusion body called Pick's body, made up of cytoskeletal elements.

Frontotemporal dementias are of special interest in psychiatry as they often present with behavioural symptoms and personality changes, and the memory is relatively preserved in the initial period.

Kluver–Bucy syndrome, characterised by hyperorality, hypersexuality, disinhibited behaviour and placidity (unusual calmness), is commonly seen in patients with frontotemporal dementia.

Three distinctive forms of FTD have been described:
a. **Frontal variant FTD:** The symptoms are primarily of loss of frontal lobe function, especially the orbitobasal structures, such as disinhibition, stereotypy, poor impulse control, apathy and loss of executive function. The memory is relatively preserved and gets impacted only in advanced cases.
b. **Semantic dementia:** The symptoms are primarily of loss of temporal lobe functions and are characterised by loss of memory for words (semantic memory). In patients, particularly those with right-sided atrophy, the semantic loss is often accompanied by prosopagnosia (inability to recognise faces).
c. **Progressive nonfluent aphasia:** The symptoms are primarily speech dysfluency, word-finding difficulties, and spelling deterioration. Gradually, symptoms worsen, and comprehension may get affected too. The left temporal lobe is atrophied primarily.

Treatment of frontotemporal dementia: There is a limited role of pharmacotherapy in managing frontotemporal dementias. Antipsychotics, selective serotonin reuptake inhibitors (SSRIs) and antiepileptic medications (e.g., Valproate) are used to manage behavioural symptoms. The procognitive medications effective in Alzheimer's disease and vascular dementia (e.g., Donepezil, Memantine) are not as effective in frontotemporal dementias. The general care and psychosocial management of frontotemporal dementia is similar to Alzheimer's disease.

LEWY BODY DISEASE (DEMENTIA WITH LEWY BODY)

It is an irreversible form of dementia, clinically similar to Alzheimer's disease. The core features include:
1. Fluctuating levels of attention and alertness
2. Recurrent visual hallucinations
3. Parkinsonian features (resting tremors, bradykinesia and cogwheel rigidity)

In addition to the core features, some patients present with syncopal attacks, falls, delusions (often patients have Capgras syndrome) and hallucinations in modalities other than visual. Patients with Lewy body dementia have severe intolerable side effects to neuroleptic medications (known as neuroleptic hypersensitivity). This is expected as the patients already have parkinsonian features. The disease often has an insidious onset and slowly progressive course.

Functional neuroimaging studies have found decreased blood flow and metabolic activity in the occipital lobe and basal ganglia, which may be responsible for visual hallucinations and parkinsonian symptoms.

Lewy body dementia is characterised by the presence of inclusion bodies in the neurons (known as Lewy body) composed of **alpha-synuclein**. Similar inclusion bodies are found in about 1/5th of the cases of Alzheimer's disease.

Treatment of Lewy body dementia: Patients with Lewy body dementia show some response to the cholinesterase inhibitors (e.g., donepezil). Behavioural symptoms (delusions, hallucinations) can be treated with quetiapine in low doses. SSRIs are useful in the management of mood symptoms associated with Lewy body dementia. General care and psychosocial management follow the same principle as for Alzheimer's disease.

DEMENTIA DUE TO HUNTINGTON'S DISEASE

Huntington's disease is associated with the development of an irreversible and subcortical form of dementia, which is primarily characterised by motor abnormalities. Choreoathetoid movements are the most common movement abnormalities seen in Huntington's disease. The classical movement abnormalities seen with Huntington's disease include "piano-playing" movement of the hand, "milkmaid" grip and "dancing-and-prancing" gait. Disturbances of speech and deglutition are also commonly seen. The cognitive deficits in Huntington's disease are characterised by poor attention and concentration, reduced processing speed, poor planning and organisational ability, but memory and language remain relatively intact in the early and middle stages of the illness.

Depression and psychosis are more common in dementia of Huntington's disease than in Alzheimer's disease.

Treatment of Huntington's disease: The choreoathetoid movements usually respond to tetrabenazine or low dose antipsychotic medications. Comorbid depression and psychosis are treated with antidepressant and antipsychotic drugs, respectively. The cognitive symptoms are mostly refractory to the antidementia medications. Supportive care is an essential component of treatment in Huntington's disease.

DEMENTIA DUE TO PARKINSON'S DISEASE

It is an irreversible form of subcortical dementia, usually seen in the elderly age group. The symptoms of Parkinson's disease are clinically evident, and features of dementia (cognitive disturbances) develop as the illness progresses. The Parkinsonian symptoms are usually present—tremors, bradykinesia and rigidity. In addition, patients may have a short-stepped, shuffling gait, stooped posture, and a tendency to fall. The cognitive symptoms are characterised by recent memory loss, poor planning and organisation, slowness in information processing, and impairment of abstract ability. Many patients develop symptoms such as emotional lability, depression, apathy, sleep disturbances, psychomotor slowing, autonomic instability and fatigability. The onset is insidious, and the illness progresses slowly.

Treatment of dementia due to Parkinson's disease: The treatment of Parkinson's disease includes conventional pro-dopaminergic drugs (Levodopa and carbidopa; Selegiline, Ropinirole, Pramipexole). These dopaminergic medications may lead to the development of psychotic symptoms (delusions and hallucinations) that may require dose adjustment. If psychotic symptoms persist, antipsychotics are used. Quetiapine and clozapine are considered the safer antipsychotics in such cases. Comorbid depressive symptoms can be treated with antidepressants, and cognitive symptoms are treated with the cholinesterase inhibitors like donepezil.

DEMENTIA DUE TO CREUTZFELDT-JAKOB DISEASE

Creutzfeldt-Jakob disease (CJD) leads to a **rapidly progressive** and irreversible form of dementia. It is a prion disease. The endogenous prion protein (PrPc, coded by *PRNP* gene located in chromosome 20) is abundant in neurones and contains a high proportion of α-helices. PrPc can convert into PrPSc, a form with more than 40% of β-pleated sheets, which forms insoluble aggregates. PrPSc is not only resistant to proteases; it also interacts with the native PrPc and facilitates its conversion to PrPSc, giving prion protein an infectious quality.

The deposition of prion protein is associated with neuronal degeneration, astrocytosis and a characteristic spongy appearance of grey matter which is at times visible to the naked eye. The 'status spongiosus' of the cortex is highly characteristic of CJD. In most cases, Creutzfeldt-Jakob disease is sporadic, but in approximately 10% of cases, it follows autosomal dominant inheritance. The clinical features include psychiatric symptoms such as insomnia, anxiety, depression and psychotic symptoms in the vast majority of patients, especially in the initial phase. Gradually the intellectual deterioration and neurological symptoms become prominent. These include aphasia, agnosia, ataxia, myoclonus, akinesia (loss of movement), and visual difficulties.

Multiple investigations help in making the diagnosis. In CSF, both 14-3-3 protein and tau are elevated. MRI findings include cortical atrophy with signal alterations in the basal ganglia and other cerebral regions. On EEG, a characteristic pattern of synchronous triphasic sharp-wave complexes at 1–2 Hz rate, emerges in later stages of the disease.

Treatment of Creutzfeldt-Jakob Disease: Extreme precautions need to be taken during the treatment as the body fluids of patients with Creutzfeldt-Jakob disease are highly contagious (due to the infective nature of the protein). There is no definitive treatment for Creutzfeldt-Jakob disease. General supportive care is recommended for Creutzfeldt-Jakob disease, like any other form of dementia.

OTHER FORMS OF DEMENTIA

The other common causes of dementia include nutritional deficiencies, traumatic brain injury, substance use, and medical conditions (e.g., Hypothyroidism; HIV infection).

Vitamin deficiencies (Vitamin B12, folate) can present with dementia. Usually, the condition reverts with specific nutritional supplementation.

Endocrine disorders like hypothyroidism, too, can be a cause of dementia.

Traumatic brain injury can lead to cognitive deficits that can progress over a period of time to dementia. Individuals (e.g., boxers), who sustain repeated head trauma may have multiple micro-bleeds in the brain parenchyma, leading to progressive neurodegeneration and dementia, commonly known as dementia pugilistica. Hypoxic brain injury may also cause dementia-like symptoms. Substance abuse can also induce dementia. Substance-induced dementia is usually associated with the use of alcohol and inhalants.

HIV infection can result in the development of dementia, commonly called AIDS dementia complex. Multiple cognitive domains (memory, visuospatial skills, attention and concentration, speech, executive function, etc.) are commonly affected. Motor abnormalities and mood symptoms are often seen in the AIDS dementia complex. Neurosyphilis too can present with dementia.

Normal pressure hydrocephalus, brain tumours, and multiple sclerosis can also present with dementia.

Dementias due to the above miscellaneous conditions needs to be treated for the underlying specific cause (if treatable). General supportive care, cognitive stimulation and psychosocial management are similar to that of Alzheimer's disease.

PSEUDODEMENTIA

Depression in elderly patients may mimic symptoms of dementia and hence is known as pseudodementia. A depressed patient may get a low score on MMSE, as a depressed individual lacks the motivation to solve the questions. Hence, low score on MMSE should be carefully interpreted if depression is suspected.

AMNESTIC DISORDERS

Amnestic disorders is a broad category that includes a variety of conditions that present with the amnestic syndrome. The amnestic syndrome is characterised by an inability to form new memories (anterograde amnesia) and the inability to recall previously remembered knowledge (retrograde amnesia). Short-term and recent memory is usually impaired with the preservation of remote and immediate memory. The memory impairment is severe relative to impairment in other cognitive domains. The major causes of amnestic disorders are:
- Thiamine deficiency (Korsakoff syndrome)
- Hypoglycaemia
- Primary brain conditions (head trauma, seizures, cerebral tumours, cerebrovascular disease, hypoxia, electro-convulsive therapy, multiple sclerosis)
- Substance-related disorders (alcohol, benzodiazepines)

Frontal lobe syndrome or frontal lobe personality is the broad term used to describe the abnormalities (usually of higher mental functions) that develop due to disturbances of the frontal lobe. Three types have been described:
1. **Orbitofrontal syndrome:** It is caused by disorders of orbitofrontal cortex and presents with:
   - Behavioural disinhibition (including inappropriate behaviours such as sexually inappropriate behaviours)
   - Impulsivity
   - Lack of insight and poor judgement
2. **Dorsolateral syndrome:** It is caused by disorders of dorsolateral prefrontal cortex and presents with:
   - Apathy, lack of motivation
   - Psychomotor retardation, impaired attention and concentration
   - The symptoms are similar to depression and often a wrong diagnosis is made initially
3. **Anterior cingulate syndrome:** It presents with executive function abnormalities primarily.

In DSM-5, rather than using the diagnosis of dementia or amnestic disorder, the diagnosis of major neurocognitive disorders is used when the cognitive decline is significant. In case the cognitive decline is modest, the diagnosis of mild neurocognitive disorder is used. DSM-5 further allows the specification of the cause. For example major neurocognitive disorder due to Alzheimer's disease or mild neurocognitive disorder due to vascular disease, etc.

CASE BASED MCQ

A 66-year-old surgeon has been facing increasing difficulties in performing surgeries for the last two years. One week back, when he could not put the sutures properly after the surgery, he got furious at the nurse and the junior surgeons and left the operation theatre. He also forgot things increasingly, such as where he kept the keys of the car, etc. A couple of weeks back, he had difficulties withdrawing money from the bank and had to take help from his assistant for the same, whereas in the past, he handled all the financial transactions by himself. The surgeon should be evaluated for which of the following conditions?
a. Depression
b. Dementia
c. Delirium
d. Schizophrenia

Ans. b. History suggestive of memory disturbances, difficulty in performing learned motor movements (having difficulties in performing surgeries and suturing) and executive disturbances (inability to withdraw money from the bank) is suggestive of dementia.

SUGGESTED READINGS

1. Mahase E. Aducanumab: European agency rejects Alzheimer's drug over efficacy and safety concerns; 2021.
2. David A, Fleminger S, Kopelman M, Mellers J, Lovestone S. Lishman's Organic Psychiatry: A Textbook of Neuropsychiatry; 2009.
3. Strub R, Black F, Geschwind N, Strub A. The mental status examination in neurology. 4th edition. Philadelphia: Fa Davis Company; 2000.
4. Geddes JR, Andreasen NC. New Oxford Textbook of Psychiatry. Oxford University Press, USA; 2020.
5. Sadock BJ, Sadock VA, Ruiz P. Comprehensive Textbook of Psychiatry, 10th edition; 2017.
6. Hategan A, Bourgeois JA, Hirsch CH, Giroux C. Geriatric Psychiatry. Springer International Publishing; 2018.

13. Personality Disorders

Padma Angmo, Praveen Tripathi

PS11.1	Enumerate and describe the magnitude and aetiology of personality disorders
PS11.2	Enumerate, elicit, describe and document clinical features in patients with personality disorders
PS11.3	Enumerate and describe the indications and interpret laboratory and other tests used in personality disorders
PS11.4	Describe the treatment of personality disorders including behavioural, psychosocial and pharmacologic therapy
PS11.5	Demonstrate family education in a patient with personality disorders in a simulated environment
PS11.6	Enumerate and describe the pharmacologic basis and side effects of drugs used in personality disorders
PS11.7	Enumerate the appropriate conditions for specialist referral

PERSONALITY

The term 'personality' refers to an individual's enduring, (i.e., long-lasting) characteristics that determine the behaviour in various circumstances. Individuals behave and react differently in a given situation, (e.g., in a conflict situation, one person may run away and the other person may escalate it). The 'personality' determines the individual's response to a particular situation.

The personality is made up of two components:
a. **Temperament:** It is the innate component, present from early childhood and remains stable throughout the life, (e.g., a person who liked taking risks in childhood continued with the risk-taking behaviours throughout the life).
b. **Character:** It is the component acquired by learning and experience as the person grows up.

Five Personality Traits

Studies have found that there are five basic dimensions of personality. These are referred to as five personality traits and include:
(*Acronym*: **OCEAN**)
1. **Openness to experience:** As the name suggests, this trait refers to the degree of curiosity and desire to indulge in new and novel experiences. Those who indulge in high-risk behaviours such as going on a dangerous expedition, or playing risky sports, often have a high openness to experience.
2. **Conscientiousness:** Conscientiousness is the trait of being self-disciplined, organised and dutiful. People with high conscientiousness are well organised. They pay their bills at the time, do their work religiously and are disciplined.
3. **Extraversion:** It refers to the tendency to be sociable, outgoing and talkative. People with high extraversion enjoy being in the company of others. They are talkative, usually comfortable around new people and make friends easily.
4. **Agreeableness:** It refers to the tendency to be cooperative and compassionate towards others. People with high agreeableness are kind, trust others and are helpful to others.
5. **Neuroticism:** It refers to the tendency to experience negative emotions (such as feeling hurt or angry) easily. It also refers to the level of emotional stability. Better emotional stability corresponds to low neuroticism.

PERSONALITY DISORDERS

Personality disorders are defined as:
a. Enduring (long-standing) and inflexible patterns of behaviours and inner experiences, (i.e., the way a person thinks, the kind of emotions he experiences and expresses, the way he handles the relationships and the way he controls the impulses) that,
b. Usually have an onset in adolescence and early adulthood and are
c. Significantly different from cultural standards, (i.e., the way a person with a personality disorder behaves and feels is quite different from other people belonging to the same culture) and
d. Result in unhappiness and socio-occupational impairment.

In other words, if an individual's personality traits are so maladaptive that they cause impairment in life, it would be called a personality disorder.

Epidemiology

The prevalence of personality disorders is around 10–20%. Personality disorders have an onset in adolescence or early adulthood, remain stable for decades, and '**maturing**' may occur later in life, usually in the forties. Maturing refers to the resolution of maladaptive ways of behaviours and inner experiences. Maturing is often seen in certain personality disorders, (e.g., antisocial personality disorder and borderline personality disorders), whereas in others (e.g., schizotypal and obsessive-compulsive personality disorder), it may never occur.

Personality disorders are '**ego syntonic**' (agreeable to self). In other words, the individuals with personality disorders do not find anything wrong in their behaviour/experiences and hence are often unwilling to take any kind of treatment.

Aetiology

The genesis of personality disorders is complex and not fully understood. The important factors that contribute to the development of personality disorders include:
A. Genetics
B. Biological factors
C. Developmental factors

A. **Genetics:** The following indicate the role of genetics in the development of personality disorders.
   1. The concordance rate for personality disorders amongst monozygotic twins is much higher than that seen amongst dizygotic twins, indicating that genes play a role in the development of these disorders.
   2. The three cluster A personality disorders, (i.e., paranoid personality disorder, schizoid personality disorder and schizotypal personality disorder) are more common in relatives of patients with schizophrenia than in control groups, with the strongest association being that for schizotypal personality disorder and schizophrenia. This suggests some degree of genetic overlap between schizophrenia and cluster A personality disorders.
   3. Monoamine oxidase A (MAOA): Low activity MAOA genetic variant has been associated with antisocial behaviour in men.

B. **Biological factors:** Studies have found certain biological factors to be associated with specific personality traits. These include:
   1. **Neurotransmitters:** Low levels of 5-hydroxyindoleacetic acid (5-HIAA), a metabolite of serotonin, has been associated with impulsivity and aggression. Low levels of 5-HIAA are associated with an increased risk of suicide.
   2. Minor injuries to the brain have been found to be associated with antisocial behaviour in men, although the evidence is weak.

C. **Developmental factors:** Certain life experiences during the growing up years have been found to be associated with the development of specific personality disorders. These include:
   1. Gross physical neglect or abuse or sexual abuse during childhood has been associated with the development of cluster B personality disorders.
   2. Physical abuse during childhood and violent parenting (use of violence to modify children's behaviour) has been associated with the development of antisocial personality.
   3. Conduct disorder in childhood has been associated with the development of antisocial personality in adulthood.

Defense mechanisms: Personality disorders are often characterised by excessive use of particular defence mechanisms. These defence mechanisms have been discussed along with the relevant personality disorders.

Classification of Personality Disorders

In DSM-5, the personality disorders have been grouped into three clusters: Cluster A, B and C personality disorders
Let's discuss each of these.

CLUSTER A PERSONALITY DISORDERS

The individuals with cluster A personality disorders are often considered 'odd and eccentric'. As mentioned above, the three cluster A personality disorders are more common in relatives of patients with schizophrenia than in control groups, with the strongest association between schizotypal personality disorder and schizophrenia.

Cluster A includes the following personality disorders:
a. Paranoid personality disorder
b. Schizoid personality disorder
c. Schizotypal personality disorder

Paranoid Personality Disorder

These individuals have a long-standing pattern of **mistrust** and **suspiciousness** towards others, which presents in the following ways:
1. Suspicion (without any basis) that others are trying to exploit or harm.
2. Doubts about the loyalty of friends and associates and inability to confide in others (due to fear that information will be leaked and used against them).
3. Tendency to keep grudges (inability to forget or forgive).
4. Intense interpersonal sensitivity: These individuals are extremely sensitive. They read hidden meanings (usually negative) in benign events or remarks of others, and even jokes may be interpreted as attacks. These individuals get hurt easily and may react with hostility and anger.
5. Recurrent suspicions about the fidelity of spouse/partner

These individuals have difficulty in forming close relationships and are often isolated. They are often hostile, argumentative and make frequent complaints. They may also have ideas of reference (they may feel that neutral events are somehow about them, but this belief is not fixed and hence is not a delusion) and may experience illusions, especially in stressful situations.

Paranoid personality disorder is more common in men than women. It is also more common in immigrants and minority groups.

Defense mechanism: According to psychoanalysis, in individuals with paranoid personality disorders, there is excessive use of defense mechanism of projection. (Details about 'projection' and other defense mechanisms is covered in the Chapter 18 'Psychoanalysis')

Individuals with paranoid personality disorder can be differentiated from those with schizophrenia and delusional disorder, as the former do not have any fixed delusions, hallucinations or formal thought disorders.

Treatment: Psychotherapy is the treatment of choice, although it is difficult to engage these individuals in therapy. They seldom seek help themselves and may resist the treatment process.

Anxiolytics and antidepressants can be used for comorbid anxiety and depressive symptoms. Low dose antipsychotics (like haloperidol) can be used for agitation and paranoid ideations.

Schizoid Personality Disorder

Schizoid personality disorder is characterised by a long-standing pattern of social withdrawal and restricted emotional expression, which presents in the following ways:

1. *Lack of interest in and discomfort with social interaction*: These individuals are uncomfortable with social interactions and do not desire close relationships. They usually do not have any close friends. They appear to be self-absorbed and engage in excessive daydreaming.
2. Preference towards solitary activities, in which they can avoid dealing with others.
3. *Emotional coldness*: These individuals show limited emotions and usually appear serious and aloof. They usually do not show joy, anger, sadness or other emotions.
4. *Indifference towards praise or criticism*: They usually are not interested in the reaction of others. They usually show no interest in everyday events and have no interest in the lives of others.
5. *Little or no interest in sexual experiences*: These individuals usually do not marry, as they don't desire companionship. Although, some may reluctantly agree to get married under social pressure.

Treatment: The individuals with schizoid personality disorder rarely seek treatment as they are usually comfortable the way they are and do not desire to become more social. Treatment involves psychotherapy, primarily. Low dose antipsychotics, antidepressants and stimulant medications have been used with variable success.

Schizotypal Personality Disorder

These individuals are often characterised as 'odd and eccentric' and have peculiarities of thinking, behaviour and appearance, such as the following:

1. Odd beliefs and **magical thinking** such as being extremely superstitious, belief in 'telepathy', belief in the 'other world' or the 'sixth sense'. The odd beliefs often impact their behaviour, e.g., they may do rituals to prevent harm by supernatural powers.
2. *Ideas of reference*: These individuals often have ideas of reference, (i.e., they may interpret neutrals event as somehow related to them. For example, if they are sitting in a class and a fellow student smiles, they may think that the student is laughing at them). However, these thoughts do not reach the level of delusions.
3. *Peculiar and odd interpersonal relationships*: These individuals (like paranoid personality disorder) may have suspiciousness towards others' intentions and less desire for intimate relationships (like schizoid personality disorder), resulting in social detachment and lack of close friends.
4. Unusual perceptions like illusions.
5. *Oddities of thinking and speech*: Their speech (which reflects their thinking) may be loose, vague and difficult to understand. However, they do not have formal thought disorders (which helps in differentiation from schizophrenia).
6. Oddities of behaviour and dressing

When under stress, they may develop psychotic symptoms (for a brief duration).

Schizotypal personality disorder is more common in relatives of patients with schizophrenia than in control groups.

Schizotypal personality is considered the premorbid personality of patients with schizophrenia, (i.e., those who go on to develop schizophrenia often have symptoms suggestive of schizotypal personality disorder before the frank onset of schizophrenic symptoms)

It is also frequently diagnosed in females with the fragile-X syndrome.

> In ICD-11, the schizotypal disorder is not considered a personality disorder; instead, it has been classified as a psychotic disorder.
> Schizotypal personality disorder can be differentiated from schizophrenia by lack of delusions, hallucinations and formal thought disorder in the former.

Treatment: Low dose antipsychotics are used along with psychotherapy. In case depressive symptoms are present, antidepressants can be used.

CLUSTER B PERSONALITY DISORDER

Individuals with cluster B personality disorders often appear to be **dramatic, erratic and too emotional**. Cluster B includes the following personality disorders:
A. Antisocial personality disorder
B. Borderline personality disorder
C. Histrionic personality disorder, and
D. Narcissistic personality disorder

Antisocial Personality Disorder

It is characterised by a **lack of regard and violation of the rights of others**. It is characterised by the following:

1. *Repeated involvement in unlawful activities*: These individuals frequently indulge in unlawful activities such as stealing, harassing others, trespassing etc.
2. *Deceitfulness*: These individuals often indulge in lying, manipulating or conning others for personal gains of profit or power. They may display a superficial charm and may appear very confident, the qualities they may use to fool other people.

3. *Impulsivity*: These individuals may take sudden decisions (about personal and professional life) that may have far-reaching consequences for themselves and their family members (e.g., suddenly shifting to a new city).
4. *Irritability and aggressiveness*: These patients may show irritability and frequently indulge in physical fights (including spouse abuse or child abuse).
5. *Disregard for the safety of self and others*: These individuals may indulge in behaviours like drunk driving, unsafe sexual practices, and high-risk substance abuse that may be unsafe for self or others
6. *Lack of responsible behaviour*: They may show irresponsible behaviours repetitively, (e.g., leaving a job despite the need for money, not taking care of a child etc.)
7. *Lack of remorse and guilt*: These individuals seldom show any remorse or guilt for the consequences of their acts.

The diagnosis of antisocial personality disorder can be made only after 18 years of age. DSM-5 criteria for antisocial personality disorder requires that there should be evidence of the presence of conduct disorder before the age of 15 years.

It is more common in men than women. It is quite prevalent in men with alcohol use disorders (around 70%) and other substance use disorders and in prison populations (prevalence may be as high as 75%).

These patients often show abnormalities in EEG and soft neurological signs (neurological signs that can be elicited only after detailed evaluation).

In the past, terms like sociopath and psychopath have been used for patients with antisocial personality disorders.

The symptoms run a chronic course but may improve with age, especially by the fourth decade of life.

These patients have higher chances of death by violent means (accidents, suicides or homicides) than the general population.

Alcohol use disorder and other substance use disorders, mood disorders like depression and somatic symptoms disorders are common comorbidities.

Treatment: Psychotherapy is used, although retaining the patient in psychotherapy is challenging. Pharmacotherapy is particularly useful for comorbid conditions. SSRIs can be effective in some patients. Anticonvulsants (valproate and carbamazepine) have been used to control impulsivity (especially if abnormal EEG is present), and beta-blockers like propranolol have been used for aggression management.

Borderline Personality Disorder

The term 'borderline' was used as these patients were earlier believed to be at the border of psychosis and neurosis. In the past, terms such as ambulatory schizophrenia and pseudoneurotic schizophrenia have also been used for these patients. Borderline personality disorder is characterised by a pattern of:
a. Unstable interpersonal relationships
b. Unstable emotions (affect)
c. Unstable self-image
d. Marked impulsivity

The following symptoms indicate the characteristic mentioned above:
1. **Fear of abandonment and extreme efforts to prevent the actual or imagined abandonment:** These individuals have an extreme fear that they would be abandoned and left alone. That is why they may go to extremes to avoid this 'abandonment'. Even trivial issues, such as the cancellation of a scheduled appointment by the therapist, can result in extreme anger and agitation. This fear of abandonment usually stems from intolerance of being alone and a strong need to have people around.
2. **A pattern of unstable and intense relationships:** The relationships of these individuals are usually unstable and short-lasting. They may swing from having extreme positive feelings towards the other person to having extreme dislike or hatred in a short period. They often use the defense mechanism of 'splitting', in which the person sees the world in black and white, i.e., either they really like a person or really hate the person. They find it difficult to accept that nobody is all good or all bad.
3. **Unstable emotions:** These individuals have frequent mood swings and may feel intense anger or panic, usually in response to relationship stressors.
4. **Anger outbursts:** They may have inappropriate anger outbursts and find it difficult to control themselves.
5. **Chronic feeling of emptiness:** They describe a chronic feeling of 'emptiness' and get bored quite easily.
6. **Impulsivity:** These individuals have marked impulsivity and may indulge in excessive spending, substance abuse, involvement in unsafe sex, reckless driving, or binge eating.
7. **Recurrent deliberate self-harm (DSH) and suicidal behaviour/threats:** These individuals may display self-mutilating behaviours such as cutting the wrist or overdosage of medications. These behaviours are usually performed to numb themselves from emotional pain. In some, self-mutilation is done to express anger or seek attention. These individuals may also display recurrent suicidal threats or behaviours. Around 8–10% of these individuals die by suicide.
8. **Micropsychotic episodes:** When under extreme stress, patients with borderline personality disorders may have short duration psychotic episodes (transient delusions or fleeting hallucinations) or dissociative symptoms (such as depersonalisation).
9. **Instability of self-image (disturbances of identity):** These individuals have an unstable self-image (image of what kind of a person they are), and there are sudden shifts in their goals, plans about career, sexual identity, values and type of friends.

In some patients, biological abnormalities, such as decreased rapid eye movement (REM) sleep latency, abnormal dexamethasone suppression test, and abnormal thyrotropin-releasing hormone tests may be present, although they are still not used to reach a diagnosis, as these findings are not consistent.

Apart from splitting, another defense mechanism seen in these individuals is projective identification (explained in the Chapter 18 'Psychoanalysis').

This disorder is more common in females than males, and the course is stable (symptoms remain stable). However, by their 30s and 40s, most individuals attain greater stability in their relationships and work. The common comorbidities include major depressive disorder, substance use disorder and eating disorder (particularly bulimia nervosa).

Treatment: A combination of psychotherapy and pharmacotherapy is preferred.
1. **Psychotherapy:** Psychotherapy is the mainstay of treatment. Various approaches have been used, which include:
   a. **Dialectical behaviour therapy:** Dialectical behavioural therapy was developed by Marsha Linehan (who herself had borderline personality disorder). This therapy focuses on reducing self-destructive behaviours and improving interpersonal skills.
   b. **Mentalisation-based therapy:** This therapy is based on the hypothesis that the symptoms of borderline personality disorder occur as patients are not aware of their own mental state, (i.e., emotions and thoughts) and the mental state of others during interpersonal interactions. This therapy aims to improve the mentalisation (awareness of mental state) to decrease symptoms.
2. **Pharmacotherapy:** The pharmacotherapy is used for specific symptoms. For example, SSRIs are used to improve mood and decrease anxiety and irritability. Antipsychotics are used for hostility and micropsychotic episodes. Anticonvulsants, too, have been found to reduce symptoms in some patients.

Histrionic Personality Disorder

This personality disorder is characterised by a pattern of (a) attention seeking behaviour and (b) excessive emotionality, as manifested by the following symptoms:
1. *Discomfort in situations in which they are not the centre of attention*: Individuals with histrionic personality disorder have a strong need to be the centre of attention, and they behave in a dramatic and flirtatious manner to draw the attention of others. If they are not getting enough attention, they may do something dramatic (like creating a scene or making a false but colourful story) to draw the attention of others.
2. *Inappropriate and sexually seductive or provocative behaviour*: While interacting with others, they often behave in a sexually seductive and provocative manner, which is usually considered inappropriate. Their appearance and dressing may be considered inappropriate too. Usually, this inappropriate behaviour and appearance are to draw the attention of others.
3. *Consistent use of physical appearance to draw attention*: These individuals often spend a lot of time, resources and energy on their appearance, again to draw the attention of others. They may get quite upset if someone makes a critical comment about their appearance.
4. *Have an impressionistic speech*: Their style of speech is impressionistic, (i.e., focuses on emotions and not on details). For example, when asked to describe the job of her husband, an individual responded, 'he is an amazing and a wonderful, wonderful person and does great and such important work'. In this response, there were no details about the work, just emotions.
5. *Exaggerated emotions and dramatisations*: They may show excessive emotions (e.g., crying uncontrollably after meeting an acquaintance after a few days), which may embarrass others. However, as their emotions rapidly change, others often feel they don't have genuine emotions. These patients have difficulty achieving emotional intimacy in relationships, and their emotions are usually shallow and change often.
6. *A high degree of suggestibility*: These patents are quite suggestible (i.e., they get easily influenced by others). They are often overly trusting.

The disorder is more common in females. With age, the symptoms gradually tend to decrease. The common comorbidities are substance use disorder, somatisation disorder and major depressive disorder.

Treatment: Psychotherapy is the mainstay of treatment. Pharmacotherapy is usually symptomatic (e.g., antidepressants for depressive symptoms, anxiolytics for anxiety symptoms).

Narcissistic Personality Disorder

This personality disorder is characterised by a long-standing pattern of (a) giving excessive importance to self, (b) excessive need for admiration, and (c) lack of empathy and is characterised by the following:
1. **Excessive self-importance:** These individuals overestimate their abilities and underestimate the contributions of others. They are boastful, consider themselves special, and want others to treat them like superiors. They only associate with whom they regard as 'top' people in their field and at par with their own presumed 'high' status.
2. **Fantasies of unlimited success and power:** These individuals are preoccupied with fantasies and imaginations of achieving great success in life.
3. **Excessive need for admiration and a sense of entitlement:** These individuals need constant attention and admiration. They want to get compliments regularly from others and may react with anger if their need for admiration is not met. They also expect to get favourable treatment from others (**sense of entitlement**) (e.g., they want to be attended first, they do not like when asked to wait for their turn) and get angry if their wishes are not met. In putting their needs first, they may end up **exploiting** others.
4. **Lack of empathy and concern for others:** These individuals don't recognise the feelings of others and appear selfish. They also show arrogance and an egotistical attitude towards others. They get envious of others easily and also believe that others are envious of them.
5. **Poor tolerance to criticism:** These individuals cannot tolerate the slightest criticism and may feel humiliated or

respond with rage. Their self-esteem is fragile, and any criticism can bring an extreme response.

This disorder is more common in males compared to females. These individuals may achieve professional success as they come out as confident individuals. However, their performance may get disrupted when faced with criticism. Their personal relationships are usually impaired. These individuals typically do not handle ageing well, as they give a lot of importance to strength, beauty and youth-fullness, making them particularly susceptible to a midlife crisis.

Treatment: Psychotherapy can be helpful, but it is difficult to engage these individuals in therapy. Pharmacotherapy is usually symptomatic (lithium for mood swings, antidepressants for depressive symptoms, anxiolytics for anxiety symptoms).

CLUSTER C PERSONALITY DISORDER

The individuals with cluster C personality disorder often appear to be anxious and fearful. Cluster C includes:
a. Avoidant personality disorder
b. Dependent personality Disorder
c. Obsessive-compulsive personality disorder

Avoidant Personality Disorder (Anxious Personality Disorder)

This personality disorder is characterised by:
a. *Extreme sensitivity to negative evaluation*: These individuals are extremely sensitive and fearful of others' negative evaluation (such as criticism, mockery or disapproval).
   Hence they often:
   1. Avoid occupational activities that involve others as they are afraid that others may not like them or, worse, may criticise them.
   2. Avoid making friends unless they are sure that they are liked and won't be criticised by them.
   3. Show restraint in intimate relationships and may find it difficult to express the intimate feelings due to fear of being ridiculed or shamed. They can establish intimate relationships only when they are assured of complete acceptance without criticism.
b. *Social inhibition*: These individuals often avoid social activities, because of the fear of not being liked, despite having a strong internal desire to socialise.
c. *Feeling of inadequacy and inferiority*: These individuals often have low self-esteem and may consider themselves incompetent or unappealing.

> Patients with schizoid personality disorder and avoidant personality disorder, both, avoid social interactions. Schizoid personality disorder patients avoid social interaction as they do not want to socialise. In contrast, patients with avoidant personality disorder have a strong desire to socialise but are too afraid of not being liked by others.
> This disorder is equally prevalent in both sexes. The symptoms tend to become less severe as the patient becomes older.

Treatment: Psychotherapy focuses on improving self-esteem and social skills. Assertiveness training, which focuses on teaching patients to express their needs clearly, is helpful.

Pharmacotherapy is used to manage anxiety and depressive symptoms, and SSRIs are commonly used. Beta-blockers (like propranolol) have also been used to control the sympathetic symptoms.

Dependent Personality Disorder

The characteristic features of this disorder include: (a) strong need to be taken care of by others (usually parents or spouse), resulting in clinging and submissive behaviour (b) fear that they would be left alone and won't be able to take care of themselves (c) lack of self-confidence and belief in their abilities.

These individuals often show the following symptoms:
1. Need for excessive advice and reassurances for making everyday decisions (e.g., inability to buy clothes for self unless approved by others).
2. Allowing others (usually parents or spouses) and wanting others to take responsibility for important decisions in their lives (e.g., in which field to pursue the career, whom to marry, how many kids to have etc.)
3. Inability to express disagreement, especially with those on whom they are dependent. These individuals have a strong fear of being left out and losing support, and hence they are not able to express their disagreement with things that they feel are not correct. In fact, they may agree to do things that they don't really like because they feel that it will help in the continuation of 'support' from others. Abuse and infidelity by a spouse may be tolerated to avoid separation.
4. Feeling of 'helplessness' when alone. These individuals believe that they won't be able to take care of themselves. If their close relationship ends (e.g., breakup), they urgently look for another relationship that can provide them with the much needed 'support'.
5. Lack of confidence in self and tendency to belittle own achievements and abilities: These individuals often cannot 'initiate' any work as they doubt their abilities. They tend to downplay their achievements and feel that others are more competent than them.

Dependent personality disorder is more common in females than males. In case individuals with dependent personality disorder lose the person on whom they are dependent, they are at risk of developing a major depressive disorder.

> In folie a deux (or shared psychotic disorder), the dependent person often develops the same delusion that the assertive partner has.

Treatment: Psychotherapy is often successful. The focus is on improving self-confidence, self-esteem, cognitive restructuring (changing the patterns of thinking) and assertiveness training.

Pharmacotherapy is usually used for symptomatic relief from symptoms of anxiety and depression. SSRIs and benzodiazepines are often used.

Obsessive Compulsive Personality Disorder (Anankastic Personality Disorder)

It is one of the commonest personality disorders and is seen more commonly in males than females. It is characterised by a pattern of excessive orderliness, perfectionism and inflexibility. The individuals with this disorder have the following symptoms:

1. *Preoccupation with rules, details and schedules*: These individuals give excessive attention to rules and regulations and spend a great deal of time making detailed lists and organising detailed schedules to the extent that major activity points may get lost. e.g., If asked to organise a college reunion, they would make multiple lists of who all are likely to attend, who should sit where, how many minutes should be given for speech, how to give reminders if someone crosses the allowed speech time, which bell to ring and how many times if someone crosses the speech time etc. While making these lists, they forget that a college reunion is all about old friends getting together and having a good time.
2. **Perfectionism** *that interferes with task completion*: These individuals want to complete the tasks 'perfectly' and set very high standards for what 'perfect' means to them. They are often unsatisfied with their work and may spend a lot of time perfecting it, leading to unnecessary delays in task completion and missing deadlines.
3. *Excessive devotion to work and exclusion of pleasurable activities and fun in life*: These individuals are involved in work excessively and may not give time to activities like pursuing hobbies, vacations, or being with family and friends.
4. *Excessive rigidity about morality and ethics and lack of flexibility*: These individuals show extreme conscientiousness and are inflexible in their approach. For example, an individual got into a big fight with his wife as she had jumped the traffic signal and later even filed a complaint against her.
5. *Difficulty in giving work to others*: These individuals often feel that only they know how to do a particular task and may find it difficult to let a subordinate do it unless he does it exactly the same way they want. They appear to be very rigid and stubborn and may insist that things be done exactly their way.
6. *Indecisiveness*: As these individuals are afraid of making mistakes and want to take the 'right' decision, the decision-making becomes difficult for them, and they often end up procrastinating.
7. *Stinginess*: These individuals often find it difficult to spend money and have a living standard far below their means; they save money for a future 'difficult situation' that may arise.

It must be remembered that obsession and compulsions do not form the criterion of obsessive-compulsive personality disorder. If along with symptoms of OCPD, the patient also has recurrent obsessions and compulsions, a comorbid diagnosis of obsessive-compulsive disorder should be made.

Many features of OCPD are similar to type A personality (described below):

Treatment: Unlike other personality disorders, individuals with OCPD are often aware of their symptoms and may seek treatment by themselves. The treatment is primarily psychotherapy, and the use of pharmacotherapy is symptomatic and for comorbid diagnosis, if any.

OTHER CLASSIFICATIONS

In the 1950s, two cardiologists, Meyer Friedman and Ray Rosenman, described two types of personalities: Type A and Type B personality.

Type A personality individuals were described as having characteristics such as competitiveness, time urgency (highly focussed on time management), hostility and **anger**. The people with type A personality were described as being ambitious, impatient and hard-working workaholics. It has been suggested that type A personality or type A behaviour patterns (especially the hostility and anger traits) are a risk factor for **coronary heart disease**.

In comparison, individuals with **type B personality** were described as easy going and relaxed, not excessively competitive and more focused on enjoyment and less on winning or losing.

Type A and B personality theory have been criticised by many researchers as the original research was found to have multiple statistical limitations. Many later studies didn't find any link between type A behaviour patterns and coronary heart diseases. Also, many studies on type A behaviour pattern were funded by the tobacco industry. For many years, the tobacco industry tried to delink tobacco consumption with an increased risk of coronary heart diseases by arguing that it was actually the type A behaviour pattern (often present in smokers) that was associated with an increased risk of coronary heart diseases and not the smoking per se. Obviously, it is now proven beyond doubt that tobacco use is a significant risk factor for coronary heart disease.

Recently new personality types, type C and type D have also been described:
- Type C personality is characterised by perfectionistic tendencies (focus on every detail) and a lack of assertiveness
- Type D personality: It is characterised by pessimism, negative affectivity (a tendency to experience negative emotions) and social inhibition (tendency to inhibit the expression of emotions). Individuals with type D personality are predisposed to the development of **coronary heart disease**.

ICD-11 UPDATES

Unlike DSM-5, the ICD-11 classifies the personality disorders based on the severity of symptoms, [i.e., depending on the number of areas of personality functioning affected (like the ability to control impulses, ability to control behaviour, having a stable sense of self, ability to maintain relationships etc.)] into:
1. Mild personality disorder
2. Moderate personality disorder
3. Severe personality disorder

According to ICD-11, depending upon the characteristic features present, a specifier of 'prominent personality traits or patterns' can be added after the diagnosis. For example, an individual who has marked impairment in all the areas of personality functioning with significant dysfunction would get a diagnosis of 'severe personality disorder'. Now, if the prominent features of the personality of this person are a disregard for the rights of others, aggression, lack of empathy etc., in that case, a specifier of 'dissociality in personality disorder' will be added, which makes the final diagnosis as Severe personality disorder (dissociality in personality disorder).

ICD-11 describes the following types of prominent personality traits that can be applied to personality disorder diagnosis:
1. *Negative affectivity in personality disorder*: It is characterised by a tendency to experience negative emotions, and emotional instability, out of proportion to the existing situation.
2. *Detachment in personality disorder*: It is characterised by a tendency to have restricted emotional attachment with others and a lack of desire to socialise. It is similar to the DSM-5 diagnosis of 'schizoid personality disorder.'
3. *Dissociality in personality disorder*: It is characterised by a disregard for the rights and feelings of others, lack of empathy and aggressiveness. It is similar to the DSM-5 diagnosis of antisocial personality disorder.
4. *Disinhibition in personality disorder*: It is characterised by a tendency to act impulsively without considering the long-term consequences of such behaviour.
5. *Anankastia in personality disorder*: It is characterised by a tendency for perfectionism, emphasis on organisation, inflexibility etc. The symptoms are similar to the DSM-5 diagnosis of obsessive-compulsive personality disorder.
6. *Borderline pattern*: It is characterised by features such as impulsivity, unstable interpersonal relationships, fear of abandonment etc. The symptoms are similar to the DSM-5 diagnosis of borderline personality disorder.

CASE BASED MCQ

A 22-year-old medical student was brought to the emergency after she cut her wrist following an altercation with her boyfriend. In the past, too, she had cut herself on many occasions, usually after similar fights. The student never had a long-lasting relationship, and most of her affairs ended in less than three months. In the hospital, the student said that her boyfriend is the 'worst human being ever', whereas she felt that the surgery resident who helped in the emergency ward was like 'an angel straight from heaven'. What is the likely diagnosis?
a. Histrionic personality disorder
b. Anankastic personality disorder
c. Borderline personality disorder
d. Schizoid personality disorder

Ans. c. History suggestive of multiple acts of deliberate self-harm, inability to have long-term relationships and seeing people in black and white (called as splitting, worst human being ever and angel from heaven) is suggestive of borderline personality disorder.

SUGGESTED READINGS

1. Shaw WS, Dimsdale JE. Type A Personality, Type B. Stress consequences: Mental, neuropsychological and socioeconomic. 2010;6:72-6.
2. American Psychiatric Association. Diagnostic and Statistical Manual of Mental Disorders. Arlington, VA: American Psychiatric Publishing, 2013.
3. Boland R, Verduin M. Kaplan & Sadock's Concise Textbook of Clinical Psychiatry. Lippincott Williams & Wilkins; 2021.
4. Harrison P, Cowen P, Burns T, Fazel M. Shorter Oxford textbook of psychiatry. Oxford university press; 2017.
5. Sadock BJ, Sadock VA, Ruiz P. Comprehensive textbook of psychiatry 10th edition.
6. World Health Organization. ICD-11 for mortality and morbidity statistics (2018).

14 Eating Disorders

Praveen Tripathi, Priyanka Goyal

Eating disorders are characterised by abnormalities in the pattern of food intake and/or the amount and nature of food intake.

ANOREXIA NERVOSA

Of all the eating disorders, anorexia nervosa perhaps gets the most attention because of its striking presentation.

Anorexia nervosa is characterised by three essential features:

1. **Restriction of energy intake leading to significantly low body weight:** In Anorexia nervosa, there is a severe restriction of energy intake as compared to the requirement. This leads to significantly lower body weight in the context of the individual's height, age and developmental stage.
2. A BMI (body mass index) **<18.5 kg/m²** is considered a significantly low body weight for adults. There may be a failure to make expected weight gain in children and adolescents, and **BMI for age under the fifth percentile** suggests significant underweight. The severity of anorexia nervosa is defined based on the BMI in adults and BMI for age percentiles in children and adolescents. For adults:
   - *Mild*: BMI ≥ 17 kg/m²
   - *Moderate*: BMI 16–16.99 kg/m²
   - *Severe*: BMI 15–15.99 kg/m²
   - *Extreme*: BMI < 15 kg/m²

   In patients with anorexia nervosa, the weight loss is achieved by a significant redution in food intake and a disproportionate reduction in high fat and high carbohydrate food consumption.
3. **Intense fear of gaining weight or becoming fat:** Patients with anorexia nervosa have a morbid fear of becoming fat. This fear continues and, in many cases, worsens, despite having significant weight loss.
4. **Disturbances in the way one's body weight or shape is experienced:** Patients often have 'body image' disturbances, which means that the way they perceive their body is disturbed. Despite being thin, they may feel that they are overweight or that certain parts of their body are 'too fat'. The self-esteem of these patients is often highly dependent on their perception of body weight and shape. If they can lose weight, they consider it an achievement and any weight gain is regarded as a failure.

In addition to the three essential features, patients with anorexia nervosa often have certain physical signs and symptoms secondary to starvation. These include:

a. **Amenorrhea:** It is quite common and is present in 68–89% of women with anorexia nervosa. In pre-pubertal females, menarche may be delayed
b. Hypotension, hypothermia, dependent oedema, bradycardia
c. Appearance of lanugo (neonatal like hair)
d. Delayed gastric emptying and gastric dilatation
e. Signs and symptoms secondary to purging behaviour.

Some of the **laboratory findings** in anorexia nervosa include:

a. Leukopenia (with apparent lymphocytosis), mild anaemia and thrombocytopenia.
b. Elevated blood urea nitrogen (secondary to dehydration), and elevated liver enzymes.
c. High serum cholesterol
d. Sinus bradycardia, ST segment and T wave changes, occasional prolongation of QTc interval and rarely arrhythmias.
e. Abnormalities on electroencephalogram.
f. Endocrine abnormalities as mentioned below:

Individuals with anorexia nervosa usually either lack insight or deny having a problem. They seldom complain about weight loss. It must be remembered that 'anorexia nervosa' is a **misnomer** as there is no 'anorexia or loss of appetite' in these patients. The food intake is restricted despite having a normal appetite. In fact, these patients often are preoccupied with the food and may spend long hours collecting food recipes, hoarding food and preparing meals for others. Patients may also show peculiar behaviours about food, such as while eating, they may cut the food into small pieces, arrange the food around the plate or hide the food in napkins.

Many adolescent patients have delayed sexual development, and adults often have markedly decreased interest in sex.

> In DSM-4 and ICD-10, amenorrhea was a necessary symptom for diagnosing anorexia nervosa in females; however, in DSM-5 and ICD-11, this criterion has been removed, and anorexia nervosa can be diagnosed in the absence of amenorrhea now.

Epidemiology

Anorexia nervosa is 10–20 times more common in **females** than males. The most common age of onset is in the mid-teens. Earlier, it was reported that it is more common in the upper socio-economic class, but recent studies have not shown any such distribution. It is more common in professions that give a lot of importance to thinness, such as ballet dancing, modelling and gymnastics. Anorexia nervosa is less common in non-western countries.

The most common comorbidity is depression, followed by social phobia and obsessive-compulsive disorder.

Subtypes

There are two clinical subtypes:
a. **Restricting type:** Present in 50% of the cases, this type is characterised by highly restricted food intake and, in some cases, excessive activity levels.
b. **Binge eating/purging type:** In this type, alternating with rigorous dieting, are episodes of binging (in a binge episode, an excessive amount of food is ingested) and purging (to compensate for calorie intake, there is self-induced vomiting and, in some cases use of laxatives, diuretics, enemas or emetics). Many of the physical findings and lab findings found in patients with anorexia nervosa are because of repeated purging episodes.

Aetiology

Genetics: The genetic contribution to the development of anorexia nervosa is evident by the heritability of 28–74%. Further, evidence is provided by the higher concordance rate in monozygotic twins than dizygotic twins in patients with anorexia nervosa.

Neurobiology: Many neurobiological abnormalities have been reported in the patients; however, it is difficult to determine whether these abnormalities are responsible for causing anorexia nervosa or whether they develop due to starvation in these patients. Some of the findings include:
a. Enlargement of CSF spaces (enlarged ventricles and sulci) during starvation. These get reversed with weight gain.
b. Endocrine abnormalities: These are believed to be caused by starvation and include:
   i. Low gonadotropin-releasing hormone, low FSH and low LH. Anorexia nervosa is often associated with hypothalamic amenorrhea.
   ii. Severe weight loss is often associated with nonthyroid illness syndrome with low T3, normal or slightly decreased T4, normal TSH and raised reverse T3 (due to increased peripheral deiodination of T4 to reverse T3).
   iii. Increased corticotropin-releasing hormone, increased cortisol and dexamethasone non-suppression. Hypercortisolaemia is believed to be due to the stress of chronic starvation and helps maintain glucose levels despite starvation.
   iv. A state of acquired growth hormone resistance, with increased growth hormone concentration but decreased systemic insulin-like growth factor 1 (IGF-1). Low IGF-1 appears to help conserve energy by decreasing expenditure on growth, and increased growth hormone also helps maintain glucose levels via gluconeogenesis.
   v. Global endocrine dysfunction is also associated with reduced bone mineral density (BMD) and increased fracture risk.
c. Abnormalities of the three neurotransmitters involved in the regulation of eating behaviour—serotonin, dopamine and norepinephrine.

Sociocultural factors: The cultural emphasis on thinness as a desirable trait also influences the development of anorexia nervosa.

Treatment

Patients with anorexia nervosa are usually secretive, deny having any problem and resist the treatment. It takes a significant effort by the psychiatrist and persuasion by family members to get the patient ready for the treatment.

The treatment setting (whether inpatient or outpatient) must be decided, keeping in mind the patient's nutritional state. The presence of dehydration, starvation and electrolyte imbalances warrants immediate measures. In general, **hospitalisation is advised** if the patient's weight is 20% below the expected (weight for height). Long term psychiatric hospitalisation is recommended if the weight is 30% below the expected weight for their height.

Daily weight monitoring and fluid intake/urine output monitoring must be done if the patient is admitted. The calorie intake should be gradually increased, as a sudden increase can cause gastric dilatation or circulatory overload. A common practice is to give patients about 500 calories above the amount required to maintain the current weight (usually 1,500–2,000 calories per day). If patients do not gain weight, one should suspect purging (self-induced vomiting) after the meals. To prevent it, nursing staff should supervise the patient for **2 hours** after the meals and make the bathroom inaccessible to the patient.

The treatment usually involves a **combination** of behavioural management (praise for healthy eating habits, restriction on self-induced vomiting and over-exercising), individual psychotherapy (e.g., cognitive behavioural therapy), family therapy and medications. Medications such as cyproheptadine, TCAs (tricyclic antidepressants), and SSRIs (selective serotonin reuptake inhibitors) have been tried with varied success.

The course of anorexia nervosa varies, from spontaneous recovery to death. Death commonly results from medical complications or suicide (the risk for suicide is high in anorexia nervosa). The prognosis of the binge-eating/purging type is better than the restricting type.

BULIMIA NERVOSA

Bulimia nervosa is more common than anorexia nervosa. The usual age of onset is in late adolescence, and it is more common in females than males (approximate female:male ratio, 10:1).

Bulimia nervosa is characterised by three essential features:

1. **Recurrent episodes of binge eating:** There are repeated episodes of binge eating (to diagnose bulimia nervosa, the frequency of binge eating should be at least once a week, for more than three months). An episode of binge eating involves:
   a. Eating a large amount of food in a short time.
   b. During the episode, there is a sense of 'loss of control', i.e., the patient feels that she just can not stop herself from eating.

   During binges, the patient often eats food that is sweet and high in calories and eats rapidly, sometimes not even chewing before swallowing. Usually, patients indulge in binge eating when they are alone, and the most common trigger for these episodes is negative emotions. The binge eating continues until the individual feels uncomfortably or even painfully–full. After the episode, the individual has feelings of shame, guilt and disgust for self, and fear of weight gain. Patients restrict their calorie intake and prefer low-calorie foods between the binge episodes.

2. **Recurrent inappropriate ways of stopping weight gain:** Most individuals with bulimia nervosa recurrently use inappropriate ways to stop weight gain, collectively referred to as 'purging' or 'purge behaviours'. The most common method is self-induced vomiting, usually induced by sticking a finger down the throat to induce the gag reflex. Other purging methods include the use of laxatives, diuretics, emetics, and use of enemas. Individuals may also use fasting or excessive exercising to prevent weight gain. The severity of bulimia nervosa is based on the frequency of inappropriate compensatory behaviour per week; the more the frequency, the higher the severity.

   As discussed above, binging and purging episodes can be a feature of both anorexia nervosa and bulimia nervosa.

3. **Excessive concern about the body shape or weight:** The self-esteem of these individuals is highly dependent on how they perceive their weight and body shape. Like anorexia nervosa, patients with bulimia nervosa also have a fear of gaining weight, a desire to be thin and general dissatisfaction with their body; however, unlike in anorexia nervosa, these patients are not able to sustain prolonged periods of semi-starvation.

The purging behaviour can lead to the following:
a. **Parotid gland enlargement** (overstimulation of salivary gland secretion due to binge-eating and/or purging behaviour).
b. **Loss of dental enamel** (mostly from lingual surfaces of the front teeth, due to recurrent vomiting) and increased frequency of dental caries.
c. **Callouses or scars on knuckles** (patients, while trying to induce gag reflex by sticking the finger down the throat, injure the dorsal surface of the hand due to repeated contact with the teeth).
d. Rarely oesophageal tears or gastric rupture (due to forceful vomiting).

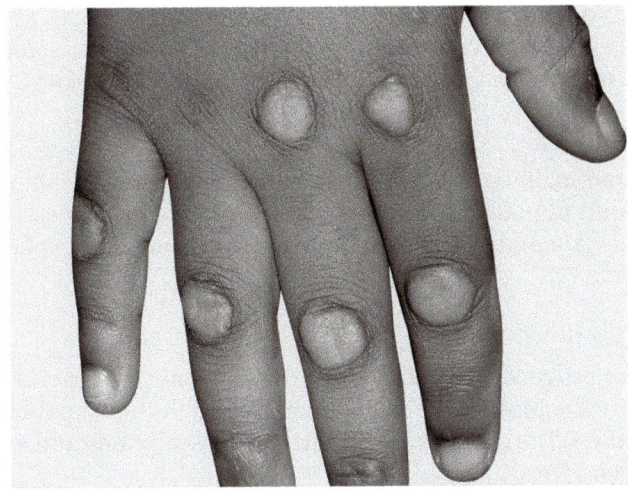

Fig. 14.1: Calluses on knuckles.

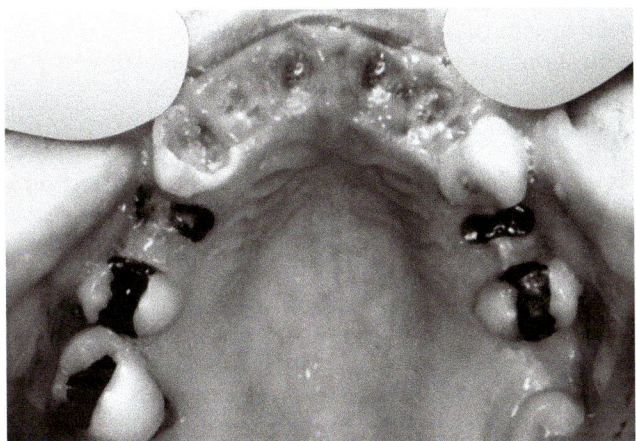

Fig. 14.2: Loss of teeth due to erosion.

Several **laboratory findings** may be present, secondary to purging, and these include:
a. Hypokalaemia (may cause cardiac arrhythmias), hyponatraemia and hypochloraemia
b. Metabolic alkalosis (loss of gastric acid due to vomiting)
c. Metabolic acidosis (in those who frequently use laxatives or diuretics)
d. Elevated levels of serum amylase (this is due to salivary isoamylase rather than pancreatic amylase)

These physical and laboratory findings, secondary to purging, are also usually present in patients with anorexia nervosa, binge eating/purging type.

Patients with bulimia nervosa have increased suicide risk and must be evaluated for the same.

In contrast to patients with anorexia nervosa, those with bulimia nervosa typically have normal body weight. Unlike anorexia nervosa, patients with bulimia nervosa are usually sexually active. Many patients with bulimia nervosa have menstrual disturbances.

Subtypes

1. **Purging type:** This type includes patients who use purging (self-induced vomiting or use of laxatives, diuretics, or emetics) as a compensatory behaviour.

2. **Non-purging type:** This type includes those who use excessive exercising or dieting as compensatory mechanisms but do not indulge in purging behaviours.

Aetiology

Abnormalities of serotonin and norepinephrine have been found in patients with bulimia nervosa. As in the case of anorexia nervosa, societal pressure for thinness, too, plays a role.

Treatment

The prognosis in bulimia nervosa is better than anorexia nervosa. Most of the patients are treated in the outpatient setting. The patients usually accept the symptoms and are open to treatment.

Cognitive behavioural therapy is considered the first-line treatment for bulimia nervosa. In pharmacotherapy, SSRIs like fluoxetine are useful. TCAs (like imipramine) are useful in some cases. In general, a combination of CBT with medications has been found to give the best results.

BINGE EATING DISORDER

It is the **most common** eating disorder. It is characterised by episodes of binge eating; however, unlike bulimia nervosa, there are no compensatory behaviours. Binge eating disorder is associated with overweight and obesity. Treatment of binge eating disorder is similar to bulimia nervosa.

PURGING DISORDER

It is characterised by recurrent purging behaviour after consuming a small amount of food (unlike bulimia nervosa, where purging follows binge eating episodes). The weight of the person is usually normal.

AVOIDANT RESTRICTIVE FOOD INTAKE DISORDER

It is a new diagnosis that has been included in both ICD-11 and DSM-5. It is characterised by the following:
1. Insufficient intake of quantity or variety of food that results in weight loss (or inability to gain weight) and nutritional deficiencies. The patient may report a lack of interest in eating or may avoid food due to sensory characteristics (e.g., not liking the smell or taste of food).
2. There are no disturbances of body image (this characteristic helps to differentiate avoidant restrictive food intake disorder from anorexia nervosa, restrictive type).

OTHER EATING DISORDER

Pica: It is characterised by—
- Regular consumption of non-food objects and materials such as soil, plaster, paper, etc., or consumption of raw food ingredients such as large amounts of salt or cornflour
- The consumption is persistent, in significant amounts and can cause damage to the health or functioning of the individual
- The consumption happens in an individual who should be able to distinguish between the edible and non-edible food by virtue of the developmental age (by two years of age, one is expected to distinguish between edible and non-edible food)

Rumination-regurgitation disorder: It is characterised by—
- *Regurgitation*: Intentional and repeated bringing up of previously swallowed up food back into the mouth
- *Rumination*: Re-chewing of the regurgitated food, which is again swallowed back or spat out
- It is diagnosed only if the patient's age is more than 2 years

Night eating syndrome: It is characterised by—
- Consumption of a large amount of food after the evening meal
- Lack of appetite during the day
- Insomnia

CASE BASED MCQ

A 14-year-old girl was brought for medical evaluation by family members as she has been eating 'too less' and becoming 'too thin'. On examination, the BMI of the girl was 17 kg/m^2, and there were callouses on her knuckles. The girl was irritable during the interview and insisted that she was doing 'just fine' and eating well. The mother reported that when she is forced to eat, she goes to the washroom later and sounds suggestive of vomiting come from the bathroom. The girl did not have menstrual periods for the last three months; what is the likely diagnosis?
a. Anorexia nervosa
b. Bulimia nervosa
c. Binge eating disorder
d. Pica

Ans. a. History of significantly reduced food intake, a significantly low body mass index, amenorrhea, history suggestive of purging episodes and signs suggestive of purging (callouses in knuckles) are also suggestive of anorexia nervosa.

SUGGESTED READINGS

1. Kaye WH, Wierenga CE, Bailer UF, Simmons AN, Bischoff-Grethe A. Nothing tastes as good as skinny feels: the neurobiology of anorexia nervosa. Trends in neurosciences. 2013;36(2):110-20.
2. Schorr M, Miller KK. The endocrine manifestations of anorexia nervosa: mechanisms and management. Nat Rev Endocrinol. 2017;13(3):174-86.

3. Hoffman ER, Zerwas SC, Bulik CM. Reproductive issues in anorexia nervosa. Expert Rev Obstet Gynecol. 2011;6(4):403-14.
4. Wolfe BE, Jimerson DC, Smith A, Keel PK. Serum amylase in bulimia nervosa and purging disorder: differentiating the association with binge eating versus purging behavior. Physiol Behav. 2011;104(5):684-6.
5. American Psychiatric Association. Diagnostic and Statistical Manual of Mental Disorders. Arlington, VA: American Psychiatric Publishing; 2013.
6. Boland R, Verduin M. Kaplan & Sadock's Concise Textbook of Clinical Psychiatry. Lippincott Williams & Wilkins; 2021.
7. Harrison P, Cowen P, Burns T, Fazel M. Shorter Oxford Textbook of Psychiatry. Oxford university press; 2017.
8. Sadock BJ, Sadock VA, Ruiz P. Comprehensive Textbook of Psychiatry, 10th edition.

15 > Sleep Disorders

Praveen Tripathi, Vijay Niranjan

Humans spend one-third of their lives sleeping. Sleep serves many functions, including restoring and repairing physical and psychological processes, memory consolidation, conservation of energy, maintenance of the immune system, and growth. Prolonged sleep deprivation can cause significant physical and psychological disturbances and even death.

PHYSIOLOGY OF SLEEP

Sleep can be divided into two stages:
A. **Nonrapid eye movement sleep (NREM) or slow-wave sleep** and
B. **Rapid eye movement (REM) sleep**

Nonrapid Eye Movement Sleep

It is further divided into four stages of increasing depth of sleep (as the depth increases, awakening the individual from sleep becomes more difficult). These include:

- **Stage 1, NREM:** In a typical night of sleep, a young adult first enters NREM sleep stage 1. In this stage, the sleep is light (individual can be easily aroused). The EEG shows **loss of alpha waves** (which predominate when an individual has eyes closed but is awake), and theta waves are **predominant**.
- **Stage 2, NREM:** Stage 2 follows stage 1 and is characterised by two typical findings on electroencephalogram:
  a. **Sleep spindles:** These are bursts of regular waves (13–15 Hz, 50 microvolts) and
  b. **K-complexes:** These are high voltage spikes that are seen intermittently.

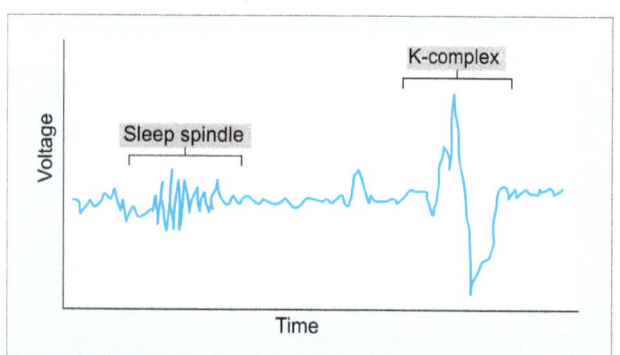

- **Stage 3, NREM:** In stage 3, the sleep deepens, and delta waves appear.
- **Stage 4, NREM:** This is deep sleep and is characterised by a predominance of delta waves on EEG.

Some authors use the term 'slow-wave sleep' exclusively for stage 3 and 4 NREM. As mentioned, stage 3 and 4 NREM are the deepest phases of NREM sleep and if a person is woken up from these stages, he may appear disoriented and may not be able to think clearly for a while.

Some important features of NREM sleep include the following:
1. There is a pulsatile release of gonadotropins and growth hormones during NREM sleep.
2. The blood pressure, heart rate and respiratory rate decreases during NREM sleep and all these parameters are quite regular during this stage of sleep.
3. Blood flow to most tissues (including cerebral blood flow) is reduced
4. Like wakefulness, there is a homeothermic condition of temperature regulation in NREM sleep, and body temperature is maintained despite changes in surrounding environment temperature.

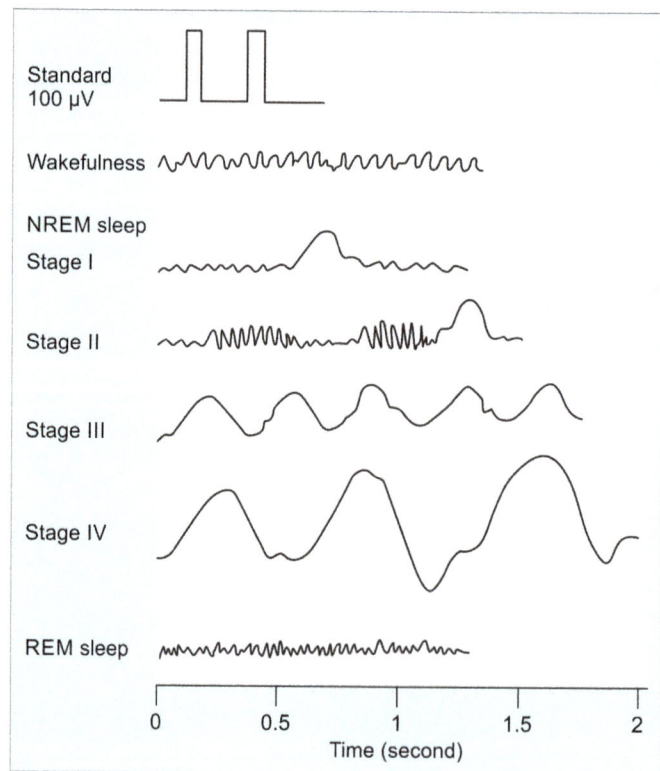

Rapid Eye Movement Sleep

It follows the NREM sleep. It is characterised by the following:
- Presence of rapid eye movements.
- Generalised **loss of muscle tone**
- **Increased rate** of metabolism in the brain
- Increase (and significant variability) in pulse rate, respiratory rate and blood pressure, at times above the awake state
- **Penile erection (partial or full) in every REM period**
- **Dreams:** People awakened from REM sleep usually report that they were dreaming. (Dreaming happens in NREM too, but is much less compared to REM sleep.)
- **REM sleep is a poikilothermic state** (i.e., body temperature changes with the ambient temperature)
- The EEG shows increased activity similar to the awake state (**beta activity**) and the return of **alpha activity. Despite sleeping, since EEG is quite similar to the awake state, REM sleep is also called paradoxical sleep.**
- **Ponto-geniculo-occipital spikes** (large phasic potentials that originate in cholinergic neurons in the pons and pass rapidly to the lateral geniculate body and then to the occipital cortex) are characteristically seen during REM sleep.

In a typical night of sleep, a young adult first enters NREM 1, followed by NREM 2, NREM 3 and NREM 4. After around 90 minutes (called as REM latency period), the individual enters REM sleep. The REM sleep occurs regularly after every 90–100 minutes, with around 4–5 REM sleeps in the entire night. Most of stage 4, NREM, occurs in the first one-third of the night, whereas most of the REM sleep occurs in the last one-third of the night.

In an 8-hour sleep, maximum time (around 6–6.5 hours) is spent in NREM sleep and the rest (around 1.5 hours) in REM sleep. Of all the stages, the **maximum time** is spent in NREM 2.

Sleep and EEG Rhythms (Table 15.1)

Assessment of Sleep Disorders

Assessment involves taking a detailed history of sleep from the patient and the partner (in many sleep disturbances patient is not aware of the problems, but the partner is).

Audio-video recordings of the patient while sleeping can help diagnose certain disturbances.

Body movements during sleep (which can provide information about the duration and quality of sleep) can be measured by using wristwatch-like motion sensing devices (this technique is called **actigraphy**).

The gold standard for the evaluation of sleep is **polysomnography**. Polysomnography involves the recording of EEG (electroencephalogram), EOG (electrooculogram) and submentalis EMG (electromyogram) while the patient sleeps overnight in a sleep laboratory. The recordings are scored for stages of sleep, and other indicators such as:

a. Sleep latency: Duration between turning off lights and the individual falling asleep as ascertained by EEG and behavioural parameters.
b. Total sleep time
c. Sleep efficiency: Total sleep time/time in bed
d. REM latency: Time from sleep onset to onset of the first REM sleep period.

SLEEP-WAKE DISORDERS

Insomnias

Insomnia occasionally affects around 33% of the population, and in around 10%, it is persistent and chronic. In older adults, the prevalence is up to 25%. Women, individuals with a medical or psychiatric disorder, and shift job workers have a higher prevalence of insomnia. Insomnia and associated daytime sleepiness is a leading cause of motor vehicle accidents (sleep-related motor vehicle accidents are more common than accidents due to drunk driving and driving under the influence of drugs combined) and even industrial accidents.

Insomnia manifests as dissatisfaction with the quantity or quality of sleep and presents with one of the following:
a. Difficulty in the onset of sleep (**sleep onset insomnia**)
b. Difficulty in the maintenance of sleep (frequent awakenings at night and difficulty in going back to sleep) (**sleep maintenance insomnia**)
c. **Early morning awakening** (getting up earlier than usual time and inability to go back to sleep)

There are often associated daytime effects of poor sleep, such as poor attention and disturbances of other cognitive functions, tiredness, sleepiness, irritability and impairment of performance.

Table 15.1: EEG rhythms.

EEG rhythms	Frequency (Hz)	Amplitude (microvolt)	Salient points	Region
Alpha (α)	8–12	50–100	Seen when individual is awake, at rest, eyes closed and mind wandering	Present maximally in occipital and parieto-occipital area
Beta (β)	14–30	5–10	Normal awake pattern, when attention is focussed beta waves appear	Predominantly in frontal area
Theta (θ)	4–7	10	Transition from wakefulness to sleep early sleep	Parietal region and temporal region (hippocampus)
Delta (δ)	1–4	20–200	Deep sleep	

> There are significant differences in the DSM-5 and ICD-10 classification of sleep disorders. In the ICD-11, sleep disorders have been removed from the section of psychiatric disorders, and a separate section has been made for the sleep-wake disorder.
>
> Arguably, the most elaborate classification of sleep disorders has been done in the International Classification of Sleep Disorders. Rather than getting confused with all these different classifications, undergraduate students must focus on the important clinical aspects of sleep disorders.

Types

1. **Adjustment insomnia:** Insomnia caused by an identifiable stressor (e.g., sudden financial trouble, shifting to a new city) or anticipation of a stressor (e.g., impending exams) is called adjustment insomnia. Such insomnia is usually associated with anxiety symptoms and resolves with the resolution of the stressor.
2. **Psychophysiological insomnia (conditioned insomnia):** It is one of the commonest types of chronic insomnia. It often occurs in combination with other types of insomnia (e.g., adjustment insomnia, insomnia due to medical or psychiatric disorders). If an individual had insomnia for many days and kept lying on the bed for hours wide awake, gradually, the bed, the pillows, the bedroom, etc., become associated with a state of being awake (through **classical conditioning**). Once this conditioning develops, it maintains insomnia. These patients often report tiredness, become preoccupied with their inability to sleep and try too hard to fall asleep. At bedtime, they become anxious with racing thoughts and somatic symptoms of anxiety, such as increased muscle tension. They often sleep well outside their bedroom (as the new bedroom is not conditioned with insomnia).
3. **Subjective insomnia (sleep state misperception):** In this type, patients complaints of sleep disturbances, but objective measures (such as polysomnography) do not show any sleep abnormality.
4. **Idiopathic insomnia:** The cause of insomnia is unknown.
5. **Insomnia due to medical disorders**
6. **Insomnia due to mental disorders**
7. **Insomnia due to drug use** (prescription medicine, caffeine, alcohol)
8. **Insomnia due to inadequate sleep hygiene** (sleep hygiene refers to healthy lifestyle practices that aid in healthy sleep, discussed more in the management section)

Earlier, it was believed that insomnia is always because of some underlying cause, but now it is well established that insomnia can be an independent condition and must be appropriately managed.

Treatment

Pharmacological treatment: Benzodiazepine receptor agonists (often referred to as the **'z' drugs**, zolpidem, zaleplon, eszopiclone) and benzodiazepines are primarily used for pharmacological management of insomnia. Benzodiazepines are avoided for long term treatment due to their dependence potential. Benzodiazepines are also avoided in elderly patients (due to increased risk of falls) and in insomnia associated with sleep-related breathing disorders due to their respiratory depressant effect.

Benzodiazepine receptor agonists offer more sustained benefits for insomnia and have lesser side effects. They have become the first choice of pharmacotherapy for insomnia.

Melatonin receptor agonist ramelteon has also been approved for sleep onset insomnia. Melatonin is often used as an over-the-counter drug and may help in reducing sleep latency, but robust data about its clinical efficacy is lacking.

Sedating antidepressants like trazodone and mirtazapine are also often used to manage insomnia.

Hypnotics should ideally not be prescribed for >2 weeks due to the potential for tolerance and withdrawal, but in clinical practice, often they are prescribed for a much longer duration.

Psychotherapy: Cognitive behavioural therapy (CBT)—CBT should be preferred over pharmacological management in severe and persistent insomnia cases. CBT is effective in patients with persistent sleep problems, and the effects are maintained for the long term. Despite the superior efficacy of CBT over medications for insomnia, the practical problems prevent the widespread use of CBT. CBT takes longer than medications to show results, and often patients want immediate relief. Also, CBT happens over multiple sessions, requires trained professionals and also requires a willingness on the part of the patient to indulge in therapy. Many different behavioural and cognitive techniques can be used, and there is no clear advantage of any one technique over another. The techniques used commonly include:

a. **Universal sleep hygiene:** Sleep hygiene includes healthy lifestyle practices that aid in sleep and include the following—
   1. Keep a regular time for going to bed and getting up
   2. Avoid heavy meals in the dinner
   3. Avoid caffeine in the afternoon and evening (remember half-life of caffeine is around 5 hours); other stimulants should be similarly avoided
   4. Keep the bedroom comfortable and conducive for sleep
   5. Do regular exercise (in the morning, late afternoon or evening). Exercise should be avoided in the late evening as it may increase arousal
   6. Try to wind down before going to bed, and do not indulge in mental tasks that may cause worry or increased anxiety
   7. Use the bed only for sleep and sex (avoid other activities like watching television, reading, eating, etc., while sitting on the bed)
   8. Do not use alcohol to help with sleep
   9. Do not look at your watch repeatedly when not able to sleep

   Avoid daytime naps (not applicable for all)

b. **Stimulus control therapy:** This therapy aims to ensure that the bed, bedroom, and nighttime are associated with sleepiness and not wakefulness. Some of the instructions given to the patient include:
   1. Go to bed only when sleepy so that chances of falling asleep quickly are high (if a person is lying in bed awake

for long periods, the bed becomes associated with a state of wakefulness gradually).
2. If not able to fall asleep in 15–20 minutes or sleep breaks and not able to go back to sleep, get out of the bed, go to some other room and do something non-stimulating till you feel sleepy again.
3. Sleeping is not allowed in areas other than the bedroom and at times other than the night.
4. Bed is to be used only for sleep (and sex). No reading, talking on the phone, or watching television is allowed in bed.
5. To improve the sleep-wake cycle, get up at the same time in the morning (irrespective of the time one was able to fall asleep).

c. **Sleep restriction therapy:** This therapy aims to increase sleep efficiency (time asleep/time in bed), particularly for those patients who lie in bed, awake, for long periods. If an individual can sleep for 5 hours only but lies in bed for 8 hours, it results in poor sleep efficiency. In this case, the person is told to go to bed around 5 hours before the fixed waking up time to improve sleep efficiency. Once sleep efficiency increases, gradually, the time in bed is increased.

d. **Cognitive restructuring:** Irrational thoughts and faulty beliefs about sleep (such as 'If I don't sleep, the next day will be a complete waste') may lead to anxiety that further increases insomnia. The patient is taught to identify and challenge these thoughts.

e. **Thought suppression:** A chain of thoughts at bedtime may lead to insomnia. Articulatory suppression, in which the patient is asked to repeat the word 'the' subvocally every 3 seconds, may help break the chain and facilitate sleep.

f. **Relaxation therapy and feedback:** Use of deep breathing exercises, progressive muscle relaxation, imagery exercises (wherein the person imagines being at a peaceful and relaxing place such as on a beach or a park), or biofeedback can be used to induce relaxation that may help with the sleep.

g. **Paradoxical intention:** It works in some cases, wherein the patient is instructed to try 'not' fall asleep (hence paradoxical). This is believed to alleviate performance anxiety and may help with sleep.

Hypersomnolence Disorder (Excessive Sleepiness)

Excessive sleepiness can be life-threatening; almost 50% of patients with excessive sleepiness report automobile accidents. It also adversely impacts concentration, attention, memory and other cognitive functions, motivation to work, and mood.

Test for Hypersomnolence

During evaluation for hypersomnolence, a detailed history from the patient and family members is necessary. The history must be supplemented with laboratory tests to make the diagnosis. Some important tests include:

1. **Multiple sleep latency test:** The basic premise of the test is that 'the sleepier the subject is, the faster he will fall asleep'. In this test, beginning 2 hours after morning awakening, the subject is provided 20 minutes nap opportunities, repeated every 2 hours (EEG, EOG and EMG are used to record the sleep stage). The mean latency (in 4 or 5 tests) to fall asleep, called the global sleepiness index, is calculated. Sleep latency of <5 minutes indicates pathological sleepiness, the latency of 10–20 minutes is considered normal, and if latency is in between, it is considered to be in a diagnostic grey zone.

2. **Maintenance of wakefulness test (MWT):** In this test, the subject sits in a comfortable chair or bed in a darkened room and is asked to try to remain awake. Four 40 minutes sessions are done at 2 hours intervals. Inability to stay awake on MWT shows some level of sleepiness, and a mean sleep latency of <8 minutes is considered abnormal (between 8–40 minutes is in a diagnostic grey zone).

3. **Polysomnography:** Traditional polysomnography or ambulatory recordings can be used to determine actual sleep time in a 24 hours period.

Types of Hypersomnia

1. **Kleine–Levin syndrome:** It is a type of recurrent hypersomnia usually seen in adolescent males. The syndrome is characterised by recurrent episodes of **hypersomnia** (sleep of 18–20 hours a day) associated with behavioural disorders such as **hypersexuality** (making inappropriate sexual advances, masturbation in public, expression of sexual desire in a socially unacceptable manner), **hyperphagia** (with binge eating) and behavioural oddities (e.g., behaving like a child). Other symptoms include disorientation, hallucinations, and feeling of unreality.

    In between the episodes, the person is asymptomatic. The patient may have amnesia for episodes, which may last from a few days to a few weeks.

    Treatment: Stimulants like modafinil or amphetamines can be used to manage hypersomnia. In severe cases, prophylactic treatment with mood stabilisers (carbamazepine, lithium, valproic acid) can be used to prevent future episodes.

2. **Menstrual-related hypersomnia:** It presents with hypersomnia that starts at or shortly before the menses, lasts around for a week and resolves with menstruation. Hormonal imbalance appears to be the cause, and treatment with oral contraceptive pills is usually effective.

3. **Idiopathic hypersomnia:** It includes two different types:
    a. **Idiopathic hypersomnia with long sleep time:** It is characterised by long sleep periods and unwanted naps, which are not refreshing. Getting up from sleep is laborious; patient often does not wake up to the alarm clock and rely on family members who use vigorous procedures to wake them up. Even after getting up, the patient may appear confused and not completely in his senses (often referred to as 'sleep drunkenness'). The EEG pattern is similar to normal individuals who are sleep deprived and remains like that despite several nights of long hours of sleep.

b. Idiopathic hypersomnia without long sleep time manifests with isolated excessive daytime sleepiness.

Some of these patients have autonomic nervous system dysfunction (and are HLA-Cw2 positive), others may develop the symptoms post viral infections (e.g., GBS, mononucleosis), and others are truly idiopathic.

The MSLT is usually <8. For treatment, modafinil is used.

4. **Behaviourally induced insufficient sleep syndrome:** Individuals who routinely obtain less than required sleep develop this syndrome which manifests with excessive sleepiness in the afternoon or early evening. Associated symptoms include poor concentration, fatigue and irritability. This syndrome is widespread among truck drivers, doctors, students, executives, and working mothers. Treatment involves increasing the duration and regularity of sleep.

5. **Narcolepsy:** Narcolepsy presents with hypersomnia and is caused by the intrusion of REM sleep into the waking state (there is a **sudden intrusion of REM sleep elements in a person who is awake**, leading to characteristic symptoms). The onset is usually in adolescence or young adulthood. Narcolepsy can be divided into two types:
   A. Narcolepsy with cataplexy
   B. Narcolepsy without cataplexy

   A. **Narcolepsy with cataplexy:** It is characterised by two cardinal features:
      i. **Irresistible sleep episodes (sleep attacks):** It is the most common symptom of narcolepsy. Patient experiences excessive daytime sleepiness, which builds up into an irresistible sleep episode (as the patient can not stop himself from sleeping, it is often referred to as a sleep attack) that usually lasts for 10-20 minutes, after which the patient feels refreshed, at least for a brief period. These attacks usually happen during passive times, such as while watching the television or attending a lecture, but may also occur while talking, driving (can cause accidents) and even during sex. Excessive sleepiness can also result in automatic behaviours such as saying inappropriate words.
      ii. **Cataplexy:** It is the most specific symptom of narcolepsy. Cataplexy is characterised by sudden bilateral loss of voluntary muscle tone, while the patient remains conscious. Usually, only some muscles are involved, such as jaw muscles (leading to jaw drop), facial muscles (leading to grimace), and thigh muscles (causing weakness of knees), but rarely there may be paralysis of all skeletal muscles (except extraocular and respiratory musculature) leading to a collapse. The patient remains conscious, although if the attack is long, it may merge with a sleep episode. The cataplexy is usually precipitated by positive environmental factors such as laughter or humour; it can also be precipitated by anger but never by fear or stress. It can be conceptualised as an intrusion of muscle atonia (which is a feature of REM sleep) into the waking state.

      Apart from the two cardinal features, there are accessory symptoms that include:
      iii. **Hypnagogic hallucinations (and hypnopompic hallucinations):** Patients may have auditory or visual hallucinations at the onset of sleep (hypnagogic hallucinations) or at the time of waking up (hypnopompic) and may be frightened by these experiences. These can be conceptualised as 'vivid dreams' (which are usually a part of REM sleep) that intrude while the patient is still conscious or partially conscious.
      iv. **Sleep paralysis:** It is seen usually while getting up in the morning, wherein the patient wakes up and is conscious but is not able to move at all (hence the term 'paralysis'). Sleep paralysis is again similar to a REM sleep element, i.e., muscle atonia. (Kindly remember, isolated sleep paralysis can occasionally occur in otherwise healthy individuals too).

      Apart from these symptoms, nocturnal sleep disruption with recurrent awakening is common. REM sleep behaviour disorder (explained later) can also be present.

   B. **Narcolepsy without cataplexy:** The rest of the symptoms are present, except for cataplexy

   The hallmark of narcolepsy is **reduced latency of REM sleep**. Usually, it takes around 90 minutes to reach REM sleep (after crossing all the NREM sleep stages); however, in patients with narcolepsy, the patient reaches REM sleep much earlier. Narcolepsy is caused by a deficiency of **hypocretin**, a neurotransmitter that promotes appetite and alertness. Hypocretin secreting neurons project from **the hypothalamus** to other parts of the brain.

   There is a strong association of narcolepsy with **human leukocyte antigens class II** (HLA-DR2 and HLA-DQB1*0602). It has been hypothesised that narcolepsy is an immune-mediated disorder and is caused by autoimmune destruction of hypothalamic neurons that secret hypocretin.

   Investigations:
   i. **Polysomnography and MSLT:** At night, a sleep-onset REM period (defined as REM sleep latency less than or equal to 15 minutes) is highly specific, and is present in 25–50% of patients with narcolepsy. MSLT shows sleep latency of <8 minutes and two or more sleep-onset REM periods.
   ii. **CSF levels of hypocretin-1:** Below 110 pg/mL is considered highly specific and sensitive for narcolepsy with cataplexy.

   Treatment:
   i. **Pharmacological treatment:** The mainstay of treatment is pharmacological.
      a. **Modafinil:** Modafinil (an α1-adrenergic receptor agonist) is considered the first-line treatment for

reducing sleep attacks. Methylphenidate is not as commonly used nowadays.

  b. **SSRIs and TCAs:** By virtue of their REM sleep suppressant actions, SSRIs and TCAs can be used to reduce cataplexy.
  c. **Sodium oxybate:** It is used for the management of sleep attacks and cataplexy.

  ii. **Non-pharmacological management:** A regimen of forced naps at regular intervals during the day often helps to reduce sleep attacks. Patients are also asked to ensure that they don't do any potentially dangerous activity (e.g., driving, swimming, handling heavy machinery) when alone.

6. **Hypersomnia due to a medical condition:** Various neurological conditions such as stroke, head trauma, Parkinson's disease, multiple system atrophy, normal pressure hydrocephalus, Arnold–Chiari malformations, and myotonic dystrophy can present with hypersomnia. Infectious diseases like Epstein–Barr disease, atypical viral pneumonia, hepatitis B, Guillain–Barré syndrome, and human African trypanosomiasis are also associated with hypersomnia.
7. **Hypersomnia due to drugs or substance use:** Hypnotics, antidepressants, antipsychotics, antihistamines, and opioids can also cause hypersomnia. Withdrawal from stimulants like cocaine, amphetamines, caffeine or nicotine can also cause hypersomnia.
8. **Hypersomnia in the context of sleep-related breathing disorder:** The most common condition amongst these is **obstructive sleep apnoea**, which is characterised by repetitive collapse or partial collapse of the upper airway while the person is asleep. Clinical features include nighttime symptoms such as loud snoring and apnoea episodes (sleep apnoea episode is defined as stopping of breathing for 10 seconds or more during sleep) which ends with sonorous breathing resumption, nocturia, and tiredness and headache at waking up. Along with these, the patient experiences excessive sleepiness, irritability, poor concentration, and depressed mood during the daytime.

Patients are often obese, but obesity is not always present. They may have a narrow upper airway due to closely set posterior tonsillar pillars, abnormally long and hypotonic soft palate, macroglossia and a hypertrophic uvula. Patients with obstructive sleep apnoea are at risk of developing systemic hypertension, arrhythmias, cardiac or cerebral ischaemia, depression and cognitive impairments.

Treatment: **CPAP (continuous positive airway pressure)** is the most widely used treatment. Weight loss can be of help. In certain cases, surgical reconstruction is done to correct the airway obstructions and malformations. In mild obstructive sleep apnoea, oral appliances can be used. These oral appliances manipulate the jaw's position, lift the palate or retain the tongue, thereby widening the upper airway.

Circadian Rhythm Sleep Disorders

These disorders are caused by a lack of alignment between an individual's internal circadian rhythm and the desired or conventional sleep-wake cycle (based on the social or professional schedule).

The intrinsic sleep-wake rhythm is slightly >24 hours (to be precise, it is 24 hours 15 minutes). It gets synchronised with 24 hours day-night rhythm by bright light, social cues such as mealtimes, and social activities. Failure to achieve this synchronisation results in circadian rhythm sleep disorders.

The circadian clock of the body that regulates the timing of sleep is in the **suprachiasmatic nucleus of the hypothalamus.**

Types of Circadian Rhythm Sleep Disorder

1. **Delayed sleep phase type (the night owls):** In this type, the biological clock runs slower than 24 hours or is delayed, and hence the major sleep period is delayed (usually by >2 hours) to desired sleep wake-up time. The patients complain of sleep onset insomnia, difficulty waking up in the morning, and excessive sleepiness in the early daytime. For example, the person does not feel sleepy till say 3 AM at night and cannot wake up before 11 AM the next morning. So, if this person works in an office which starts at 10 AM, he is likely to face significant difficulties.
2. **Advanced sleep phase type (early birds):** In this type, the biological clock is faster than 24 hours or shifted early. These individuals have the major sleep period earlier (usually by >2 hours) than the desired sleep wake-up time. They feel sleepy in the evening, retire to bed early and are up early morning.
3. **Irregular sleep-wake type:** Here, there is a lack of proper circadian rhythm. The sleep is fragmented into 2–3 sleep periods, and there is no major sleep period. There are complaints of insomnia at night and excessive sleepiness in the daytime. It is typically seen in patients with neurodegenerative disorders like Alzheimer's disease or neurodevelopmental disorders in children.
4. **Non-24-hour sleep wake type:** As discussed above, the internal circadian rhythm is slightly more than the 24-hour day-night rhythm and needs to be reset every day. Failure to do so can result in non-24-hour sleep-wake disorder. In this disorder, the sleep onset keeps on getting delayed progressively, resulting in worsening sleep onset insomnia and daytime sleepiness. Gradually, the sleep onset gets shifted to the daytime, and the person is unable to sleep at night. As the cycle continues, the sleep onset again starts moving towards the normal time, resulting in a short duration when the individual's circadian rhythm matches with the 24-hour day-night cycle. The whole cycle repeats itself. This disorder is commonly seen in the blind and can also be seen in patients with traumatic brain injury.
5. **Shift work type:** It is seen in individuals doing shift work and is worse with frequent shift rotations. The symptoms include excessive sleepiness at work and impaired sleep at home, resulting in a profound sleep loss.
6. **Jet lag type:** Air travel to a different time zone can lead to a desynchronisation between the person's circadian rhythm and the environmental day-night cycle leading to sleep disturbances. It has been observed that a shift of one to two time zones does not cause much disturbance as the body is able to adapt, but if the transition involves

more time zones, the body takes longer to adapt, and in the intervening period, sleep disturbances may ensue.

Treatment

1. **Chronotherapy:** The goal of chronotherapy is to synchronise the individual's circadian rhythm with the desired sleep-wake cycle. To do so, the individual's sleep is progressively delayed by 2–3 hours a night till the two rhythms get synchronised. During the treatment, odd sleeping hours can interfere with the work significantly. Hence, nowadays, light therapy is preferred over chronotherapy.
2. **Light therapy or phototherapy:** Bright light (>10,000 lux) and particularly blue part of the light spectrum can be used to alter the internal circadian rhythm. This can be used to synchronise the circadian rhythm with the desired sleep-wake schedule. For example, in patients with delayed sleep phase, bright light can be given early morning to advance the phase and match with the desired schedule. Similarly, in patients with advanced sleep phase, bright light can be given in the evening to delay the phase. Such treatment can also be used in shift work type and jet lag type disorders.
3. **Melatonin:** Melatonin release is related to the dark-light cycle. It gets secreted by the pineal gland during darkness (increased secretion from dusk till dawn), and its secretion is inhibited by bright light. Melatonin influences circadian rhythm via the suprachiasmatic nucleus. Over-the-counter, melatonin or synthetic melatonin agonist (ramelteon) can be used for sleep-onset insomnia and other circadian rhythm disorders.

Parasomnias

Parasomnias are a group of sleep disorders characterised by **undesirable physical or behavioural phenomena** that occur during sleep or are potentiated by sleep. These can emerge while falling asleep, during sleep or at arousal from any stage of sleep. Objective diagnosis of parasomnias can be made by polysomnography.

Parasomnias can be conceptualised as loss of boundary between wakefulness, NREM sleep and REM sleep with elements from one of these stages intruding into the other, resulting in the characteristic features.

NREM Sleep Arousal Disorders (NREM Sleep Parasomnias)

These are 'disorders of arousal' from sleep and usually occur during NREM-3 and 4 (slow-wave sleep). The following are the types:

1. **Sleepwalking (somnambulism):** In this condition, the individual who was asleep, gets up from the bed and aimlessly wanders without getting fully awake. The individual may carry out more complex behaviours like carrying objects from one place to another, rearranging furniture, going outdoors and rarely even driving a car. During the episode, the eyes are usually wide open, and the individual is able to maintain basic interaction with the environment, e.g., the individual is able to dodge the objects in the way while walking; however, communication with the sleepwalker is usually not possible. The sleepwalker may show poor judgement (e.g., may try to walk out of the window or walk in the middle of the road), which may lead to accidents. Rarely there may be aggression during the episode. No attempt should be made to wake up the sleepwalker by shouting or shaking, as that might be misconstrued as an attack by the sleepwalker, who may respond violently. Gently leading the sleepwalker back to the bed is the better approach. There is no memory of the sleepwalking episodes the next day. Sleepwalking is quite common in children and is rarely seen in adults. In some cases of sleepwalking, there may be eating during the episode (called sleep-related eating) or sexual behaviour in the form of masturbation, sexual advances or even intercourse (called sex-related sleep behaviour or sexsomnia) for which the patient has no recollection.
2. **Sleep terror (pavor nocturnus):** It is characterised by a sudden arousal from sleep (from NREM 3 or 4 sleep), wherein an individual gets up with a scream and appears fearful. There are accompanying somatic symptoms of anxiety (such as tachypnoea, tachycardia, etc.). The person is usually unresponsive and, if awakened, looks confused. Occasionally there are movements like jumping out of bed, during which injury may happen. Unlike in nightmares, in which the person sees an elaborate dream, in sleep terrors, usually, the individual does not see any images or may see some static images. The person has amnesia for the event. Sleep terror is more commonly seen in children.

   Both sleepwalking and sleep terror can be provoked by sleep deprivation.
3. **Sleep talking (somniloquy):** As the name suggests, the person talks during sleep with varying degrees of comprehensibility in this disorder. It is by far the most common parasomnia, with a prevalence of >50% in children aged 3–13 years. Its frequent comorbidity with sleepwalking and sleep terrors suggests common pathophysiology for the three disorders.

Treatment: In children, usually, treatment is not required. **Reassuring** the parents that these episodes would disappear as the child grows up while ensuring that the child does not injure self during the episodes is required. In cases, there are injuries/likelihood of injuries during the episode and further episodes need to be stopped, treatment with benzodiazepines like clonazepam is usually effective.

Parasomnias Associated with REM Sleep Disorders

1. **REM sleep behaviour disorder:** As previously discussed, one of the features of REM sleep is muscular atonia. Even vivid dreams, in which an individual is running, fighting, jumping, etc., do not elicit any body movement in the dreamer as the muscles are in a state of atonia. In cases the atonia fails to develop, the person may end up enacting the dreams and may make violent movements ending up in injuries to self or the bed partner. This is what happens in REM sleep behaviour disorders. It is more common in older males. Around 50% of cases are

associated with neurological disorders, predominantly neurodegenerative disorders (especially parkinsonism).

Treatment involves the use of clonazepam and ensuring the safety of the patient and partner by modulating the sleep environment.

2. **Nightmare disorder:** Nightmares are scary dreams that cause sympathetic activation and finally wake up the dreamer. After waking up, the individual can recall the dream (unlike sleep terror, where the person is not able to recall the dream). Frequent nightmares are distressing, and the person may become afraid of sleep, resulting in insomnia. Sleep deprivation is in itself a risk factor for nightmares, and hence a vicious cycle may ensue. Nightmares are quite common in young children and rare in adults. Most patients with nightmares do not have any psychiatric disorder. In some cases, e.g., in patients with PTSD, nightmares are a part of the symptomatology. Treatment involves the use of benzodiazepines and behavioural techniques such as universal sleep hygiene and cognitive behavioural therapy.
3. **Nocturnal enuresis:** Discussed in child psychiatry

SLEEP-RELATED MOVEMENT DISORDERS

1. **Restless legs syndrome (Ekbom syndrome):** It is characterised by an unpleasant, "creepy crawly sensation" (sensation of ants crawling on the skin) in the lower extremities during times of inactivity, such as while trying to fall asleep. These sensations are relieved by movement of the legs, squeezing or rubbing the legs, or walking; however, making such movements causes disturbances in sleep and leads to insomnia. Dopaminergic agonists (pramipexole and ropinirole) are FDA approved for the treatment of restless legs syndrome.
2. **Periodic limb movement disorder:** It is characterised by sudden, repetitive movement of limbs, usually, legs, during NREM sleep. The movement involves the extension of the big toe and partial flexion of the ankle, knee or even hip joint. The movement may cause partial arousal and disturbance of sleep, and there may be excessive sleepiness the next day. The sleep of the partner often gets disturbed. Treatment involves the use of benzodiazepines or opiates.
3. **Sleep-related bruxism:** It is characterised by grinding or clenching of teeth during sleep. It may damage the teeth, cause jaw pain, or the sound may disturb the bed partner. It usually occurs in NREM 2, but it can also occur in other stages. It was formerly classified as a parasomnia. Treatment involves wearing an oral appliance to protect the teeth during sleep. Benzodiazepines can be used for the treatment.

CASE BASED MCQ

A 30-year-old female complained of excessive daytime sleepiness along with episodes of irresistible urges to sleep, due to which she slept once in the middle of a conversation and once in the grocery store. She also had a jaw drop while laughing on a few occasions, which was very embarrassing for her. The patient also reported hearing strange voices when she is about to fall asleep; what is the likely diagnosis?
a. Narcolepsy with cataplexy
b. Narcolepsy without cataplexy
c. Obstructive sleep apnoea
d. Pavor nocturnus

Ans. a. History of sleep attacks, cataplexy (sudden loss of muscle tone manifesting as jaw drop in the patient) and hypnagogic hallucinations (hearing strange voices while falling asleep) is suggestive of narcolepsy with cataplexy.

SUGGESTED READINGS

1. Walker M. Why we sleep: Unlocking the power of sleep and dreams. Simon and Schuster; 2017.
2. American Psychiatric Association. Diagnostic and Statistical Manual of Mental Disorders. Arlington, VA: American Psychiatric Publishing, 2013.
3. Boland R, Verduin M. Kaplan & Sadock's Concise Textbook of Clinical Psychiatry. Lippincott Williams & Wilkins; 2021.
4. Sadock BJ, Sadock VA, Ruiz P. Comprehensive textbook of psychiatry 10th edition.
5. World Health Organization. ICD-11 for mortality and morbidity statistics (2018).

16 Sexual Disorders

Sujita Kumar Kar, Praveen Tripathi

PS13.1	Enumerate and describe the magnitude and aetiology of psychosexual and gender identity disorders
PS13.2	Enumerate, elicit, describe and document clinical features in patients with magnitude and aetiology of psychosexual and gender identity disorders
PS13.3	Enumerate and describe the indications and interpret laboratory and other tests used in psychosexual and gender identity disorders
PS13.4	Describe the treatment of psychosexual and gender identity disorders including behavioural, psychosocial and pharmacologic therapy
PS13.5	Demonstrate family education in a patient with psychosexual and gender identity disorders in a simulated environment
PS13.6	Enumerate and describe the pharmacologic basis and side effects of drugs used in psychosexual and gender identity disorders
PS13.7	Enumerate the appropriate conditions for specialist referral

NORMAL HUMAN SEXUALITY

Sexuality has many aspects. Four interrelated factors determine human sexuality. These include:
1. **Sexual identity:** Sexual identity refers to the individual's biological sexual characteristics (chromosomes, hormones, internal genitalia, external genitalia and secondary sexual characteristics).
2. **Gender identity:** Gender identity is the individual's sense of being a male or a female. Biological factors (genes, hormones, physical characteristics like genitalia, body shape, etc.) and psychosocial factors (e.g., the differential way in which parents and society at large behave with a child depending upon the gender) play a role in the development of the gender identity. By the age of 3 years, the child can appreciate his or her gender, and gradually the child learns to behave in a distinct gender-specific manner. Usually, an individual's gender identity and anatomical sex are congruent, (e.g., a person with male anatomical sex considers himself to be a 'man'); however, if they are not congruent, it may result in the development of gender dysphoria.
3. **Sexual orientation:** It describes whether the individual is sexually attracted to the opposite sex (heterosexual), same-sex (homosexual) or both (bisexual).
4. **Sexual behaviour:** Sexual behaviour of an individual is impacted by various factors that include biological, psychological and socio-cultural factors.

SEXUAL RESPONSE CYCLE

William Masters and Virginia Johnson studied the physiological response to sexual stimulation in both men and women, called as sexual response cycle.

The sexual response in normal individuals goes through a series of steps, during which specific physiological changes occur. Specific hormones and neurotransmitters mediate the physiological processes during each step.

The sexual response cycle is divided into four phases:
1. **Desire phase:** This phase is characterised by sexual fantasies, wishes for having sex and feeling the need to develop a sexual bond with the partner.
2. **Excitement phase:** This phase is characterised by psychological and/or physiological stimulation resulting in penile intumescence and erection in males and vaginal lubrication in females. In this phase, in males, a few drops of mucoid secretion (which may contain viable sperm) from the Cowper's gland may appear in the urethral aperture, and some individuals may confuse it with premature ejaculation. Similarly, during the excitement phase in females, erection of nipple, congestion and engorgement of labia, vaginal lubrication, and retraction of shaft of clitoris into prepuce occurs. The excitement phase can last from several minutes to several hours. Some authors describe the final part of the excitement phase as a separate phase called the, plateau phase, and it is characterised by intensified sexual tensions before orgasm.

3. **Orgasm phase:** In this phase, there is a peaking of sexual pleasure, followed by the release of sexual tension and ejaculation of semen. In females, orgasm is characterised by involuntary contraction of the lower third of the vagina and contractions from the fundus downward to the cervix. An increase in respiratory rate, heart rate and blood pressure is observed in the excitement and orgasmic phase in both genders. The orgasm phase lasts for 3–15 seconds, and it is the **shortest phase** of the sexual response cycle.
4. **Resolution phase:** It is the last phase of the sexual response cycle, in which there is a return to the pre-excitement level. This phase lasts for 10–15 minutes. If there is no orgasm, it may last from half to a full day. Penile detumescence, the disappearance of flushes and cessation of uterine contraction occur during this stage. Males often go into a **refractory state** (a state of nonarousal to any form of sexual stimuli), which may last from a few minutes to a few days depending on age and other factors.

Various neurotransmitters and hormones play a crucial role in different stages of the sexual response cycle. These are summarised in the **Table 16.1** below.

Table 16.1: Hormones and neurotransmitters role in different stages of sexual response cycle.

Hormones/Neurotransmitters	Effect on sexual response cycle
Dopamine	Increases desire (both gender)
Serotonin	Decreases desire (both gender)
Testosterone	Increases libido (both gender)
Estrogen	• Increases lubrication (in females) • Increases sensitivity for stimulation (in females)
Progesterone	Decreases desire (in both gender)
Prolactin	Decreases desire (in both gender)
Cortisol	Decreases desire (in both gender)
Oxytocin	Increases pleasure (in both gender), i.e., enhances orgasm

MASTURBATION

Masturbation, which involves self-stimulation, is usually a precursor of partner-related sexual behaviour. Following puberty, boys and girls feel sexual urges and tensions. To derive sexual pleasure, they may indulge in self-stimulating sexual activities, which helps in releasing the sexual tension. Research suggests that almost all males and three-fourths of females masturbate sometime during their lives. People may continue to masturbate even when in a sexual relationship. Contrary to widespread myths in society, masturbation has not been found to cause any physical or sexual disorder.

Masturbation is, however, considered pathological if it is **compulsive** (beyond a person's willful control), is done at a socially inappropriate place, (e.g., masturbating in a public place) or if it becomes the predominant mode of sexual activity and is preferred over sex with the stable partner, leading to distress in the relationship.

HOMOSEXUALITY

Homosexuality is **not considered an illness**. It is considered a normal variant of human sexuality. Often terms such as gay (for men) and lesbian (for women) are used to denote homosexual orientation. Research suggests that the prevalence of homosexuality is 2–4% in the general population. Most individuals with homosexual orientation report that they had an onset of same-sex attraction during adolescence or even before that; however, typically, it takes a few years before individuals are able to accept and become comfortable with their sexuality. Many individuals with a homosexual orientation (both men and women) have had heterosexual experiences too. Also, it has been found that homosexual relationships tend to be more stable in females (female-female relationships) than in males (male-male relationships).

Biological and genetic factors contribute to the development of homosexual orientation, and it is not a matter of choice. The concordance rate for homosexual orientation is higher in monozygotic twins than in dizygotic twins. Also, there is a familial distribution, with the prevalence of homosexual orientation higher in the brothers of homosexual men compared to heterosexual men.

The impact of genetic factors appears to be different in male and female homosexuality. Female homosexuality has been found to be more linked to hormonal and epigenetic mechanisms. The prenatal exposure to androgens has been found to play a role, and women with congenital adrenal hyperplasia (CAH), who get exposed to high levels of testosterone during the prenatal imprinting, have been found to have a higher rate of homosexual orientation in comparison to nonCAH women. Some studies have found lower levels of androgens in males with homosexual orientation than heterosexual males.

Few studies have found evidence of linkage between the Xq28 allele (on the X chromosome) and male homosexuality.

> In September 2018, in a landmark ruling, the Supreme Court of India decriminalised adult consensual same-sex relationships. Many countries around the world have similarly decriminalised consensual same-sex relationships.

GENDER DYSPHORIA (GENDER INCONGRUENCE)

Gender dysphoria is characterised by **incongruence** between the experienced gender (the gender with which an individual identifies with, gender identity) and the one they were born with (referred to as assigned gender). It is more commonly seen in males (assigned gender) than females.

A. **Gender dysphoria (gender incongruence) in children:** The disorder usually first manifests in preschool years. The following are the characteristic features:
   1. The child shows a preference for the dress and play activities that are typically associated with the opposite gender, (e.g., a male child shows a preference towards skirts and may play exclusively with dolls and reject the

cars and other toys which boys usually prefer. Also, the child prefers girls as playmates).
2. The child expresses a strong desire to be of the opposite gender.
3. Some children may express dislike for one's sexual anatomy, (e.g., a male child may repeatedly assert that the penis and testicles are disgusting and will disappear in due course of time) and may express a strong desire for secondary sexual characters of the opposite gender.
4. The symptoms do not necessarily carry into adulthood, and >50% of these children start identifying with their assigned gender by the time they become adults.

B. **Gender dysphoria (gender incongruence) in adolescents and adults:** It is characterised by the following features—
1. There is a significant discomfort with one's primary and secondary sexual characteristics and a desire to get 'rid' of them. Sometimes, individuals with gender dysphoria use phrases like '**I am a man trapped in a woman's body**' or vice versa to express how they feel.
2. A strong desire to get the primary and secondary sexual characteristics of the opposite gender.
3. A desire to live and be treated as the other gender.

Most of the adults with gender dysphoria report that they identified with the other gender from the very childhood. These individuals frequently have a homosexual orientation.

The diagnosis of gender dysphoria is only made when the individual is significantly distressed or impaired. In cases of gender dysphoria in children, the distress of the caregiver is not enough to make the diagnosis. A diagnosis should be made only if the child has significant distress and impairment.

> **Few important terms:**
> 1. **Transgender:** Its a broad term used to describe all the individuals who identify with a different gender than the one they were born with (assigned sex).
> 2. **Transsexuals:** Transgender people who want to have their bodies changed and have the body of the opposite sex are called transsexuals.
> 3. **Genderqueers:** These are the individuals who do not identify with either gender. They may feel that they belong to both, or feel that they are in between the genders, or may identify with neither gender.

Aetiology of Gender Dysphoria

Certain biological and psychosocial factors are known to play a role in the development of gender dysphoria. Though the gender-specific hormones in individuals with gender dysphoria are usually normal; however, there is a hypothesis that significant alterations in these hormones at crucial periods of embryonic development could result in disrupted brain development (especially in the hypothalamus, particularly the preoptic nucleus) that may lead to the development of gender dysphoria in later life.

Genetic factors also play a role in the development of gender dysphoria. Abnormalities in the development of sexual organs may also contribute to the development of gender dysphoria. In-utero exposure to phthalates increases the fetal testosterone level and increases the risk of developing gender dysphoria.

Psychosocial factors like socio-cultural perception about the gender of the individual play a crucial role in the development of gender identity. Abuse and neglect during childhood, sexual abuse and maltreatment may contribute to the development of gender dysphoria.

> In older versions of DSM and in ICD-10, the diagnosis of 'Gender Identity Disorder' was used, and it corresponds to the diagnosis of 'Gender dysphoria' in DSM-5. ICD-11 uses the term '**gender incongruence**' instead of 'gender dysphoria'.

Treatment

In children, treatment focuses on providing psychotherapy to the child and parents and guiding the child in exploring the gender identity further.

Sometimes in adolescents (particularly those who have significant anxiety about impending physical changes during puberty), puberty-blocking endocrine treatment (GnRH agonists) is used to provide more time to the patient and the family to make a decision.

In adults, psychotherapy is offered to help the individuals explore the issues and the available options. The use of hormonal treatment and surgical procedures helps in improving the quality of life.

Hormonal treatment: Individuals who identify with the male gender can be helped with testosterone treatment. Testosterone injections help increase muscle mass, and cause cessation of menses and later on, with continued treatment, there are changes like deepening of the voice, increase in body hair, and the enlargement of the clitoris.

Individuals who identify with the female gender are offered estrogen, progesterone, and testosterone blockers. This helps with the redistribution of fat in the female pattern and breast tissue growth. However, voice change does not happen as testosterone permanently deepens the voice. Erection and ejaculation get decreased.

With hormone therapy, fertility is reduced (or lost) in both sexes.

Surgery: Sex reassignment surgeries help individuals with gender dysphoria in transition to their desired gender. Most commonly, surgery involves the construction of either a male contoured chest or breast augmentation (the '**top surgery**').

Surgery on genitals, the sex reassignment surgeries are less common and include:
a. *Metoidioplasty*: Freeing the clitoris from ligament and increase in the length and girth of the clitoris (giving it a look more similar to the penis)
b. *Scrotoplasty*: Placement of testicular implants
c. *Phalloplasty*: Creation of penis, using skin from other parts
d. *Vaginoplasty*: Involves removal of testes, reconstruction of the penis into a clitoris, and creation of a vagina.
e. *Orchiectomy*: Removal of testes.

In both DSM-5 and ICD-11, gender dysphoria (gender incongruence) has been described separately from sexual disorders. In this book, for the sake of convenience, this topic has been clubbed with sexual disorders.

SEXUAL DYSFUNCTIONS

Sexual dysfunctions are characterised by impairment in the subjective need and experience, or objective performance related to sex. Sexual dysfunction may affect isolated phases of the sexual response cycle or may involve the entire cycle. Sexual dysfunctions can be:

a. Lifelong (present since the individual became sexually active) or acquired (developed later after a period of normal functioning).
b. Generalised (not limited to any partner or situation) or situational (limited to specific partners or situations).

DISORDERS OF DESIRE PHASE

Male Hypoactive Sexual Desire Disorder

It is characterised by decreased to an absent desire for sexual activity. The patient may have reduced to absent sexual fantasies too. It is more prevalent in older individuals. Male hypoactive sexual desire disorder is often comorbid with other sexual dysfunctions (erectile disorder, ejaculatory disorders).

Aetiology

The presence of chronic stress or psychiatric disorders like anxiety disorders, depression or alcohol use can decrease sexual desire. Poor relationship with the partner, hostility towards the partner, and lack of sex for long periods, are some of the factors known to decrease sexual desire. Negative attitude towards sex (considering sex as sinful or dirty), early life adversities, inadequate sex education, medical conditions (hyperprolactinaemia, hypogonadism) and increasing age can also result in a decreased desire for sex.

Treatment

Treatment primarily involves psychological management that includes general behavioural management in the form of relaxation, sex education, clarification of myths about sexuality and sensate focus techniques (discussed later in the Chapter) and individual cognitive-behavioural therapy.

Pharmacological management includes Apomorphine (a centrally acting D1 and D2 receptor agonist, which is also available in sublingual form) and Bupropion (an antidepressant).

Female Sexual Interest/Arousal Disorder

Unlike males (who have desire before arousal/excitement), in females, both desire and arousal often happen simultaneously. Hence, the interest and arousal disorders have been clubbed in a single entity. This disorder is characterised by:

a. Most common complaint is lack of pleasure during sexual activity.
b. Absent or reduced sexual fantasies, interest in sex and lack of receptivity to partner's initiation.

Often comorbidities like inability to achieve orgasm and dyspareunia are present in patients with female sexual interest/arousal disorders.

Aetiology

Poor relationship with the partner (marital discord) is one of the commonest causes of the disorder. Other factors include a negative attitude towards sexuality, chronic stress, and comorbid medical conditions like diabetes, abnormal thyroid function and alterations in levels of sex hormones.

Treatment

The mainstay of treatment is psychotherapy. Different techniques such as sensate focus techniques (discussed later in the Chapter), cognitive behavioural therapy, systematic desensitisation and couples therapy have been used with varying success.

Pharmacological treatments include:

a. *Flibanserin*: It is a 5HT1A receptor agonist [also known as norepinephrine dopamine disinhibitor (NDDI)] that is postulated to increase dopamine and norepinephrine and decrease serotonin levels in the prefrontal cortex. It has been approved by FDA for the treatment of hypoactive sexual desire disorder in premenopausal women.
b. *Bremelanotide*: It is a nonselective agonist of the melanocortin receptor. The *subcutaneous injection* of bremelanotide has been approved for use in premenopausal women with hypoactive sexual desire.

DISORDERS OF EXCITEMENT (AROUSAL) PHASE

Erectile Disorder (Erectile Dysfunction)

The term 'impotence' was used for erectile disorders in the past, but its use must be avoided due to its derogatory nature. Erectile disorder can present with:

a. Difficulty in achieving erection during sexual intercourse.
b. Difficulty in maintaining the erection with loss of erection before completion of sexual intercourse.
c. Marked decrease in the rigidity achieved during the erection.

Erectile disorder is one of the commonest sexual disorders, and its prevalence increases with age, particularly after 50 years.

Aetiology

On the basis of aetiology, the erectile disorder can be divided into two subtypes:

a. **Organic erectile disorder:** Organic erectile disorder is diagnosed when there is a physiological basis for poor erection. It can be caused by vascular disorders, (e.g., Peyronie's disease, focal arterial occlusive disease, subclinical endothelial dysfunction), neurogenic disorders (e.g., multiple sclerosis, spinal cord injury, pelvic trauma), endocrine disorders (e.g., hypo/hyperthyroidism, low testosterone levels etc.) and medication side effects (antipsychotics, finasteride, antidepressants etc.). Risk factors for erectile dysfunction include diabetes, hypertension, dyslipidaemia, smoking, lack of exercise, cardiovascular disorders and chronic kidney disease.
b. **Psychogenic erectile disorders:** When psychological factors like stress, performance anxiety, and relationship

problems lead to the development of erection disturbances, the diagnosis of psychogenic erectile disorder is made.

Lifelong erectile disorder and erectile disorder in older people are usually due to organic causes, whereas erectile disorder in young adults and that of acquired type (often with sudden onset) is usually due to psychological causes. Earlier it was believed that most of the cases of erectile disorder in younger individuals are psychogenic in origin, but the recent data suggest the role of organic factors in a large number of younger patients too.

Detailed history, as well as investigations, help differentiate organic erectile disorders from that of psychological origin. The history of **nocturnal and morning erections**, in particular, is often used to differentiate between the two. Men have spontaneous erections during REM sleep. If the cause of the erectile disorder is psychogenic, these spontaneous nocturnal and morning erections should be present. Lack of spontaneous nocturnal and morning erection points towards an organic cause.

Rather than relying on history alone, tests such as nocturnal penile intumescence testing (which uses a device to measure erections while the patient is asleep) can be done and help in the diagnosis.

The table below highlights the clinical differences between organic and psychological erectile disorder.

Clinical characteristics	Organic erectile disorder	Psychological erectile disorder
Onset	Lifelong and acquired variant of elderly onset	Acquired variant in young adults
Spontaneous erections (in the absence of sexual activity)	Mostly absent	Mostly present
Nocturnal/Morning erections	Mostly absent	Mostly present
Erection during masturbation	Mostly absent	Mostly present
Erection with other partner(s) than the usual one	Mostly absent	Mostly present
Evidence of vascular, neurogenic or endocrine dysfunction	Mostly present	Mostly absent
Nocturnal penile tumescence testing	Impaired testing	Normal results
Penile duplex Doppler ultrasonography	May give evidence of arterial or venous insufficiency	Normal results

Treatment

Pharmacological Treatment

1. **Phosphodiesterase-5 inhibitors (PDE-5 inhibitors):** PDE-5 inhibitors are considered the first-line treatment for erectile disorder. Sildenafil, vardenafil, tadalafil, and avanafil all have similar efficacy. Tadalafil has the longest duration of action (remains effective till 36 hours after dosing), and avanafil has the most rapid onset of action.

   Mechanism of action: Understanding the physiology of erectile response is essential to understanding how PDE-5 inhibitors work. Sexual excitement in men leads to the release of nitric oxide, which increases cGMP, resulting in cavernosal smooth muscle relaxation. This increases the blood flow in the penis and results in an erection. The detumescence (loss of erection) is mediated by the catabolism of cGMP by the phosphodiesterase-5 enzyme.

   Phosphodiesterase-5 inhibitors decrease the breakdown of cGMP and hence improve erection. It must be remembered that sufficient sexual stimulation and arousal are required to generate enough nitric oxide in the first place, for PDE-5 inhibitors to work.

   Phosphodiesterase-5 inhibitors are contraindicated in individuals taking nitrates and should be used very carefully in those taking alpha-adrenergic blockers, as concomitant use of PDE-5 inhibitors with nitrates/alpha-adrenergic blockers may precipitate severe hypotension.

   A small number of cases of development of **non-arteritic ischemic optic neuropathy (NAION)** after using sildenafil have been reported. NAION may lead to permanent vision loss.

2. Oral phentolamine (decreases sympathetic tone and relaxes smooth muscles of corpora cavernosa) and apomorphine (causes vasodilatation) are occasionally used in the management of erectile disorder.

3. Alprostadil (used transurethrally or injected into corpora cavernosa) contains prostaglandin E and results in vasodilatation and consequently erection. With alprostadil use, erection can happen even without sexual arousal, is experienced within 2–3 minutes of use and may last for an hour. The method of use of alprostadil is cumbersome and is not liked by a majority of patients.

4. Vacuum pump: These are mechanical devices that create a vacuum around the penis, leading to the blood flow into the penis and hence, erection. Once erection has been achieved, a ring is placed at the base of the penis to maintain the erection (by preventing the blood outflow).

5. Penile prosthetic implants: Surgical implantation is reserved for those who do not respond to other treatment methods. Semi-rigid rod prosthesis (that result in a permanent erection) and inflatable types (that can be inflated and deflated) are the two options available for prosthetic implants.

Psychotherapy:

A. **Dual-sex therapy:** It was developed by Masters and Johnson. This therapy treats the **"couple"** and **not the individual.** The couple is taught ways to improve their communication. The couple is also taught exercises to increase their sensory awareness. These exercises are called sensate focus exercises. Initially, the couple is asked to touch, rub, and kiss each other's body parts, excluding breasts and genitals (this stage is called the **nongenital sensate focus).** In the next stage, the same activities are done on breasts and genitals (called the **genital sensate focus**). The whole purpose is to make the couple aware that pleasure can be given and received by methods other

than sexual intercourse. The sex therapy is effective not only for erectile dysfunction but other sexual disorders like premature ejaculation.
B. Other techniques, such as behavioural therapy, cognitive therapy, relaxation training, hypnotherapy and psychoanalysis have also been used with varying success rates.

DISORDERS OF ORGASM PHASE

Female Orgasm Disorder

Female orgasm disorder (*anorgasmia*): It is characterised by a persistent delay or absence of orgasm after a phase of normal excitement. Inadequate stimulation during sexual activity may also result in an inability to achieve orgasm, but that does not qualify for female orgasm disorder. The causes of female orgasm disorder include stress, fear and apprehension about pregnancy, negative attitude towards sex, socio-cultural causes (e.g., orthodox beliefs such as 'good women shouldn't enjoy sex), as well as medical causes (conditions that cause pain during sex).

Treatment: Females with orgasm disorder should be evaluated for any underlying medical condition. If the orgasmic dysfunction is due to an underlying medical condition, it needs to be treated adequately. If present, psychosocial issues are addressed with psychotherapy or behaviour therapy. Psychodynamic sex therapy may also be useful in certain cases.

Premature Ejaculation

It is characterised by a persistent pattern (for at least 6 months duration) of ejaculation with minimal sexual stimulation. According to DSM-5, if the ejaculation occurs within approximately 1 minute following vaginal penetration **(IELT, intravaginal ejaculatory latency time <1 minute)** and before the individual wishes for it, it would qualify for the diagnosis of premature ejaculation, provided that early ejaculation occurs on all or almost all (75–100%) occasions of sexual activity.

The severity of premature ejaculation is classified as:
a. Mild (if ejaculation occurs within 30–60 seconds of penetration),
b. Moderate (if ejaculation occurs within 15–30 seconds of penetration) and
c. Severe (if ejaculation occurs within 15 seconds of penetration or before penetration).

As one can see, these specific duration criteria have been defined only for vaginal intercourse, albeit the diagnosis of premature ejaculation can be made for individuals indulging in nonvaginal sexual activities too.

Premature ejaculation can further be classified as:
a. *Lifetime premature ejaculation*: If the individual always had early ejaculation as defined above.
b. *Acquired premature ejaculation*: If the individual developed symptoms of early ejaculation later in life, after a period of normal sexual functioning.

Patients with PE often develop anticipatory anxiety (they are anxious that whenever they have sex next, they will again ejaculate early and won't be able to satisfy their partner). Anticipatory anxiety often worsens sexual performance.

Premature ejaculation is the most common sexual disorder in men, and around one-third of patients with PE have comorbid erectile difficulties.

Aetiology
The aetiology of premature ejaculation is multifactorial. Genetics plays a role, and in some studies, an association has been found between ejaculation latency and serotonin transporter gene polymorphism. Some patients may have early ejaculation because of shorter nerve latency time, but no clear-cut neurobiological cause can be found in most cases.

Psychological factors (such as behavioural conditioning) appear to play an important role. Early sexual experiences (e.g., in parental home, or with a commercial sex worker) wherein there was pressure to complete the act quickly might lead to conditioning towards rapid ejaculation. Relationship difficulties with the partner and partners with sexual problems (such as sexual pain or sexual avoidance) are also commonly seen in patients with premature ejaculation.

Treatment
Pharmacological treatment: SSRIs (particularly paroxetine) have been found to be effective in increasing ejaculation latency.

Dapoxetine, a SSRI, has been developed specifically for the management of PME. It has a rapid onset of action and is taken 1–2 hours before sexual activity to improve ejaculatory control.

Tricyclic antidepressants like clomipramine can also increase ejaculation latency but have more adverse effects than SSRIs.

Topical anaesthetics such as lidocaine or prilocaine can be used to decrease penile sensitivity and increase ejaculatory control.

Psychotherapy: Specific behavioural techniques have been developed for the management of PME. These include:
a. *Squeeze technique*: In this technique, when the man gets the feeling of impending ejaculation, the female partner (or the man himself) squeezes the coronal ridge of the glans penis. This results in the inhibition of ejaculation.
b. *Stop-start technique (Semans technique)*: Here, when the man gets the feeling of impending ejaculation, the thrusting is stopped for some time, and once the excitement has decreased, it is restarted.

Apart from these techniques, dual sex therapy (as described earlier), cognitive therapy, and other behavioural techniques have also been used to treat premature ejaculation.

Delayed Ejaculation

Individuals with delayed ejaculation complain of either significant delay in ejaculation or an inability to ejaculate during partnered sexual activity without any desire for the same. These patients may have normal ejaculation during masturbation. The incidence of delayed ejaculation is less than that of premature ejaculation.

Treatment: Currently, there is no approved medication for delayed ejaculation. Evidence suggests possible roles of cabergoline, amantadine, bupropion, cyproheptadine, buspirone, oxytocin, bethanechol and yohimbine. Similarly, several other pro-dopaminergic agents like apomorphine, pramipexole, and ropinirole have been tried with variable success rates.

Genito-pelvic Pain/Penetration Disorder

It is also known as sexual pain disorder. It may present with one or more of the following symptoms:
1. Marked difficulty in vaginal penetration during intercourse or attempted intercourse.
2. Marked vulvovaginal pain or pelvic pain during vaginal intercourse or attempted intercourse.
3. Marked anxiety that vulvovaginal pain or pelvic pain will happen if intercourse is done.
4. Marked tensing of muscles of pelvic floor when vaginal penetration is attempted.

The term **dyspareunia** is used to describe "painful coitus", and *the term vaginismus* is used to describe "painful vaginal contraction during penile penetration". Recurrent episodes of vaginismus may lead to dyspareunia. Various psychosocial factors (childhood sexual trauma, childhood traumatic experience involving surgical procedures, interpersonal issues with partner) may contribute to the development of genito-pelvic pain disorder. Various genito-pelvic pathologies like vulvar dermatoses, neuropathic conditions, endometriosis, bladder pathologies, vulvodynia and atrophy resulting from hormonal disorders may also result in the development of genito-pelvic pain disorder.

Treatment: Treatment involves management of the underlying medical cause and use of medications (local anaesthetics), physical therapy (nonintercourse penetration), stress coping skill training, relaxation techniques, and, if required, surgical intervention may be useful in the management of genito-pelvic pain disorder.

Substance/Medication Induced Sexual Dysfunction

Use of certain substances during or soon after intoxication or withdrawal can disturb sexual functioning. Similarly, certain medications can also cause sexual disorders.

Substances that are commonly associated with sexual dysfunctions include:
- Alcohol
- Opioids
- Sedatives and hypnotics
- Anxiolytics
- Stimulants (including cocaine)

Medications that commonly cause sexual dysfunctions include:
- Antidepressants
- Antipsychotics
- Hormonal contraceptives

Antidepressants commonly affect the phase of orgasm and ejaculation, though other phases of the sexual response cycle like desire may also get impacted adversely. Similarly, antipsychotics may cause impairment of desire, erection, vaginal lubrication, orgasm as well as ejaculation. Mood stabilisers may affect the desire phase of the sexual response cycle. The medications that are relatively spared from sexual side effects are: antidepressants like Bupropion, Mirtazapine, antipsychotics with prolactin sparing properties and mood stabilisers like Lamotrigine.

Name of the medication	Nature of sexual dysfunction
Tricyclic antidepressants	Erectile disorder, Delayed ejaculation
Selective serotonin reuptake inhibitors (SSRIs), Venlafaxine	Reduced drive for sex, anorgasmia, delayed ejaculation and retrograde ejaculation
MAO inhibitors, Bupropion	Increased sexual drive
Trazodone	Priapism (prolonged and painful erection of penis)
Stimulants (amphetamine, methylphenidate)	Increased sexual drive
α-adrenergic antagonist and β-adrenergic antagonist	Erectile disorder, retrograde ejaculation
Anticholinergic agents	Erectile disorder, reduced vaginal lubrication

Management of substance/medication-induced sexual dysfunction: If the sexual dysfunction is related to the use of addictive substances, the substance use disorder must be treated adequately. If the sexual dysfunction is psychotropic medication-induced, the offending medication is usually replaced by a safer medication. For example:
- Individuals reporting sexual dysfunction due to antipsychotic medications may be shifted to aripiprazole, which is a partial agonist at D2 receptors.
- Cyproheptadine can be used to reverse the sexual dysfunction induced by SSRIs.
- Individuals having sexual dysfunction due to antidepressant use (commonly TCAs, SSRIs or SNRIs) can be shifted to bupropion or mirtazapine.

Also, the specific treatment modalities suggested for individual subtypes of sexual dysfunctions (as mentioned above) may be followed in substance-induced sexual dysfunction too.

OTHER FORMS OF SEXUAL DYSFUNCTION

- **Postcoital dysphoria:** It is a disorder of mood that manifests during the resolution phase of the sexual response cycle (after the coitus), characterised by anxiety, depression and irritability. There is no specific treatment for it. However, psychological management of anxiety and fear related issues in the individual may be helpful.
- **Postcoital headache:** Headache that occurs following coitus, usually of throbbing type and may last for hours. The treatment is usually with analgesics.

PARAPHILIC DISORDERS (TABLE 16.2)

Paraphilias are disorders of sexual preference, also known as sexual perversions. In patients with paraphilias, sexual arousal and orgasm are achieved by sexual stimuli or acts that are deviations from normal sexual behaviour. Just having a deviant fantasy is not enough for the diagnosis; the person must have acted on the paraphilic fantasy or urges before the diagnosis can be made.

Paraphilias are seen predominantly in males, with peak paraphilic behaviour being expressed between ages 15 and 25 years, followed by a gradual decline.

Many factors contribute to the development of paraphilic disorders, including biological factors such as genetic abnormalities, neurological disorders, head injury, hormonal disorders, and severe mental disorders (e.g., schizophrenia, mania). Psychological factors (such as modelling of behaviour on the behaviour of others) too play a role.

Among the paraphilic disorders, the pedophilic disorder is targeted towards children (human figures), whereas fetishistic disorder and transvestic disorder are directed towards nonhuman objects for sexual gratification. Paraphilia is diagnosed as a disorder when it causes significant distress to the individual and poses the risk of harm to self or others. Individuals may present with one or more paraphilic disorders.

Apart from these, some other paraphilias include:
- *Scatologia*: Sexual arousal and gratification are achieved by making obscene phone calls.
- *Necrophilia*: Sexual arousal and gratification is achieved by indulging in sexual acts with dead bodies.
- *Zoophilia*: Sexual arousal and gratification are achieved by indulging in sexual acts with animals.
- *Coprophilia*: Sexual arousal and gratification are achieved from faecal matter.
- *Klismaphilia*: Sexual arousal and gratification are achieved from enemas.
- *Urophilia*: Sexual arousal and gratification are achieved from urine.
- *Partialism*: Sexual arousal and gratification are achieved by concentrating on one part of the body to the exclusion of all others. Oral–genital contact—such as cunnilingus (oral contact with a female's external genitals), fellatio (oral contact with the penis), and anilingus (oral contact with the anus), can be a part of normal foreplay, but if these activities are the only way of achieving sexual gratification, it is considered as a paraphilia. It is also called *oralism*.

Diagnosis of paraphilic disorders needs persistence of symptoms for more than 6 months.

Management: As comorbid psychiatric conditions may contribute to the development of the paraphilic disorder, adequate treatment of any comorbid psychiatric disorder is important. Usually, the paraphilic disorder is associated with increased sexual drive, which can be controlled by the use of SSRIs or antiandrogens (e.g., cyproterone acetate and medroxyprogesterone acetate). Psychological interventions like cognitive behaviour therapy, social skill training, sex education, relaxation methods, imaginal desensitisation and aversion therapy have been found to be effective in the management of paraphilic disorders.

Table 16.2: Characteristic features of paraphilic disorders.

Paraphilic disorders	Characteristic features
Voyeuristic disorders (Voyeurism)	Sexual arousal and gratification are achieved through observation of an unsuspected person during undressing, in the naked state or while engaged in sexual activity
Exhibitionistic disorder (Exhibitionism)	Sexual arousal and gratification are achieved by exposing one's genitalia to an unsuspected person
Frotteuristic disorder (Frotteurism)	Sexual arousal and gratification are achieved through touching or rubbing against a nonconsenting person, usually in public places such as a bus or in the metro
Sexual masochism disorder (Masochism)	Sexual arousal and gratification are achieved from acts of being tortured, bound, beaten, bitten or otherwise made to suffer
Sexual sadism disorder (Sadism)	Sexual arousal and gratification are achieved by inflicting physical or psychological suffering on another person
Pedophilic disorder	Sexual arousal and gratification are achieved through sexual activity with a prepubescent child or children (generally below 13 years of age)
Fetishistic disorder (Fetishism)	Sexual arousal and gratification are achieved through the use of nonliving objects, (e.g., clothing or attires used by the opposite gender) or non-genital body parts
Transvestic disorder (Transvestism)	Sexual arousal and gratification are achieved through cross-dressing

---

CASE BASED MCQ

A 27-year-old male is quite distressed as he loses his erection whenever he tries to have sexual intercourse with his wife. These symptoms started 6 months back and have been worsening with time. The patient reports that he gets good morning erections, and there is no medical history of hypertension, diabetes or any other medical illness. The patient is not a smoker and doesn't use any other drugs. The patient reports, 'during sex, I am always worried that the erection would be lost, and eventually, I always end up losing the erection; this is so humiliating for me'. What is the likely diagnosis?
a. Psychogenic erectile dysfunction
b. Organic erectile dysfunction
c. Premature ejaculation
d. Hypoactive sexual desire disorder

Ans. a. History of normal morning erections and difficulty in maintaining erections during sexual intercourse in a young male with no medical comorbidities is suggestive of the diagnosis of psychogenic erectile dysfunction.

SUGGESTED READINGS

1. American Psychiatric Association. Diagnostic and statistical manual of mental disorders (DSM-5®). American Psychiatric Pub; 2013 May 22.
2. Sadock BJ, Sadock VA, Ruiz P (Editors). Kaplan & Sadock's Comprehensive Textbook of Psychiatry, 9th Edition, Lippincott Williams & Wilkins; 2009.
3. Sadock BJ, Sadock VA. Kaplan and Sadock's synopsis of psychiatry: Behavioral sciences/clinical psychiatry. Lippincott Williams & Wilkins; 2011.
4. Balon R, Segraves RT (Editors). Handbook of sexual dysfunction. CRC Press; 2005.
5. Nilamadhab K, Kar GC, (Editors). Comprehensive Textbook of Sexual Medicine. Jaypee Brothers Medical Publishers; 2014.
6. Jannini EA, Burri A, Jern P, Novelli G. Genetics of Human Sexual Behavior: Where We Are, Where We Are Going. Sex Med Rev. 2015;3(2):65-77.
7. Beemer BR. Gender dysphoria update. Journal of psychosocial nursing and mental health services. 1996;34(4):12-9.
8. Garg G, Marwaha R. Gender Dysphoria (Sexual Identity Disorders). InStatPearls [Internet] 2018.
9. Ludwig W, Phillips M. Organic causes of erectile dysfunction in men under 40. Urol Int. 2014;92(1):1-6.

17 Child Psychiatry

Hiral Kotadia, Praveen Tripathi

PS14.1	Enumerate and describe the magnitude and aetiology of psychiatric disorders occurring in childhood and adolescence
PS14.2	Enumerate, elicit, describe and document clinical features in patients with psychiatric disorders occurring in childhood and adolescence
PS14.3	Describe the treatment of stress related disorders including behavioural, psychosocial and pharmacologic therapy
PS14.4	Demonstrate family education in a patient with psychiatric disorders occurring in childhood and adolescence in a simulated environment
PS14.5	Enumerate and describe the pharmacologic basis and side effects of drugs used in psychiatric disorders occurring in childhood and adolescence
PS14.6	Enumerate the appropriate conditions for specialist referral in children and adolescents with psychiatric disorders

ATTENTION DEFICIT HYPERACTIVITY DISORDER

Attention deficit hyperactivity disorder (ADHD) is a neuropsychiatric disorder that causes significant educational, social, and interpersonal impairments. The older name for ADHD was **"minimal brain dysfunction"**. It is a common disorder with a prevalence of 7–8% in school-age children, with males being affected 5–8 times more than females. ADHD may have an onset in infancy but is rarely diagnosed before 3–4 years of age.

Clinical Features

As the name suggests, the main clinical features in ADHD include: (a) Inattention, (b) Impulsivity, and (c) Hyperactivity.

A. **Inattention:** It may manifest in the following ways:
   1. Inability to give attention to closer details resulting in difficulties at school or work.
   2. Difficulty sustaining attention resulting in disturbances such as inability to follow a lecture or read a long text. This may result in a loss of interest and a tendency to run away from tasks that demand sustained attention.
   3. Difficulty in following the instructions and completing the task. The child may find it difficult to complete the sequential tasks (tasks requiring multiple but interconnected steps).
   4. Tendency to get easily distracted and forgetfulness. The child may look lost during the conversation.

B. **Hyperactivity and Impulsivity:** Hyperactivity and impulsivity may manifest with the following symptoms:
   1. Difficulty in sitting in one place. The teachers may complain that the child often gets up from the seat and roams around in the class, disturbing other students too.
   2. While sitting, the child looks fidgety (keeps on moving) and restless.
   3. Child is often 'on the go'. The child may start running or walking around at places such as restaurants or meetings where it is expected to stay still for prolonged periods.
   4. Child has difficulty waiting for the turn and often breaks the queue and demands to be attended to first.
   5. Answers even before the question is complete. When others are conversing, the child may intrude in between.

Diagnosis is made using history (teacher's report and parent's report) and clinical observation.

Based on predominant symptoms, ADHD is divided into three subtypes:
1. Combined presentation (where significant symptoms of both inattention and hyperactivity/impulsivity are present),
2. Predominantly inattentive presentation
3. Predominantly hyperactive/impulsive presentation.

To diagnose ADHD, symptoms must be present for at least 6 months and in at least two different settings (e.g., at home, at school/work, with friends/relatives). According to DSM-5, the symptoms must have an onset before 12 years of age for the diagnosis.

Around 65–75% of children with ADHD have one or more co-morbid conditions such as oppositional defiant disorder (ODD), conduct disorder (CD), learning disorders, anxiety disorders, mood disorders, tics or Tourette's syndrome, and autistic spectrum disorders.

In most children with ADHD, there are no gross signs of central nervous system damage. However, the examination may reveal **soft neurological signs** (soft neurological signs are fine abnormalities that can be elicited only with detailed neurological examination, such as difficulty in copying age-appropriate figures, difficulty in performing rapid alternating movements, difficulty in right-left discrimination, etc.).

In around 40% of cases, symptoms of ADHD remit by puberty. However, symptoms may continue into adolescence and adulthood in many patients. Hyperactivity may significantly decrease with age, but inattention and impulsivity may persist. If ADHD remits, hyperactivity is usually the first symptom to go and distractibility the last.

In patients where symptoms do not remit, or there is only partial remission, there is an increase in vulnerability to the development of antisocial personality disorder, substance use disorder, and mood disorders like depression.

Aetiology

Attention deficit hyperactivity disorder has multifactorial causation.

Genetics plays a strong role, and the heritability in ADHD is around 75%. The monozygotic concordance rate is higher than the dizygotic concordance rate, and the prevalence of ADHD in immediate family members of patients is higher than in the general population. Studies have found an association of ADHD with the dopamine transporter gene *(DAT1)* and dopamine 4 receptor gene *(DRD4)*, but these findings need to be replicated.

Neurotransmitters such as dopamine and norepinephrine have been found to play a role in the development of ADHD symptoms.

Dysfunction in brain circuits, specifically cortico-basal ganglia-thalamo-cortical circuit, has been hypothesised as a cause for the development of ADHD. Also, the prefrontal cortex, given its role in attention and impulse regulation, also appears to play a significant role in developing symptoms.

Finally, many developmental factors have been found to be associated with ADHD. These include prematurity, maternal infections, perinatal insults, maltreatment or neglect during growing up.

Management

Both pharmacotherapy and psychosocial interventions play an important role in the management of ADHD.

Pharmacotherapy: Pharmacotherapy with stimulants is considered the **first-line treatment**.
- Stimulants: **Methylphenidate** (dopamine norepinephrine reuptake inhibitor) is considered the **drug of choice** for the treatment of ADHD; it is effective in about 75% of children with ADHD. It is FDA approved for treatment in children above six years of age. Long-acting forms and methylphenidate patches are available now and help in improving compliance. In cases of ADHD with tics, methylphenidate can increase tics and must be used carefully. Other stimulants available include amphetamine, dextroamphetamine and dextroamphetamine/amphetamine combination. Stimulants are usually well-tolerated and have mild side effects. Short term adverse effects include loss of appetite, weight loss, delayed onset of sleep, headache and abdominal pain. Long term use of stimulants may result in growth suppression, which can be managed by instituting drug holidays (on weekends or during holidays). Children tend to eat more during the drug holidays and catch up with the growth. Modafinil is another CNS stimulant that is occasionally used to manage ADHD but is not FDA approved.
- Non-stimulants like atomoxetine (a norepinephrine reuptake inhibitor) and clonidine (alpha-adrenergic agonist) are also approved for the treatment of ADHD in children above six years of age. Other medications that can be used include guanfacine, bupropion, and venlafaxine.

Psychosocial interventions: Non-pharmacological treatment is an integral part of managing ADHD. The techniques used include environmental modifications (structuring of routine, minimisation of external distraction), parent training, cognitive behavioural therapy and social skills training.

A combination of medications and psychosocial interventions is the preferred approach for managing ADHD in children.

AUTISM SPECTRUM DISORDER

Autism spectrum disorder (ASD) (previously known as pervasive developmental disorders) is characterised by an impairment in social communication and restricted and repetitive behaviours. ASD is four times more common in males than females. The prevalence of ASD is not dependent on socioeconomic class, as was earlier thought.

> In older classifications, five separate disorders, autistic disorder, Asperger's syndrome, childhood disintegrative disorder, Rett syndrome and pervasive developmental disorder not otherwise specified, were described under the broader category of pervasive developmental disorders. In DSM-5 and ICD-11, these subtypes have been removed, and a single diagnosis of autism spectrum disorder has been described.

The disorder is usually evident by the second year of life, but the diagnosis may be missed for many years in milder cases.

The symptoms of ASD can be divided into "core symptoms" and "associated behavioural symptoms".

Core symptoms of ASD: The presence of core symptoms (current or historically) is necessary to diagnose ASD. There are two core symptoms of ASD:
- **Persistent deficits in social communication and interaction:** Children with ASD have impaired social

skills and non-verbal social interactions. It results in the following manifestations:
- As infants, they may not develop a **social smile**.
- There may be a lack of anticipatory posture (the posture that the kid assumes when he wants to be picked up by a caretaker)
- Poor eye to eye contact, which usually continues as the child grows up
- Lack of imaginative and interactive play, limited interest in other children
- Lack of attachment to parents/caregivers, the child may not acknowledge their presence (e.g., when the father comes back home from the office, the child does not come running to meet him and may not show any reaction to his presence)

Children with ASD have difficulty understanding the feelings, desires, intentions and beliefs of others (also called "**theory of mind**"). They cannot empathise with others which further limits their ability for social interaction.

As they grow older and enter school, they have difficulty making friends due to limited social skills; they face difficulties in having a fluent conversation, are not so spontaneous, and struggle with the use of gestures.

Individuals with ASD desire friendships, and as they turn into adolescents and young adults, they also seek romantic relationships, but limited social skills make it difficult for them.

Restricted, Repetitive Patterns of Behaviour, Interests, and Activities: The children with ASD tend to have repetitive behaviours as manifested by the following:
- Repetitive or stereotyped movements such as hand wringing, finger flicking, etc.
- Using toys and objects in a repetitive manner (e.g., spending hours spinning a coin or lining up the toys). The exploratory play (play in which the child uses the sensations to explore the world around them) is minimal. Overall, the play behaviour is restricted, and the child repeatedly plays in the same manner.
- There is an insistence on following the same routine, even small changes such as a change in the food packing, or clothing or change in furniture may lead to excessive anxiety and distress in the child.
- The interests are highly restricted, and there may be an extreme attachment to certain inanimate objects such as a toy or a household item, like a photo frame.
- There may be hypo- or hyper-reactivity to sensory input. For example, the child may be extremely fascinated with the sound of the ticking of the clock. On the other hand, there may be hyposensitivity to pain and other sensations, e.g., the child may not feel giddy despite running in circles for long periods.

Associated Symptoms of ASD

These are the symptoms that are not necessary to diagnose ASD but nonetheless are important in the overall clinical picture. These include:
- **Language disturbances:** Language development is often delayed. In up to 25% of cases, there is a history of some language development that is subsequently lost. Some children make stereotypical sounds which are not meant for communication. Even when children with ASD have enough vocabulary, they still struggle to put meaningful sentences together. Their speech may consist of echolalia, stereotyped phrases repeated without context, and pronoun reversal (using 'you' in the place of 'i').
- **Intellectual disability:** Around 30% of children with ASD have co-morbid intellectual disability (severe to profound intellectual disability is more common than mild to moderate), and the presence of intellectual disability makes the **prognosis worse**.
- **Irritability:** It is a problematic symptom, more so when it is associated with aggression and self-injurious behaviour (like biting self, head banging or skin picking)

Hyperactivity and inattention, insomnia, a higher rate of minor infections and gastrointestinal symptoms may also be present.
- **Precocious skills (splinter skills/savant skills):** In certain domains, children with ASD may show skill levels far better than their peers, like exceptionally well rote memory, hyperlexia (better ability to read), calculation skills and musical skills.
- **Physical abnormalities:** Children with ASD have higher rates of minor physical anomalies such as **abnormal dermatoglyphics** (fingerprints) and ear malformations. The establishment of dexterity (being right handed or left handed) may be delayed by many years.

> **CARS (CHILDHOOD AUTISM RATING SCALE)**
> It is a widely used rating scale for the detection and diagnosis of autism.

Aetiology

As suggested by family and twin studies and high heritability rates, there is a significant genetic component in the aetiology of autism spectrum disorder.

Autism spectrum disorder is associated with rare single-gene disorders such as **fragile X syndrome (most common)**, tuberous sclerosis, and neurofibromatosis. These associations provide a window into the possible mechanisms of the development of autism spectrum disorder, as discussed below.

Fragile X mutation is characterised by CGG repeats on the X chromosome, which leads to decreased production of FMR protein (FMRP). FMRP represses gene translation and contributes to neural plasticity. It is known that many genes that carry a risk for ASD are targets of FMR protein, and this may explain the observed association between ASD and Fragile X syndrome.

In tuberous sclerosis, there is a mutation in the genes coding either TSC1 (Tuberous sclerosis complex 1) or TSC2 (Tuberous sclerosis complex 2) proteins. These proteins are members of the mTOR (mammalian target of rapamycin)/Akt (protein kinase B) intracellular signalling pathway, which is involved in multiple cellular processes like proliferation, growth, cell survival and mobility. Some ASD risk genes like PTEN (phosphatase and tensin homolog) are also members of this pathway, which may explain the observed association between ASD and Fragile X syndrome.

The recent focus of research is on the role of **copy number variations (CNVs)** in the aetiology of ASD. A copy number variation is when the number of copies of a particular gene varies from individual to individual. Cumulatively, the CNVs may account for 15–20% of cases of ASD. These CNVs disrupt the coding region of one or more genes. Multiple genes that carry CNVs have been studied and reported in individuals with ASD. These genes are involved in the development of neurons, synaptic plasticity, and chromatin re-modelling, which helps maintain the integrity of the synapse and structure of the DNA within neurons.

One of the consistent findings in patients with ASD is **increased serotonin levels** in the platelets. Platelets pick serotonin as they pass through intestinal circulation. The transporter that mediates this process is SERT (serotonin transporter), and the gene *SLC64A* encodes it. This gene encodes the same protein in the brain too. It has been hypothesised that the variation that leads to increased serotonin uptake in platelets in the intestine causes a similar impact in the brain too, which may be responsible for alteration in neuronal migration and growth in the brain.

Neuroimaging studies have shown both structural and functional abnormalities in the brain of patients with ASD. One of the consistent findings is increased brain volume (primarily due to increased volume in the frontal lobe and anterior temporal region) in children younger than four years of age, whose neonatal head circumferences were either normal or below normal. Interestingly, studies in children aged between 5–16 years did not find increased brain volumes. It appears that there is an increase in brain volume in the first few years, followed by a decrease.

Functional MRI studies that measure brain activity during different tasks have found a different activation pattern in individuals with autism spectrum disorders compared to control subjects. For example, Studies have found that while scanning faces, individuals with autism focus more on the mouth region than the eye region, and they focus on individual features of the face more rather than scanning the entire face multiple times.

Patients with autism spectrum disorder have EEG abnormalities, and the frequency of seizure disorders is more than the general population.

Environmental factors like increased maternal and paternal age (**paternal age more important than maternal age**), prenatal exposure to thalidomide and valproic acid, and obstetric complications are all associated with the increased likelihood of autism spectrum disorder development.

> A fraudulent research paper published in 1998 claimed a link between the administration of the MMR vaccine and the development of autism, but this claim was found to be untrue. Research has clearly shown that the MMR vaccine is not associated with the development of autism.

Course and Prognosis

ASD is generally a lifelong disability, with a majority of patients requiring social and family support. Children with IQ >70 and development of communicative language by 5–7 years have a relatively better prognosis.

Treatment

The management of ASD involves both non-pharmacological and pharmacological treatment.

1. **Non-pharmacological treatment:** Non-pharmacological treatment is the mainstay for managing the core symptoms of autism. The following psychosocial interventions have been found to be useful:
   - **Early Intensive Behavioural and Developmental interventions:** In these interventions, the focus is on teaching adaptive skills (skills necessary for daily living), relationship skills and play skills to the children using positive reinforcement. Examples of such intervention include ESDM (Early Start Denver Model) and Parent Training approaches.
   - **Social skills training:** The core deficit in autism is the lack of social skills and the inability to understand social situations properly. In social skills training, the child is trained in a graded and stepwise manner on behaving in a socially appropriate way. Also, the child is taught the identification and labelling of emotions and social problem-solving techniques. This helps the child make friends too, which is otherwise a challenge for children with ASD.
   - **Educational interventions like TEACHH** (Treatment and education of Autistic and related Communication-handicapped Children) involve structured teaching that incorporates many visual supports and a picture schedule to help learn academic subjects and socially appropriate responses.
2. **Pharmacological treatment:** Pharmacological interventions in ASD are primarily for managing associated behavioural symptoms rather than core features. Irritability can be treated with the use of second-generation antipsychotics.
   - **Risperidone and aripiprazole** have been FDA approved for managing irritability in autism. Hyperactivity/Impulsivity and Inattention can be managed by using stimulant medications (Methylphenidate) or non-stimulant medications (Atomoxetine, clonidine). For repetitive/stereotypical behaviours, second-generation antipsychotics or Selective Serotonin Reuptake Inhibitors (SSRIs) can be used. Insomnia can be managed by melatonin, clonidine or low dose benzodiazepines.

In the ICD-10 and DSM-IV, in addition to autism, other types of pervasive developmental disorders were described. As many clinicians continue to use these diagnoses, a brief description is being provided here.

Rett's disorder (Rett's syndrome): It is much more common in females than males. The most common mutation seen in these patients is in the *MECP2* gene.

Rett's syndrome is characterised by normal development until 5 months. Between 5–48 months, the child starts to lose acquired hand skills (such as fine motor skills), and there is a loss of acquired speech. Also, there is a deceleration of head circumference resulting in microcephaly. The child gradually develops stereotyped hand movements such as hand wringing, licking, or biting fingers. The language function remains impaired, and there is also a loss of social interaction. The child also develops poorly coordinated gait or trunk movements. Along with these symptoms, around 75% of children have seizures. The disorder is usually progressive, and treatment is symptomatic (physiotherapy for muscular dysfunction; anticonvulsants for seizures; behavioural therapy for self-injurious behaviours).

Rett's syndrome is not considered part of autism spectrum disorder in DSM-5 and is diagnosed separately.

Childhood disintegrative disorder (Heller's syndrome): It is characterised by normal development until 2 years. Between 2–10 years, there is a loss of acquired motor skills, social skills, language skills, and bowel/bladder control. The child develops the symptoms of impaired communication, impaired social interaction and repetitive, stereotyped behaviour. The course is usually progressive though some patients may show improvement, and the treatment is symptomatic.

Asperger's syndrome: It is characterised by impairment of social interaction and restricted, repetitive and stereotyped behaviour. However, no language delay or disturbance is seen. The treatment is usually supportive.

MOTOR DISORDERS

Motor disorders include: (i) Tourette's disorder (ii) Persistent (Chronic) Motor or Vocal Tic disorder (iii) Developmental Coordination disorder, and (iv) Stereotypic Movement disorder.

Tic Disorder

Tics are brief, sudden, rapid, repetitive, non-rhythmic motor movements (motor tics) or vocalisations (vocal tics), which are typically performed in response to irresistible premonitory urges (internal urges). Though tics are involuntary, they can at times be voluntarily suppressed for a while.

A. **Motor tics:** Motor tics usually affect the muscles of the face and neck and can be further divided into simple and complex types, based on the muscle groups involved in the movement:
   - **Simple motor tics:** These are repetitive, rapid contractions of functionally similar muscle groups, resulting in movements such as eye-blinking, neck-jerking, shoulder-shrugging, and facial-grimacing.
   - **Complex motor tics:** These involve multiple muscle groups resulting in complicated movements such as grooming behaviours, jumping, touching behaviours, echopraxia (imitation of observed behaviour), and copropraxia (display of obscene gestures).

B. **Vocal tics:** These are sounds made using the voice (vocalisations), such as throat-clearing, grunting, snorting, and coughing. Vocal tics are further divided into simple and complex types.
   - **Simple vocal tics** include coughing, throat-clearing, sniffing, and barking.
   - **Complex vocal tics** include repeating words or phrases out of context, coprolalia (use of obscene words or phrases), palilalia (repeating own words), and echolalia (repetition of the last-heard words of others).

Tics typically emerge at the age of 5–6 years and reach the greatest severity between 10 to 12 years. In about half to two-thirds of children, there is improvement or remission by adolescence or early adulthood.

The most widely studied and severe tic disorder is Gilles de la Tourette syndrome, also known as **Tourette's disorder**. Males are affected three to four times more than females.

There is a strong genetic contribution to the development of tic disorders. Neurobiologically, a dysfunction in the basal ganglia region of the brain, particularly of dopaminergic transmission in the cortico-striatothalamic circuit, has been hypothesised to play a role. The role of infections (Group A beta-hemolytic *Streptococcus*) and autoimmune process in the causation of Tourette's disorder is controversial and is highly unlikely.

CLINICAL FEATURES AND DIAGNOSIS

To make the diagnosis of Tourette's disorder.
- Both, multiple motor and one or more vocal tics should be present at some point of time during the illness, though they may not be present concurrently.
- The tics should be present for >1 year since the first tic onset.
- The onset of illness should be before 18 years of age.
- The tics usually first appear in the face and neck and later progress to other body parts. Motor tics appear before vocal tics. Echolalia, palilalia and coprolalia are characteristic of Tourette's disorder. Tics should be differentiated from other movement disorders (e.g., dystonia, choreoathetosis, myoclonus) and neurological diseases such as Huntington's disease, Parkinsonism, Sydenham's chorea, and Wilson's disease). Obsessive-compulsive and related disorders are a common comorbidity in patients with Tourette's disorder.

COURSE AND PROGNOSIS

Tourette's disorder develops in early childhood, and generally, a reduction in symptom severity or remission occurs by adolescence or adulthood.

MANAGEMENT

A combination of psychotherapy (behavioural treatment) and pharmacological treatment is preferred in the management of Tourette's disorder.

Psychotherapy (Behavioural Therapy)

Behavioural therapy is the first line of treatment. Both habit reversal training and exposure and response prevention are effective in decreasing tics.

In **habit reversal**, the patient learns to identify the urge (premonitory urge) that develops before the tics. The patient is trained to replace the tic movement with a voluntary behaviour (such as slow rhythmic breathing) whenever he senses the premonitory urge.

In exposure and response prevention, the patient is asked to voluntarily suppress the tic whenever he feels the premonitory urge. The principle is similar to exposure and response prevention in OCD, where the patient is asked to not indulge in compulsive behaviour in response to obsessions. The goal of exposure and response prevention therapy is to break the association between premonitory urges and tics. If the patient can resist the tic for long enough, the premonitory urge becomes more tolerable in due course of time.

In pharmacotherapy, noradrenergic agents such as clonidine and guanfacine are often used as **first-line agents** due to better side effect profiles. Atypical antipsychotics, particularly risperidone, have been found to be effective. Haloperidol and Pimozide, which are typical antipsychotics, are FDA approved for the treatment of Tourette's disorder but not used as often due to significant side effects.

Persistent (Chronic) Motor or Vocal Tic disorder

Tic disorders are called chronic (persistent) if either motor or vocal tics (but not both) persist for at least 1 year, with an onset before 18 years. The management is on the same lines as Tourette's disorder.

DEVELOPMENTAL COORDINATION DISORDER

Historically known as **clumsy child syndrome**, developmental coordination disorder is a neurodevelopmental disorder in which a child's fine and/or gross motor coordination is slower and less as compared to children of the same age. Children with this disorder show delayed and erratic development of motor milestones. Children with this disorder have difficulty performing daily activities requiring fine and gross motor skills like jumping, hopping, running, catching a ball, tying the shoelaces, or writing. Management includes: (a) sensory integration programs which aim to increase sensory and motor function awareness by indulging the child in various kinds of physical activities, and (b) neuromotor task training.

STEREOTYPIC MOVEMENT DISORDER

This disorder is characterised by repetitive, seemingly driven, and apparently purposeless motor behaviours that interfere with social, academic, or other activities. These motor behaviours usually emerge in the early developmental period. Examples of stereotypic movements include hand flapping, body rocking, hand waving, lip-licking, skin picking, or self-hitting. These movements often appear to be self-soothing or self-stimulating, but in some cases, they may cause injury to the self. Nail-biting, thumb-sucking, and nose-picking are included in this disorder only if they cause impairment. Treatment includes: (1) Behavioural therapy—habit reversal (in which the child is trained to replace the undesired repetitive behaviour with a more acceptable behaviour) and differential reinforcement (reinforcing the desired behaviour and not reinforcing the undesired behaviour) are effective in the management of stereotypic movement disorder (2) Pharmacological interventions—Selective serotonin Reuptake Inhibitors (SSRIs) and second-generation antipsychotics (risperidone) are used primarily to reduce the self-harming stereotyped movements.

DISRUPTIVE BEHAVIOUR DISORDERS

Oppositional defiant disorder and CD are the two major disruptive behaviour disorders.

OPPOSITIONAL DEFIANT DISORDER

The onset of ODD is usually by 4–8 years of age; it is more common in males before puberty and equally common in males and females after puberty. The prevalence of ODD decreases after 12 years of age.

Clinical Features and Diagnosis

Oppositional defiant disorder is characterised by a consistent pattern of **disobedience and hostility** towards the authority figures (parents, elders, teachers). It is characterised by a pattern of angry or irritable mood, argumentative or defiant behaviour or vindictiveness as manifested by the following symptoms:

- **Angry/irritable mood:** The child loses temper easily, gets annoyed easily, and is often angry or resentful.
- **Argumentative/defiant behaviour:** The child often argues with authority figures such as parents and teachers, often breaks the rules and refuses to comply with the requests of authority figures. The child deliberately annoys others and often blames others for his own mistakes.
- **Spiteful/vindictive:** The child manifests a revengeful attitude and behaviour.

These children generally do not resort to physical aggression or significantly destructive behaviour (unlike children with CD).

Oppositional defiant disorder should be differentiated from normal developmental oppositional behaviour such as the terrible twos (at 2 years of age) and adolescence, as during these periods, some amount of oppositional behaviour is considered developmentally normal.

Aetiology

Difficult temperament (temperament determines how an individual regulates the emotions and responds to various situations) as a toddler and during preschool is commonly associated with ODD at a later age.

Various psychosocial factors like difficult parenting, neglect, and maltreatment may also lead to the development of ODD.

Course and Prognosis

Around 25% of children with ODD show resolution of symptoms by adolescence. Children with angry and vindictive symptoms are at high risk of developing CD.

Treatment

The management involves primarily family intervention and behavioural therapy.

In family intervention, the parents are trained to manage the child in a more adaptive manner with a goal to increase prosocial behaviours in the child while decreasing the undesired behaviours. In behavioural therapy, desired behaviours are reinforced using rewards, and undesired behaviours are not reinforced.

CONDUCT DISORDER

The disruptive behaviours seen in children with CD are more severe than in children with ODD. Conduct disorder is more common in boys than girls, and the sex ratio ranges from 4:1 to as much as 12:1.

Clinical Features and Diagnosis

Conduct disorder is characterised by a persistent pattern of behaviour that **violates the basic rights of others** and breaks societal norms. The disruptive behaviour present in these children can be divided into the following four categories:

1. **Physical aggression or threat of harm to people:** Child bullies or threatens others; initiates fights, has used a weapon such as a knife or a bat that can cause serious physical harm, has shown physical cruelty towards people or animals, has stolen while confronting a victim such as mugging and has forced someone into sexual activity.
2. **Destruction of property:** Child has indulged in fire setting or has used other means to damage the property.
3. **Theft or acts of deceit:** Child has indulged in acts of stealing or conning others.
4. **Frequent violation of age-appropriate rules:** Child has stayed out of home at night despite parental prohibitions, was involved in truancy (running away) from school or home; these behaviours should be present before 13 years of age to be considered as age-inappropriate.

Conduct disorder is generally diagnosed before 18 years of age. It can be diagnosed after 18 years of age, provided that the criteria for Antisocial Personality Disorder are not met.

Aetiology

Multiple factors are involved in the development of CD. Genetic factors are involved, and the role of the X-linked monoamine oxidase A gene in the development of CD is under investigation. Neurotransmitter disturbances have been found, such as low levels of plasma dopamine β-hydroxylase in children with CD. Since β-hydroxylase converts dopamine into norepinephrine, it has been hypothesised that decreased noradrenergic functioning may play a role in the development of CD. Studies have also found high plasma serotonin levels in children with CD (plasma serotonin levels are inversely correlated with 5-HIAA levels in CSF, and low CSF 5-HIAA levels are associated with increased impulsivity and aggression). Psychosocial factors such as punitive and harsh parenting, neglect, maltreatment, child abuse, hostility between parents, and exposure to violent video games also contribute to aggressive behaviour in children.

Course and Prognosis

Children with CD have a high risk of developing substance use disorder, delinquency, and criminal behaviour in adulthood. Good prognostic factors are mild severity and absence of comorbidities.

Treatment

Treatment of CD involves pharmacotherapy, psychosocial interventions and management of comorbidities.

A. **Pharmacotherapy:** Atypical antipsychotics like risperidone and quetiapine and mood stabilisers like valproate have been found to decrease aggression. SSRIs like sertraline and paroxetine are used to manage anger, irritability, and impulsivity.
B. **Psychosocial interventions** like problem-solving skills training (how to respond to a problem or stress in an acceptable and non-harmful way); parent management training (teaching parents how to handle children with CD using behavioural reinforcement techniques), and cognitive behaviour therapy are commonly used for the management of CD.
C. Identification and management of co-morbid disorders such as ADHD, learning disorders, mood disorders and substance use disorders is important to improve the outcomes.

ELIMINATION DISORDERS

Mastering control over bowel and bladder function involves motor and sensory functions, coordinated by the frontal lobe and regulated in the pons and midbrain area. The bowel and bladder control develops in the following sequence: (a) development of nocturnal (at night) faecal continence, (b) development of diurnal (during the day) faecal continence, (c) development of diurnal bladder control, and (d) development of nocturnal bladder control.

Inability to achieve bowel or bladder control results in elimination disorders. Enuresis and encopresis are the two elimination disorders.

ENURESIS

Enuresis is diagnosed when a child who has reached the developmental age for urinary continence (i.e., 5 years of age) repeatedly voids urine in clothes or the bed.

Enuresis could be primary if bladder control was never achieved or secondary if enuresis emerged after at least 1 year of bladder control.

Various factors can result in the development of enuresis. The majority (3/4th) of children with enuresis have a first degree relative with a history of enuresis, indicating the role of genetics in the aetiology.

Various psychosocial stressors such as abuse, poor parenting, disrupted families, sibling rivalry, death of a parent also play a role.

Medical disorders such as urinary tract infections, obstructions, spina bifida occulta, cystitis, diabetes mellitus, diabetes insipidus and seizures must be ruled out before making the diagnosis of enuresis.

Enuresis is usually a self-limiting disorder that spontaneously remits. The prevalence of enuresis is relatively high, between 5 to 7 years of age, and then reduces significantly. Only a few remain enuretic in adulthood.

Treatment

Treatment involves non-pharmacological and pharmacological interventions.

Non-pharmacological Interventions

Non-pharmacological treatment of enuresis includes the following:
1. Day-time bladder holding exercises supplemented by positive reinforcement.
2. Restriction of fluid intake after 7 PM
3. Waking up the child from sleep just before the expected time of bedwetting and making him pass urine in the toilet (the child should be fully aware of passing the urine).
4. Bell (or buzzer) and pad (or alarm) apparatus, which works on the classic conditioning principle. The bedwetting leads to the alarm ringing, awakens the child and interrupts the micturition. Gradually, the child starts waking up in response to the bladder distension before the micturition starts. Bed alarms are considered the **treatment of choice** in patients with nocturnal enuresis.

Pharmacotherapy

1. **Imipramine** (Tricyclic antidepressant): It is useful in enuresis because of its anticholinergic action. However, one should be cautious of the cardiac side effects (arrhythmias, sudden death) and it should not be used in children below 6 years of age.
2. **Desmopressin** (an antidiuretic compound): It is also used in the treatment of enuresis. The use of intranasal formulation of desmopressin is no longer indicated by FDA. The most severe side effect of desmopressin is hyponatremic seizures.

The rebound of enuresis after stopping pharmacotherapy is common. Desmopressin is considered the **drug of choice** for nocturnal enuresis. However, non-pharmacological interventions are usually preferred over pharmacological interventions.

ENCOPRESIS

Encopresis is diagnosed when a child who has reached the developmental age for faecal continence (i.e., 4 years of age) repeatedly passes faeces at inappropriate places. Males are affected three to six times more as compared to females.

Aetiology

Children with encopresis typically try to delay the passing of stools by contracting the external anal sphincter and gluteal muscles. In many cases, it is because of past experience of painful bowel movements due to hard stools. This results in eventual overflow passage of stools and, in some cases, faecal impaction.

Various psychosocial factors can cause secondary encopresis (encopresis starting after some period of bowel control). These include loss of a parent, abuse, birth of a sibling etc. In about 5–10% of cases, the condition is caused by medical conditions like abnormal innervation of the anorectal region, Hirschsprung disease, neuronal intestinal dysplasia, or spinal cord damage, and these must be ruled out before making a diagnosis of encopresis.

Like enuresis, encopresis, in some cases, is self-limiting. Encopresis becomes difficult to treat if it is associated with factors like poor gastric motility and an inability to relax anal sphincter muscles.

Treatment

Appropriate toilet training prevents most cases. If encopresis develops, it should be treated with judicious use of laxatives, behaviour therapy and supportive psychotherapy (to lessen anxiety and emotional disturbances). A focus on preventing constipation and reinforcing appropriate toileting behaviours usually works well.

SPECIFIC LEARNING DISORDERS (DEVELOPMENTAL LEARNING DISORDERS)

Specific learning disorders (SLD) are characterised by significant and persistent difficulties in learning academic skills and may manifest as disturbances in reading, writing, arithmetic or a combination of these. The impairment in the academic skill(s) is significant in the context of the child's age and **out of proportion to the general level of intellectual functioning.** These are neurodevelopmental disorders that result from the inability of the brain to perceive (understand, decode, comprehend) or process verbal (language) and non-verbal (gestures, body language) information properly.

According to the deficits, three types of specific learning disorders have been described:
1. **With impairment in reading:** It is characterised by difficulties in reading, such as omissions, substitutions, distortions, or additions of words or parts of words while reading; slow reading rate; long hesitations or reversals

of letters within words while reading; and difficulties in reading comprehension.
2. **With impairment in written expression:** It is characterised by difficulties in writing such as the poor ability to use punctuations, making grammar mistakes while writing, inability to organise paragraphs, difficulty in clearly articulating the ideas in writing, and making frequent spelling mistakes.
3. **With impairment in mathematics:** It is characterised by difficulty in learning mathematics such as difficulties in learning number names, remembering the signs such as for addition or subtraction, learning multiplication tables, translating word problems into computations, and performing calculations.

Diagnosis of specific learning disorders is made by using psychometric tests such as **NIMHANS SLD Battery**.

SLD generally persists in adolescence and adulthood. Mild severity of the disorder and early intervention improves the prognosis.

Treatment: Treatment involves the use of remedial education, with intensive, individually tailored and one to one classes. The management of the associated comorbidities improves the clinical outcome.

INTELLECTUAL DISABILITY (DISORDERS OF INTELLECTUAL DEVELOPMENT)

DSM-5 uses the diagnosis of 'intellectual disability (ID)' whereas ICD-11 uses the diagnosis of 'disorders of intellectual development'. In the older editions of ICD and DSM, the corresponding diagnosis was 'mental retardation'.

The prevalence of Intellectual disability in developing countries ranges from 1%-1.5%. Intellectual disability is 1.5 times more common in males than females.

Intellectual disability is characterised by deficits in both **intellectual functioning** and **adaptive functioning** (as confirmed by the clinical assessment and standardised tests) with onset during the developmental period.

Intellectual functioning refers to cognitive functions like reasoning, problem-solving, planning, academic learning, learning from experience, and judgement. Adaptive functioning refers to the ability to adapt to the environment and meet the usual demands of life. The performance rather than ability measures adaptive functioning.

As per the current recommendations, the severity of ID is diagnosed based on adaptive functioning.

However, many clinicians still use intellectual functioning to assess the severity of ID. Intellectual functioning is usually measured by calculating the IQ (intelligence quotient).

$$IQ = \text{mental age}/\text{chronological age} \times 100$$

In this formula, the **maximum denominator is 15**, even if the assessment of an older individual is being performed.
- IQ testing is also used to certify the range of disability for children with ID. This is in line with the "rights of persons with disability (RPWD) act, 2016".
- IQ for average intelligence ranges between 90 to 110.
- IQ ranging from 80–90 is 'Dull normal intelligence'
- IQ ranging from 70 to 80 is termed as "Borderline Intellectual functioning".
- IQ below 70 is diagnosed as "Intellectual disability".

Degrees of severity of ID: The severity of ID ranges from mild to profound.
- **Mild ID:** It is the commonest type of ID, present in about 85% of the cases. Children with mild ID can study till 6th grade, after which they are likely to face academic difficulties. They have minimal impairment in social interaction. They can make and sustain friendships and relationships. Individuals with mild ID have age-appropriate personal care but require some support in complex tasks like banking, money management, transportation, etc. Many individuals with mild ID can live independently and raise families with some support. IQ of individuals with mild ID ranges from 50 to 70.
- **Moderate ID:** Around 10% of individuals with ID have moderate severity. These individuals require support in academics beyond 2nd to 3rd grade. They face socialisation difficulties. They may develop adequate personal care after some training. However, they need rigorous support in complex tasks. They may be able to do some trivial jobs, but only if there is adequate support from co-workers. IQ of individuals with moderate ID ranges from 35 to 50.
- **Severe ID:** Around 4% of individuals with ID have severe ID. These individuals have poor academic skills (minimal understanding of numbers, money, and time) and poor socialisation skills. They require significant support for even basic personal care and decision making. IQ for severe ID ranges from 20 to 35.
- **Profound ID:** Around 1-2% of individuals with ID have profound ID. These individuals have almost no concept of numbers, money, and time and have poor socialisation skills. They are dependent on others for activities of daily living. IQ of individuals with profound ID is <20.

Diagnosis

Diagnosis of intellectual disability is made based on the following:
- History and clinical examination (including detailed neurological examination)
- Specific investigations like blood tests (to identify inborn errors of metabolism); chromosomal studies (to identify disorders like Down syndrome, Fragile X syndrome); neuroimaging studies (for tuberous sclerosis, unexplained seizures etc); EEG (for seizures); Thyroid function tests and enzymatic sequencing (for storage disorders).

Following tests can be done to determine the IQ:
- Seguin form board test
- Wechsler Intelligence Scale for Children (WISC)
- Malin's Intelligence Scale for Indian Children (MISIC)
- Stanford–Binet or Binet-Kamath tests
- Bhatia's battery of performance tests

The adaptive functioning of an individual can be assessed using the following scales:
- Vineland Social Maturity Scale (VSMS)
- Vineland Adaptive Behaviour Scale (VABS)
- Behavioural Assessment Scales for Indian Children with Mental Retardation (BASIC-MR)

Comorbidities

Up to 65% of children with ID have associated comorbidities. The prevalence of comorbidities is co-related with the severity of ID, and it has been found that with an increase in severity, the prevalence of comorbidities increases. The common psychiatric comorbidities include neurodevelopmental disorders (ADHD, Autism, communication disorders), CD, mood and anxiety disorders and schizophrenia. Seizure disorder is the commonest neurological comorbidity in patients with intellectual disorders.

Aetiology

The following are the common causes of intellectual disability:

Category	Type	Examples
Prenatal	Chromosomal disorders	Down syndrome, Klinefelter syndrome, Turner syndrome, Cri-du-chat syndrome
	Single gene disorders	• Inborn errors of metabolism: Galactosaemia, phenylketonuria, • Others: Fragile X syndrome, Rett syndrome, Tuberous sclerosis, and neurofibromatosis
	Adverse maternal/ environmental influences	• Iodine deficiency, folate deficiency • Severe malnutrition in pregnancy • Using substances: alcohol (maternal alcohol syndrome), nicotine • Maternal infections: Rubella, syphilis, toxoplasmosis, cytomegalovirus, herpes and HIV
Perinatal	Third trimester	Eclampsia; Maternal Diseases: cardiac, renal, diabetes, Placental dysfunction/deprivation of supply
	Labour	Severe prematurity, very low birth weight, hypoxic ischemic encephalopathy (birth asphyxia), difficult and/or complicated delivery, birth trauma
	Neonatal	Septicaemia, severe jaundice, hypoglycaemia
Postnatal		• Brain infections: tuberculosis, bacterial meningo-encephalitis; • Head injury; Chronic lead exposure; Severe and prolonged malnutrition; Gross understimulation and experiential deprivation

Management of Intellectual Disability

Management of ID can be understood in terms of primary prevention, secondary prevention and tertiary prevention.

Primary prevention: This includes measures to prevent the development of ID. Primary prevention is done by (a) Health promotion and (b) Specific protection (against specific causes of ID). Health promotion includes measures like health education, adequate perinatal care and routine health services utilisation and improvement of the nutritional status of the community. Specific protection measures include universal iodisation of salt, folic acid administration in early pregnancy, rubella immunisation for women before pregnancy, prevention of Rh iso-immunisation and universal immunisation for children.

Secondary prevention: This includes measures to halt the progression of the disorder. Early diagnosis and treatment is important for secondary prevention. Secondary prevention for intellectual disorders involves measures like neonatal screening for treatable disorders (e.g., hypothyroidism, phenynlketonuria, galactosaemia, homocysteinuria, congenital hydrocephalus), early detection of developmental delay and "at-risk" children, along with relevant interventions and treatment of associated comorbidities.

Tertiary prevention: Tertiary prevention measures help prevent complications and maximise the functioning of an individual with Intellectual disability. It includes disability limitations and rehabilitation. The following measures are used (a) Parental counselling, (b) Parent training and (c) Providing educational and vocational opportunities to the child.

Parental counselling helps educate the parents about ID, address their doubts, alleviate their anxiety, enhance family and social support and enhance coping skills.

Parent training is basically training the parents, who in turn train the child with intellectual disability. The parents are trained how to teach various skills to the child (social, language, motor, emotional) along with the reinforcement of accepted and good behaviour.

Appropriate educational support (regular school or special school) should be provided based on the level of support required. As far as possible, children with intellectual disability should be integrated into routine education (inclusive education). Children should be provided appropriate vocational training (based on the level of adaptive functioning and level of support required).

Individuals with ID have the right to live with dignity and respect, just like other members of society.

Pharmacotherapy is used to manage comorbidities such as ADHD and depression. In the presence of behavioural problems (such as aggression and self-injurious behaviours), antipsychotics such as risperidone can be used. Behavioural therapy is often helpful in the management of behavioural disturbances.

CASE BASED MCQ

The school referred a nine-year-old boy with complaints of inability to complete the classwork and lagging behind other students. The teacher specifically reported that he would write a couple of lines in his notebook and then start doing other activities, such as drawing or playing with pencils. The teacher was particularly upset as the boy would often leave his seat, go to the desks of other students, and disturb the entire classroom. The performance of the boy in academics was also below par. What is the likely diagnosis?
a. Attention deficit hyperactivity disorder
b. Autism
c. Oppositional defiant disorder
d. Conduct disorder

Ans. a. The history is suggestive of inattention and hyperactivity and the likely diagnosis is attention deficit hyperactivity disorder.

SUGGESTED READINGS

1. Thapar A, Pine DS, Leckman JF, Scott S, Snowling MJ, Taylor EA. Rutter's child and adolescent psychiatry. 6th edition. West Sussex, UK: John Wiley and Sons; 2015.
2. Martin A, Bloch MH, Volkmar FR. Lewis's child and adolescent psychiatry – A comprehensive textbook. 5th edition. Philadelphia: Lippincott Williams and Wilkins; 2018.
3. Sadock BJ, Sadock VA, Ruiz P. Kaplan and Sadock's Comprehensive textbook of psychiatry. 10th edition. Philadelphia: Lippincott Williams and Wilkins; 2017.
4. Boland RJ, Verduin ML, Ruiz P. Kaplan and Sadock's Synopsis of psychiatry. 12th edition. Philadelphia: Lippincott Williams and Wilkins; 2022.
5. Shah R, Grover S, Avasthi A. Clinical practice guidelines for the assessment and management of attention-deficit/hyperactivity disorder. Indian J Psychiatry. 2019;61(Suppl S2):176-93.
6. Kishore M T, Udipi GA, Seshadri SP. Clinical practice guidelines for assessment and management of intellectual disability. Indian J Psychiatry. 2019;61(Suppl S2):194-210.
7. Subramanyam AA, Mukherjee A, Dave M, Chavda K. Clinical practice guidelines for autism spectrum disorders. Indian J Psychiatry. 2019;61(Suppl S2):254-69.
8. Shah HR, Sagar JK, Somaiya MP, Nagpal JK. Clinical practice guidelines on assessment and management of specific learning disorders. Indian J Psychiatry. 2019;61(Suppl S2):211-25.
9. Taylor DM, Barnes TR, Young AH. The Maudsley Prescribing Guidelines in psychiatry. 14th edition. West Sussex, UK: John Wiley and Sons; 2021.

18 Psychoanalysis

Praveen Tripathi, Priyanka Goyal

The term 'psychoanalysis' is used to describe various things. Psychoanalysis is:
1. A **psychological theory** that explains how the mind works (especially how unconscious mental processes work).
2. It is also a **method of investigation** of psychological functioning; in other words, psychoanalysis is an investigation tool to find out what is causing the psychological disturbance.
3. And it's also a **method of treatment** for psychological disorders.

The term "psychoanalysis" was coined by **Sigmund Freud**, who is also known as the **"father of psychoanalysis"**. **Freud (1856–1939)** was born in Freiburg, Moravia (now in the Czech Republic) and lived most of his life in **Vienna**. He died in London in 1939.

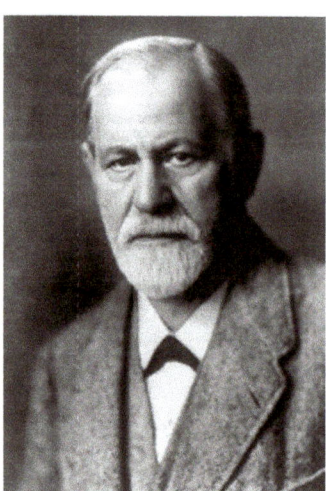

Fig. 18.1: Sigmund Freud.

According to psychoanalysis, **childhood experiences and memories, and unconscious mental activity** (activity of mind which we are not aware of) plays an important role in determining human behaviour and emotions and the development of psychiatric disorders. As discussed above, the term "psychoanalysis" is used to refer to this theory and the treatment method based on this theory.

The theory of psychoanalysis was developed by Freud while working with patients with hysteria (the term hysteria is no longer used, those patients will get a diagnosis of "dissociative disorder" or "conversion disorder" according to the current classification).

Freud came to know about a patient Anna O, who had developed multiple unexplained neurological symptoms, including paralysis of limbs, after her father's death. Whenever she could recall how a particular symptom originated, that symptom would improve. For example, she recalled that once while sitting at her sick father's bedside, she had a daydream that a snake was crawling towards her father, and while she wanted to ward off the snake, she couldn't do it as her arm had gone into sleep. As soon as Anna O was able to recall this event, the paralysis of her arm improved.

This case provided Freud with a strong demonstration that unconscious memories (memories that an individual had forgotten but were present in the unconscious mind) play an essential role in developing psychological symptoms.

Freud started treating patients with hysteria, wherein he would try to retrieve the unconscious memories during the treatment procedure. Initially, Freud used hypnosis and found that patients in a state of trance (an altered state of consciousness) could recall forgotten traumatic events. In many patients, this leads to the abreaction.

Abreaction is a process by which repressed material (forgotten material) is remembered back and relived along with the expression of associated emotions. Abreaction helped improve symptoms in a few patients with hysteria.

Later Freud developed a technique called "**free association**", in which the patient was asked to say whatever came into her mind without censoring the thoughts. Freud analysed the material obtained during free association. Freud gave a lot of importance to **the patient's slips of the tongue** (which he called **parapraxis**). Freud believed that these "slips of tongues" were not simple mistakes and that these slips actually conveyed **important information** about the content of the unconscious mind. With the help of 'free association,' Freud could understand what was going on in the patient's unconscious mind.

The psychoanalytic treatment also uses the phenomenon of transference and countertransference to get important information.

Transference is the feeling that the patient develops for the doctor. This feeling is a combination of the feelings patient had for figures from the past and the real feeling for the clinician. For example, suppose the doctor reminds the patient of his dominating and insensitive father. In that case, the patient will develop a negative feeling towards the doctor, even though the doctor has not done anything to offend him.

Countertransference is the feeling that the clinician develops for the patient.

TOPOGRAPHICAL THEORY OF MIND

In **1900**, Freud published a book called **"The Interpretation of Dreams"**. In this book, Freud said that dreams were meaningful, and by understanding dreams, one can understand the unconscious mind of an individual. In this book, Freud proposed a theory of mind, called the **topographical theory of mind**. According to this theory, the mind has three parts:

A. The conscious
B. The preconscious, and
C. The unconscious

A. *The conscious:* It is the part of the mind which is accessible to us. We are aware of the contents of the conscious mind. Everything you know about yourself is a part of the conscious mind.

B. *The preconscious:* The content of the preconscious mind is not usually available to us but can be recalled or brought into awareness by focusing attention on it. For example, you may not distinctly remember what your 5th class teacher looked like; however, if you try to focus and remember hard, you might be able to recall her face. If that is the case, her appearance was in the 'preconscious' and could be accessed by giving attention.

The preconscious separates the conscious and unconscious mind. The preconscious mind has a barrier called '**repression**', which normally does not allow the contents of the unconscious mind to reach the conscious mind. If any unconscious memory has to reach conscious awareness, it must find a way to overcome the force of "repression". Freud reported that the repression force becomes lax during sleep, and many unconscious memories and desires can reach the conscious in the form of dreams. That's why Freud believed that the interpretation of dreams could reveal the contents of unconscious memories and desires. Further, when a person indulges in "free association", some unconscious content can cross the barrier of repression and come out as "slips of the tongue".

C. *The unconscious:* The unconscious mind is not accessible to the individual. The unconscious mind contains **the instinctual drives** (i.e., the drives and desires one is born with), such as sexual instinct and aggressive instinct. Further, distressing childhood memories and distressing desires are also buried inside the unconscious. This content is not available to the conscious mind due to the barrier of "repression". Freud believed that by not allowing these memories to reach consciousness, repression causes the development of psychiatric symptoms and disorders.

The unconscious mind is characterised by **"primary process thinking"**. This is a primitive way of thinking in which the mind wants immediate "wish fulfilment" and instinctual discharge (wants all desires and instincts to be fulfilled immediately without considering the consequences). The primary process thinking is **illogical** and **contradictory**.

In "The Interpretation of dreams", Freud postulated that dreams are a way by which unconscious impulses get expressed consciously. He believed that unacceptable desires and impulses, which are a part of the unconscious mind, usually are not allowed to enter the conscious mind by the barrier of 'repression'. However, during sleep, this barrier allows certain such desires and impulses to enter the conscious mind after being transformed. This transformation is necessary as the content of these desires and impulses is usually unacceptable. If allowed to enter the conscious mind in their original form, they will cause significant distress to the sleeping person and may awaken him. This transformation process is called '**dream work**' and transforms '**latent content**' (original content) of dreams to '**manifest content**' (content after modification that one sees) of the dream.

In dream work, the unconscious desires and impulses are attached to images from the dreamer's current experience and, hence, are transformed so that they no longer remain unacceptable. For example, Say, a person has an unconscious impulse of aggression against his father; if he sees a dream in which he is hitting his father, it may result in so much distress that he is likely to wake up. So the dream work process will attach this aggressive impulse with the image of a teacher whom the dreamer met in the morning, and during the dream, the dreamer will see himself hitting the teacher.

This dream allowed the expression of aggressive impulse, and it was modified so that the dreamer did not get distressed and didn't wake up. The mechanisms that are involved in dream work are as follows:

A. *Condensation:* This mechanism allows several unconscious desires and impulses to be combined in a single image in the manifest dream content. The opposite, called 'irradiation or diffusion, involves breaking a single desire or impulse into various parts.

B. *Displacement:* This involves displacement of impulse from an original object to a substitute object. For example, the aggression was displaced from the father to the teacher in the example mentioned above.

C. *Symbolic representation:* Here, a strong or complex emotion towards an individual is symbolised by a simple image. For example, a strong homosexual impulse towards a person may be represented as a snake (snake symbolises 'penis' here).

STRUCTURAL THEORY OF MIND

Later in his life, Freud replaced the topographical theory of mind with a newer theory called the structural theory of mind. According to this theory, there are three components of the mind: id, ego and superego.

A. **Id**: It is the most primitive part of the mind with which an infant is born. The id consists of instinctual drives. It is the part of the mind which wants to have pleasure and that too immediately. Id does not care much about the external world reality or any consequences, and Id works on the **"pleasure principle"**. Id uses the primary process thinking. Id is completely in the **unconscious domain** of the mind.

B. **Ego**: It is the part of the mind that deals with the external world. The part of your mind which is reading this book is "ego". Apart from dealing with the external world, another important function of the ego is to deal with the "id" and "superego" and maintain a balance between the two and the external world. Since the ego maintains a balance and helps in dealing with the realities of the outside world, it is said to work on the **"reality principle"**. The ego is said to be the **"executive organ"** of the mind. Ego has **both conscious and unconscious** components. The "defense mechanisms" are a part of the **unconscious component** of the ego.

C. **Superego**: It is the part of the mind that follows moral principles and wants to do the "right thing". The voice of conscience, which scolds you when you are not studying, comes from the superego. Superego is **mostly unconscious** but also has a **conscious component**. To understand how the different parts of the mind work, let's take an example.

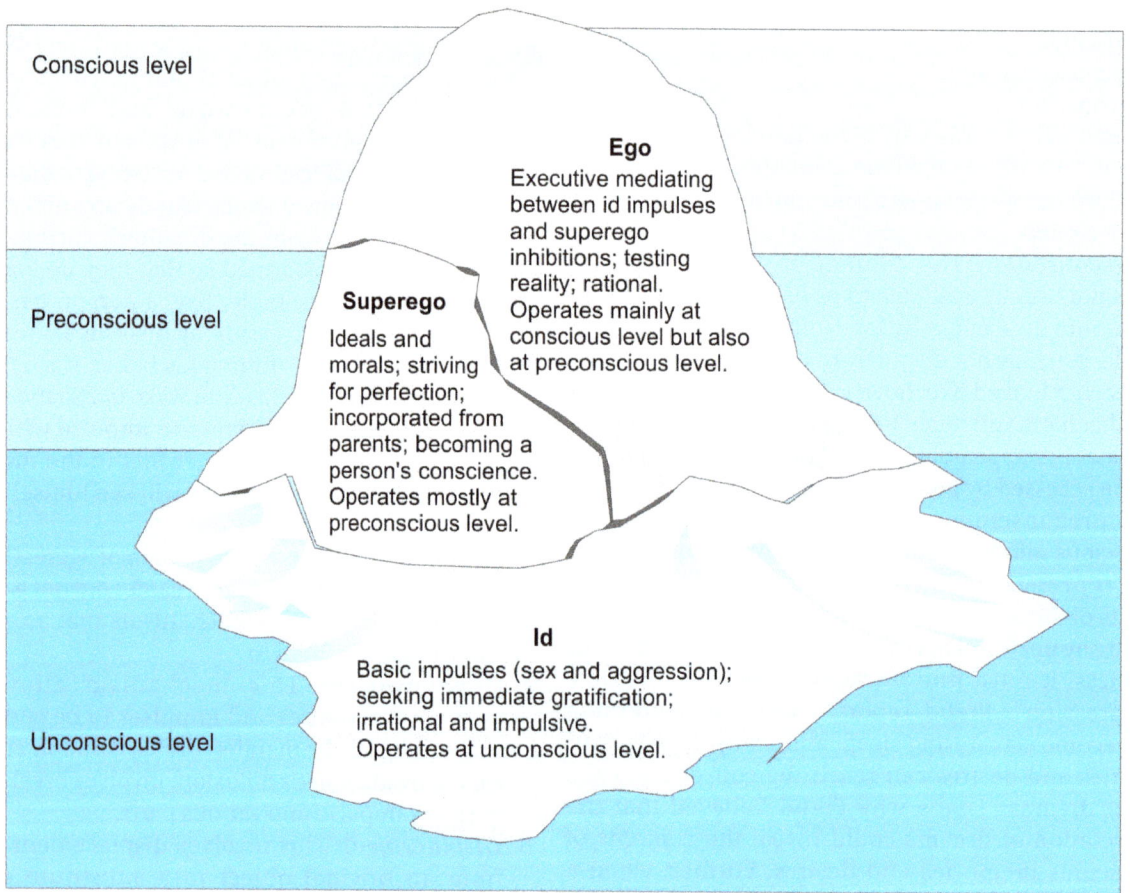

Fig. 18.2: Three components of mind: Id, ego and superego.

While you are studying, your id wants you to throw away the books and instead go out and have fun and indulge in some pleasurable activity. On the other hand, your superego wants you to study very hard without taking any breaks and stay away from all distractions. Finally, your ego does a balancing act, and you decide that you will study for 1 hour, and after that, you will take a break and watch a movie. This is how the ego tries to maintain a balance.

As mentioned in this example, conflicts keep on cropping up in the mind (between id, ego and superego), and these **unconscious conflicts** in mind are believed to be one of the causes of psychiatric disorders according to the psychodynamic (or psychoanalytic) theories.

DEFENSE MECHANISMS

An important function of the ego is to prevent a build-up of excessive and unbearable anxiety, and defence mechanisms are the tools used by the "ego" for this purpose. The defense mechanisms have been divided into four groups: narcissistic, immature, neurotic and mature defense mechanisms.

Following are the important defense mechanisms:

Narcissistic Defenses

A. ***Denial*:** It is the refusal to acknowledge reality. The person continues to behave as if nothing has happened. For example, on being given the news of the death of son in an accident, a mother refused to accept that her 7-year-old son had died and insisted that everything was okay with him and he would be back for dinner.

B. ***Projection*:** Projecting "own" unacceptable feelings about others onto others. For example, a husband with an unacceptable wish of indulging in infidelity starts accusing his wife of indulging in infidelity. Here, the husband has "projected" his own wish onto the wife. This defense mechanism is responsible for the development of **delusions and hallucinations**.

C. ***Distortion*:** It involves grossly reshaping the experience of external reality to match the internal requirements. For example, after failing an exam that most other students passed, one student insisted that he failed because the exam was extremely tough.

Immature Defenses

A. ***Acting out*:** Acting on unconscious desires without becoming aware of them. For example, a person suddenly steals an item from a shop without prior planning. In this case, this person had an unconscious desire to steal. His mind, however, did not allow this feeling to enter the conscious, as that would have resulted in the person feeling bad about himself. Hence, this person resorts to acting on the unconscious desire straight away without even becoming aware of the same. This defense mechanism is involved in the development of **impulse control disorders**.

B. ***Passive-aggressive behaviour*:** Indirectly expressing anger towards others. For example, a young boy was forced to bring a glass of water by his father. While bringing the water, the boy accidentally tripped and dropped the glass. Here, the child expressed his anger indirectly by dropping the glass.

C. ***Regression*:** Attempt to return to an earlier development phase (i.e., childhood) to avoid the tensions and conflicts of the present development phase (i.e., adulthood). For example, extremely stressed about an upcoming entrance examination, a medical student goes to the park and starts playing cricket with the children. In this example, the medical student is trying to return to his childhood days, when he could play cricket freely without worrying about the entrance exams. Regression is involved in the development of **neurosis**.

D. ***Projective identification*:** In this defense mechanism, intolerable aspects of self are projected onto another person; that person is induced to play the projected part, and the two persons then act in unison. For example, a wife who has lots of aggression can project her aggression onto the husband and make him behave aggressively, and finally, a system develops where the husband indulges in aggression, and the wife is the recipient of aggression. Please remember all of this happens unconsciously without entering into awareness of either the wife or the husband. Projective identification is seen in patients with **borderline personality disorder**.

Neurotic Defenses

A. ***Displacement*:** Shifting emotions about one object/individual onto another object/individual. For example, after being scolded by the consultant, a senior resident came to the ward and started shouting at the intern. Here, the senior resident is actually angry at the consultant, but he is displacing his anger on the intern. Displacement is involved in the development of **phobias**.

B. ***Intellectualisation*:** Excessive use of intellectual processes to avoid painful emotions. For example, a doctor diagnosed with pancreatic cancer has a long discussion about the pathophysiology of cancer with his treating physician. Here, the doctor is trying to avoid the painful emotion of being diagnosed with cancer by discussing the pathophysiology of cancers in detail.

C. ***Isolation of affect*:** Removing the feelings associated with a stressful life event. For example, a woman tells her family members that she has been diagnosed with advanced-stage cholangiocarcinoma without showing any emotions.

D. ***Repression*:** It is one of the most important defense mechanisms, often referred to as the "primary" defense mechanism. It is unconsciously forgetting something which cannot be retrieved later. For example, a young girl who was sexually abused by her father "forgets" this incidence of sexual abuse. Now, even if she wants to recall it, she cannot do it in normal circumstances.

E. ***Rationalisation*:** Offering rational explanations to justify own unacceptable behaviour. For example, a person with heavy alcohol use blamed the family environment for his excessive drinking habit. It is a commonly used defense mechanism in **substance use disorders**.

F. ***Dissociation*:** Splitting of a single (e.g., memory, identity) or group of mental functions from the remaining mental functions. It is seen in disorders like **dissociative identity disorder**, where e.g., the identity of an individual gets split from the rest of the mental functions.

G. ***Reaction formation*:** Transformation of feelings into their exact opposite. For example, a man who is infatuated with an office colleague tells his friend that he 'really hates' her. Here, the actual feeling is that of infatuation, but it is being transformed into the feeling of "hatred".

H. ***Undoing*:** An act that is done to nullify a previous act. For example, a husband brings gifts for the wife the day after fighting with her. The defense mechanism of undoing is used in **obsessive-compulsive disorder**.

I. ***Aim inhibition*:** Placing a limitation upon instinctual demands, accepting partial or modified fulfilment of desires. For example, a student who wanted to become a doctor but could not clear the pre-medical tests takes admission in a veterinary course and becomes a veterinary doctor.

Mature Defenses

A. **Altruism:** Satisfying internal needs by helping others. For example, while driving in a drunk state, a man had an accident and lost his son, who was travelling alongside him. Later, he started a campaign against drunk driving and started educating people about the ills of drunk driving.

B. **Anticipation:** Planning in advance to deal with an uncomfortable event. For example, a student plans all his arguments comprehensively before going home after a bad exam result.

C. **Humour:** Using comedy to deal with unpleasant feelings and situations. For example, two medical students joked and laughed at themselves after getting humiliated by the examiner during the viva.

D. **Sublimation:** Expression of unacceptable feelings in a socially acceptable manner. For example, a middle-aged man with unacceptable sexual desire becomes a painter and starts making nude paintings. Here, sexual desires are getting an outlet, and it's socially acceptable, too, since painting nudes is considered an art form.

E. **Suppression:** It is the only voluntary or conscious defense mechanism. It involves a voluntary decision not to think about an event for some time and avoid the accompanying emotions. For example, a medical student who is extremely stressed out about an upcoming entrance exam decides to take a one day break during which he won't think at all about the exam.

Defense Mechanisms in Psychiatric Disorders

All the defense mechanisms are used at times by all of us. However, when used excessively, they can cause the development of psychiatric disorders. Following is a list of a few defense mechanisms and associated disorders:

- **Obsessive-compulsive disorder:** Reaction formation, displacement, undoing, isolation of affect and inhibition
- **Phobia:** Displacement and inhibition
- **Dissociative disorder:** Dissociation
- **Neurosis:** Regression

PSYCHOSEXUAL STAGES OF DEVELOPMENT

Sigmund Freud proposed that sexuality develops in multiple stages. Freud used the term "sexuality" as a broader concept that includes other forms of pleasure also and not only genital sexuality. He proposed five stages of development. Freud further proposed that the development may get arrested at a particular stage (called **"fixation"**) and may result in the development of psychiatric disorders:

A. *Oral stage (0–1.5 years):* This is the first stage of development wherein the pleasure is derived from the oral cavity. The child derives pleasure in cutting, biting, chewing, etc.

B. *Anal stage (1.5–3 years):* The site of pleasure is the anal region. The child gets a sense of achievement by getting toilet trained. If the psychosexual development gets arrested at this stage (called **fixation at the anal stage**), it can result in the development of **obsessive-compulsive disorder.**

C. *Phallic stage (3–5 years):* The site of pleasure is the genital area. According to Freud, the penis becomes the organ of principal interest for children of both sexes. The male child develops what is known as **the Oedipus complex**, in which he starts developing sexual feelings towards the mother and wants to replace the father. However, the male child also becomes fearful that if the father finds out, he might castrate him (hence the child develops **castration anxiety**). The Oedipus complex in male child gets resolved once the child shifts his affection away from his mother to some other female and starts identifying (starts imitating his father and trying to become like him) with the father. In females, the Oedipus stage unfolds differently (at times, the term used for the phenomenon in the female child is **"Electra complex"**). The girl child develops a sexual desire for the father. At the same time, she becomes aware that she does not have a penis and desires to get one (known as "penis envy"). The female child believes that she was castrated, and that's why does not have a penis and holds her mother responsible for it, developing anger against the mother. The stage gets resolved when the female child starts identifying with the mother. Failure to resolve the Oedipus and Electra complex can result in the development of neurotic illnesses (like hysteria). Hence, **neurotic illness develops due to fixation at the phallic stage.**

D. *Latent stage (5–12 years):* During this stage, there is relative quiescence or inactivity of sexual drive, and the child focuses on learning and gaining skills.

E. *Genital stage (12 years onward till young adulthood):* This stage is characterised by the maturation of genital functioning and gradual achievement of a mature sexual and adult identity.

The theory of psychoanalysis and the methods of psychoanalytic treatment have all been questioned in recent years. Nowadays, evidence-based medicine has become the standard, and it is difficult to test the theory of psychoanalysis and validate it. The psychoanalytic treatment methods have also been found to be of limited efficacy in the treatment of most psychiatric disorders. Hence the practical utility of psychoanalysis has shrunken over the years.

Nonetheless, the sheer genius of Sigmund Freud that went into the creation of psychoanalysis is admirable, and different psychotherapies continue to borrow some aspects of psychoanalysis and use them in the treatment processes.

CASE BASED MCQ

A 21-year-old medical student was desperate to go on a date on the upcoming Valentine's day. He tried asking out many girls from his class, but they all refused. The student was later found to be carrying a placard that read, 'Medical student should not celebrate Valentine's day and anyone found violating this rule should be suspended from the college'. Which defence mechanism is the medical student using?

a. Displacement
b. Reaction formation
c. Undoing
d. Altruism

Ans. b. It is the transformation of feelings into their exact opposite.

SUGGESTED READINGS

1. Geddes JR, Andreasen NC. New Oxford textbook of psychiatry. Oxford University Press, USA; 2020.
2. Hall, C.S., 2016. A primer of Freudian psychology. Pickle Partners Publishing.
3. Boland R, Verdiun M, Ruiz P. Kaplan and Sadock's Synopsis of Psychiatry. Lippincott Williams and Wilkins; 2021.

19 Other Somatic Therapies

Praveen Tripathi, Priyanka Goyal

PS18.2	Enumerate the indications for modified electroconvulsive therapy
PS18.3	Enumerate and describe the principles and role of psychosocial interventions in psychiatric illness including psychotherapy, behavioural therapy and rehabilitation

In this chapter, we will discuss certain somatic therapies that are used in the treatment of psychiatric disorders.

ELECTROCONVULSIVE THERAPY

Convulsive therapies have long been used for the treatment of major psychiatric disorders. An interesting finding by Von Meduna, a Hungarian Neuropsychiatrist, played an essential role in the widespread use of convulsive therapies. Meduna observed that patients with epilepsy had more glial cells in the brain than others, whereas patients with schizophrenia had fewer glial cells in the brain. He hypothesised that there might be a **biological antagonism** between convulsions and schizophrenia.

And the corollary of this hypothesis was that if seizures could be induced in a patient with schizophrenia, the symptoms of schizophrenia should improve. In 1934, using intramuscular injections of **camphor** to induce therapeutic seizures, the first patient with psychosis was successfully treated.

Later, Lucio Bini and Ugo Cerletti used electricity to induce convulsions and it was called "**electroconvulsive therapy (ECT)**." The use of ECT has decreased in the last few decades, as effective pharmacological agents have been developed for most psychiatric disorders. However, in cases where rapid improvement is required, ECT continues to be the first-line treatment.

Types

1. **Direct ECT**: In Direct ECT, anaesthetic agents and muscle relaxants are not used. Hence, the induced, generalised convulsions can result in fractures or teeth dislocations. Due to the higher incidence of side effects, this technique is rarely used nowadays. The Mental Health Care Act, 2017 has banned the use of direct ECT in India.
2. **Modified ECT (Indirect ECT)**: Here, anaesthetic agents and muscle relaxants are administered before inducing seizures. As muscles are in a state of deep relaxation, there are no generalised convulsive movements, and the risk of bone fractures and other injuries gets minimised.

Electrode Placement

Various configurations have been developed for electrode placement. Most practitioners use bilateral electrode placements; however, unilateral ECT is gradually becoming more popular because of its better side effect profile.

1. **Bilateral ECT**: It involves the placement of electrodes on both sides of the skull. Different configurations can be used, with the **bifrontotemporal** electrode placement being the most commonly used and the bifrontal electrode placement being the other configuration. The bilateral ECT is associated with more side effects, particularly the cognitive side effects.
2. **Unilateral ECT**: In an attempt to decrease the side effects of ECT, unilateral electrode placements have been introduced. The right unilateral ECT (also called **d'Elia placement**) has been found to have a better side effect profile than the bilateral ECT and is being increasingly used.

The older ECT machines used a sine wave electrical stimulus, delivering excessive electricity and leading to more cognitive side effects. Modern machines use a brief pulse waveform to administer electrical stimulus, resulting in lesser side effects.

Following medications are used while administering modified ECT:

a. **Muscarinic anticholinergics**: Atropine is often administered before ECT to reduce the oral and respiratory secretions. It also helps to prevent bradycardias and asystoles.
b. **Anaesthetic agents**: Methohexital is the anaesthetic agent of choice and preferred over thiopental because of its short duration of action and lower association with postictal arrhythmias. Etomidate, propofol, ketamine and alfentanil can be used too but are less preferred.

c. **Muscle relaxants: Succinylcholine** is usually used to achieve profound muscle relaxation. This helps avoid fractures due to motor activity during the seizures. Before administering the muscle relaxants, a sphygmomanometer cuff is applied to the arm/ankle and inflated above the systolic BP. This allows the observation of tonic-clonic movements in the forearm/foot to monitor the duration of seizures.

In patients with pseudocholinesterase deficiency, atracurium or curare can be used.

Mechanism of Action

The induction of a bilateral generalised seizure is considered necessary for the beneficial effect of ECT. To be therapeutically effective, the seizure must last at least **25 seconds**.

Earlier it was believed that the response to ECT was an "all or none" phenomenon; however, of late, it has been found that at least in right unilateral ECTs, a dose-response relationship is present.

The mechanism of action of ECT is still not completely understood. Studies on neurotransmitter receptors have found that ECT impacts almost all neurotransmitter systems, with the downregulation of postsynaptic β-adrenergic receptors being a consistent finding.

ECT also impacts second messenger systems and has been found to affect the coupling of G-proteins to receptors and the activity of adenylyl cyclase and phospholipase C.

The latest research has suggested an increase in brain-derived neurotrophic factor, **BDNF**, to be an important mechanism of action of ECT. ECT has also been found to promote neurogenesis in areas like the hippocampus.

Indications

Electroconvulsive therapy has a rapid onset of action and hence is considered first-line treatment in life-threatening conditions such as high suicide risk, homicide risk, catatonia, poor oral intake, and risk of physical exhaustion (especially in the manic phase).

A. **Depression (Major depressive disorder)**: The ECT was originally used to treat schizophrenia and other psychotic illnesses; however, currently, the most common indication for ECT is depression. ECT is the most effective treatment of depression (in both major depressive disorder and bipolar disorder). The clearest indication for ECT is depression with suicide risk. The indications of ECT in depression include the following:
   - **Depression with suicide risk** (ECT is the treatment of choice in acutely suicidal patients due to its immediate onset of action)
   - Depression with stupor
   - Depression with psychotic symptoms (psychotic depression or delusional depression)
   - In case of failed medication trials or intolerance to medications.

   For depression, usually 6-12 ECT sessions are administered.

B. **Manic episode**: Electroconvulsive therapy is effective in acute mania; however, since pharmacotherapy for mania is in itself quite effective, ECT is rarely used for this indication. ECT is used in mania, in case of either intolerance/unresponsiveness to pharmacotherapy or when there is a risk of homicide/suicide or danger of physical exhaustion and immediate control of symptoms is required.

   ECT should not be administered to a patient on lithium, as lithium decreases the seizure threshold and may increase the chances of ECT induced delirium.

C. **Schizophrenia**: Electroconvulsive therapy is effective in acute schizophrenia, particularly against the **catatonic** symptoms. It is also effective for positive symptoms. However, as antipsychotics are quite effective in schizophrenia, ECT is used only if the patient is unresponsive/intolerant to medications or needs immediate symptom control to avoid harm to self/others. Electroconvulsive therapy is not effective in chronic schizophrenia.

D. **Other indications**: ECT is occasionally used for intractable seizures (ECT increases the seizure threshold and hence acts as an anticonvulsant), neuroleptic malignant syndrome, delirium, the on-off phenomenon of Parkinson's disease, and obsessive-compulsive disorder.

Adverse Effects

1. **Memory disturbances:** It is the most common side effect of ECT. Both retrograde and anterograde amnesia can be present; however, **retrograde amnesia** is much more common. Memory disturbances are usually mild, and recovery occurs within 1-6 months after the treatment.
2. Other side effects include delirium, headache, muscle aches, fractures (very rare with modified ECT), nausea and vomiting.
3. **Prolonged seizures:** After administration of ECT, if the seizure continues for more than **180 seconds,** it is called a prolonged seizure and must be terminated to prevent progression to status epilepticus.

Contraindications

There are **no absolute contraindications** of ECT. Earlier, raised intracranial tension was considered an absolute contraindication (due to increased risk for oedema and brain herniation after ECT); however, it is now considered a relative contraindication. Pregnancy is not a contraindication for ECT. The following are the relative contraindications of ECT:

1. Raised intracranial tension (space-occupying lesion in CNS)
2. Recent myocardial infarction
3. Severe hypertension
4. Cerebrovascular disease
5. Severe pulmonary disease
6. Retinal detachment.

Legal Status of ECT in India

Mental Healthcare Act, 2017 has banned direct ECT in India. Also, the use of ECT in minors has been banned. However, a provision has been made according to which if, in a rare case, the psychiatrist in charge considers ECT is required for the treatment of a minor, he will have to take informed consent of the guardian and prior permission from the mental health review board.

ECT carries a considerable stigma as a treatment modality, and patients and family members get scared alike at the mere mention of ECT as an option. It is the responsibility of the treating psychiatrist to provide scientific and detailed information on the benefits of ECT and help the patient make an informed decision. ECT can be life-saving, and in conditions where it is indicated, the efficacy of ECT remains unparalleled even today.

TRANSCRANIAL MAGNETIC STIMULATION

Electroconvulsive therapy involves direct electrical stimulation of the brain (through the scalp); recently, techniques have been developed that use indirect methods for electrical brain stimulation.

Transcranial magnetic stimulation (TMS) uses **rapidly changing magnetic fields** to induce small electric currents (called eddy currents) in the cerebral cortex. The devices used for TMS, deliver magnetic pulses via a coil held on the scalp, and TMS can provide more localised stimulation of the brain in a non-invasive manner.

While single pulses of TMS have a short-lived effect, repetitive pulses of TMS (also called rTMS or repetitive TMS) can result in long-lasting changes, likely related to neuroplasticity. Also, high-frequency rTMS has an excitatory effect, whereas low-frequency rTMS is inhibitory.

It has been hypothesised that depression is caused by reduced activity in the left dorsolateral prefrontal cortex. High frequency rTMS applied over the left dorsolateral prefrontal cortex has been found to be effective in treating patients with depression.

The side effect profile of rTMS is quite favourable, with seizures being one of the rare but significant side effects.

rTMS has been FDA approved for the treatment of depression (in patients who have failed a trial of one or more antidepressants), obsessive-compulsive disorder (as an adjunct treatment) and recently, in August 2020, as a smoking cessation aid.

VAGUS NERVE STIMULATION

This technique involves direct electrical stimulation of the left cervical vagus nerve. The electrode is wrapped around the left vagus nerve and is connected to a pulse generator implanted in the left chest wall. The left vagus nerve primarily contains afferent fibres, and their persistent stimulation is hypothesised to stimulate specific areas of the brain.

Although vagus nerve stimulation (VNS) is approved for long term adjunctive treatment of chronic or recurrent depression (in patients who had no response to four or more antidepressant trials), its invasive nature and limited efficacy have limited its use.

DEEP BRAIN STIMULATION

Deep brain stimulation (DBS) is an invasive modality for direct electrical stimulation of the brain. It involves the placement of small 'leads' into subcortical nuclei or specific white matter tracts. These leads are connected to a pulse generator implanted subdermally in the upper chest wall. Due to its invasive nature, this technique has limited use in clinical psychiatry.

OTHER MODALITIES

Few other modalities are currently in the experimental stage. These include:

a. **Transcranial direct current stimulation:** This technique uses a weak direct current applied to the scalp, which polarises the neuronal membrane. The exact mechanism of action is unknown.
b. **Cranial electrical stimulation:** In this technique, a weak alternating current is administered by applying electrodes on the earlobes. This technique has shown some efficacy in the treatment of anxiety disorders, but is still in the experimental stage.
c. **Magnetic seizure therapy (MST):** Like ECT, seizures are induced for therapeutic effect in magnetic seizure therapy. However, instead of direct electrical stimulation, alternating magnetic stimulation is used to induce an electrical current in the brain (similar to rTMS). MST can be used to induce a more localised electrical current with better control over its spread.

PSYCHOSURGERY

The surgical techniques for the treatment of psychiatric disorders are rarely used. They are reserved for only the chronic and severe cases which have not responded to other treatment methods. The psychosurgeries involve creating a lesion in the limbic system or its connecting fibres (the limbic system is responsible for normal and abnormal emotional reactions). The lesions are nowadays produced with precision using stereotactic methods. The following are the types:

A. **Stereotactic subcaudate tractotomy:** *It produces a subcaudate lesion and is used in chronic, severe and intractable cases of depression, obsessive-compulsive disorder and schizoaffective disorder.*
B. **Stereotactic limbic leucotomy:** *Small lesion is made in the subcaudate, and also a lesion is made in the cingulate bundle. It is used in the treatment of chronic, severe and intractable obsessive-compulsive disorder and schizophrenia.*
C. **Amygdalotomy:** *A lesion is made in the amygdala in patients with severe, uncontrolled aggression.*

Mental Healthcare Act, 2017 has banned psychosurgeries in India. However, a provision has been made according to which if, in a rare case, the psychiatrist in charge considers psychosurgery is required for the treatment, he will have to take informed consent of the patient and prior permission from the mental health review board.

SUGGESTED READINGS

1. Cohen SL, Bikson M, Badran BW, George MS. A visual and narrative timeline of US FDA milestones for Transcranial Magnetic Stimulation (TMS) devices. Brain Stimulation: Basic, Translational, and Clinical Research in Neuromodulation. 2022;15(1):73-5.
2. Boland R, Verdiun M, Ruiz P. Kaplan & Sadock's Synopsis of Psychiatry. Lippincott Williams & Wilkins; 2021.
3. Sadock B, Sadock V, Ruiz P. Kaplan & Sadock's comprehensive textbook of psychiatry. 10th ed. Philadelphia: Wolters Kluwer; 2017.

20 Psychological Theories and Interventions

Meha Jain, Snehanky Chattopadhyay, Sujita Kumar Kar, Praveen Tripathi

Before discussing the various types of psychotherapies, let's briefly discuss a few important theories in psychology.

COGNITIVE DEVELOPMENT STAGES

Cognition refers to the inner processes of the mind that lead to knowing. It includes all mental activities such as attention, remembering, symbolising, categorising, planning, reasoning and problem solving, creating and fantasising. **Jean Piaget** gave a stage theory, proposing that all humans move through an orderly and predictable series of changes during cognitive development. It is a general theory of development; the stages are universal and invariant.

The stages of cognitive development, along with their salient features, have been described below:

A. **Sensorimotor stage (birth to 2 years):** This is the first stage. During this stage, the child learns through sensory observations and gradually gains control of his motor functions. Initially, the child thinks that if he cannot see an object, it means that the object has ceased to exist. For example, if a rattle with which a child is playing is taken away and is covered so that the child can no longer see it, the child will think that the rattle no longer exists and will not try to look for it. This type of thinking is called the **"out of sight, out of mind"** and **"here and now"** type of thinking. At the end of the sensorimotor stage, the child develops "object permanence", which is the development of the concept that objects continue to exist even if they are not visible currently. In the above example, once the child develops object permanence, he will try to search for the rattle by removing the covering cloth as he now knows that the rattle continues to exist though he cannot see it. Another important development at around 18 months is a process known as **"symbolisation"**, wherein the infant starts developing mental symbols and using words for objects. For example, they make a mental symbol to represent the ball and use a word for it. The development of **"object permanence"** indicates the transition to the next stage of development, i.e., stage of preoperational thought.

B. **Preoperational stage (2-7 years):** In this stage, the thinking is still rigid, limited to one aspect of a situation at a time and strongly influenced by the way things appear at the moment. However, the capacity for mental representation increases. Language, make-believe play and drawings are the other developments during this stage. The children also develop the power of language to represent their thoughts. In this stage, children are usually **"egocentric"**, which means they cannot think from the other person's perspective and are only concerned about themselves. This egocentric thinking is also responsible for animistic thinking in children–the belief that inanimate objects have life-like qualities like thoughts, wishes, feelings and intentions. The thinking process is characterised by **"intuitive thought"**, which is thinking without the use of reasoning and an inability to use logicality.

C. **Concrete operational stage (7-11 years):** This stage extends from age 7 to 11 years and marks a major turning point in cognitive development. In this stage, egocentric thought is replaced by **"operational thought"**, and hence the children start to see things from other's perspectives also. The thinking is concrete (concrete thinking is the literal thinking). For example, when asked about the meaning of the proverb "people who live in glass houses should not throw stones", the child responded that "if my house is of glass, I should not throw stones as it will break my house". The child is not able to understand the deeper meaning. Logical thinking starts to develop, and children are able to understand and follow the rules and regulations. The cognitive accomplishments in this stage include conservation, reversibility, classification, seriation and spatial reasoning.
- **Conservation** is the ability to understand that despite changes in shape, the object remains the same. For example, water may be transferred from a cup to a glass and may appear different in shape; however, the amount will remain the same.
- **Reversibility** is the capacity to understand that one thing can turn into another and back again, e.g., water and ice.
- **In classification**, children become aware of hierarchies and become aware of relationships between categories.
- The ability to order items along a quantitative dimension, such as weight and length, is called **seriation**.

- Piaget also found that children have an understating of directions by this age and can form mental representations of familiar places.
D. **Formal operational stage (11 years and older):** Piaget believed that the capacity for abstract and scientific thinking develops at this stage. Abstract thinking is the ability to understand the deeper meaning and deduce the larger meanings. For example, when asked to explain the meaning of the phrase "pen is mightier than the sword", a child with concrete thinking will say that the pen is heavier and stronger than the sword, whereas a child who has achieved abstract thinking will say that "power of knowledge is stronger than the power of the brute force". In this stage, the thinking becomes logical; the child understands the concept of permutation and combination, and probability.

Two important developments in this stage include:
a. **Hypothetico-deductive reasoning:** When adolescents face a problem, they start with a general theory of all possible factors and then deduce a specific hypothesis about the outcome. They then test such hypotheses in an orderly fashion to see which ones work in real life.
b. **Propositional thought:** Adolescents can evaluate the logic of propositions or verbal statements without referring to real-world circumstances.

LEARNING THEORY

Learning is defined as acquiring new behaviour patterns often produced by experience. It is a permanent change in behaviour potential. There are three kinds of learning:
A. Classical conditioning
B. Operant or instrumental conditioning
C. Observational conditioning

A. **Classical conditioning:** The principles of classical conditioning were first described by Ivan Pavlov, a Russian scientist who was initially studying the digestive system of dogs. The Pavlovian experiment included the following:

Under normal circumstances, a dog would salivate to the smell of food, and the ringing of the bell would not produce any salivation response. In the experiment, a bell was rung every time before the food presentation.

Pavlov found that with the repeated pairing of the bell and the food, the dogs started salivating to the sound of the bell, even before the food was presented. This was an important discovery that gave a deeper insight into behavioural processes.

Important elements in classical conditioning are as follows:
Unconditioned stimulus: Any stimulus that naturally elicits a response, without any prior learning. For example, smell of food elicits salivation in dogs naturally.
Unconditioned response: Any reaction which is elicited naturally in response to the unconditioned stimulus. For example, salivation produced by the sight or smell of delicious food.
Conditioned stimulus: Any stimulus that, when repeatedly paired with the unconditioned stimulus, starts eliciting a response. For example, the ringing of a bell usually does not elicit any response. However, when repeatedly paired with food (unconditioned stimulus), it starts eliciting salivation.
Conditioned response: The response (salivation) which results from pairing the conditioned stimulus (the bell) with the unconditioned stimulus(the food). Thus, the response of salivation evoked by the ringing of the bell is a conditioned response.
Extinction: If the conditioned stimulus (ringing of bell) is presented repeatedly without the unconditioned stimulus (smell of food), the response (salivation) will decrease and eventually disappear. This is called extinction.
Stimulus generalisation: Any stimulus resembling the conditioned stimulus is able to generate the same conditioned response. For example, in addition to the bell, similar other sounds such as the phone's ring also started eliciting salivation.
Stimulus discrimination: The ability to discriminate between similar types of stimuli so as to respond to some but not the others. For example, being afraid of one breed of dog due to a bad experience but not being afraid of the other dog breeds.

B. **Operant conditioning:** The principles of operant conditioning were founded by BF Skinner. It is a process of learning in which an individual learns to repeat behaviours that either have a positive outcome or can help them escape or avoid negative outcomes. In other words, the frequency of a behaviour is determined by its consequences. Hence, according to this theory, any behaviour can be learned or unlearned, and its frequency can be changed by modifying the consequences of that behaviour. If a behaviour is followed by a pleasant consequence (called reward), that behaviour will get reinforced, i.e., its frequency will increase. For example, if a child is given chocolate when he studies for a particular duration of time, the frequency of studying is expected to increase. Similarly, if the consequence is negative, the frequency of behaviour will decrease. For example, if a child is punished whenever he uses foul language, the frequency of that behaviour is likely to decrease.

Types: The frequency of a behaviour is increased by positive or negative reinforcement and decreased by punishment or extinction (**Table 20.1**).

Table 20.1: Types of operant conditioning.

Type	Effect	Example
Positive reinforcement	Behaviour is increased by a positive consequence (reward)	A child increases his study hours as every study session is rewarded with a chocolate
Negative reinforcement	Behaviour is increased to avoid a negative consequence	A child increases cleaning of his room to avoid scolding by the mother

Cont'd...

Cont'd...

Type	Effect	Example
Punishment	Behaviour is decreased by a negative consequence	A child stops using foul language after getting slapped for the same
Extinction	Behaviour is decreased due to lack of reinforcement	An intern who used to work very hard in the ward, becomes inefficient as he was never praised by his seniors

C. **Observational learning:** It was described by Albert Bandura and his colleagues. They emphasised that one of the ways of learning a behaviour is through observing others and imitating that behaviour. To elucidate this point, they did an experiment, commonly referred to as the **"Bobo Doll"** experiment. In this, they showed two groups of children two different movies. In the first group, they showed a movie in which an adult is aggressive with a large inflatable bobo doll, while the other group of children were shown a movie with an adult who behaved in a non-aggressive way. Later it was observed that the children exposed to the aggressive role model also behaved in a violent way towards their toys.

PSYCHOTHERAPY

Woolberg defined psychotherapy as the treatment by "psychological means of problems of an emotional nature in which a trained person deliberately establishes a professional relationship with the patient with the object (1) of removing, modifying or retarding existing symptoms, (2) of mediating disturbed patterns of behaviour and (3) of promoting positive personality growth and development". Types of psychotherapy are discussed in **Table 20.2**.

Table 20.2: Types of psychotherapy.

Types of treatment	Objective	Approaches
Supportive therapy	Therapy aims to reduce intrapsychic conflicts by strengthening the client's healthy and adaptive behaviours	Guidance, reassurance, emotional catharsis and desensitisation, suggestive hypnosis
Re-educative therapy	Therapy aims to make the client live up to existing creative potential with or without insight into unconscious conflicts	Behaviour therapy, cognitive behaviour therapy, client centred therapy, rational emotive behaviour therapy, family therapy
Reconstructive therapy	Therapy aims to provide insight into unconscious conflicts so that there is change in character	Psychoanalysis, transactional therapy, existential therapy, play therapy, art therapy

APPROACHES OF PSYCHOTHERAPY

The following types of therapies are commonly used in practice:

Cognitive behaviour therapy (CBT): Aaron T Beck developed the cognitive-behavioural model of psychotherapy. This therapy uses the concepts of cognitive therapy (primarily focused on correcting the thoughts) as well as behaviour therapy (primarily focused on correcting the behaviour). It describes cognition and behaviour as two interconnected constructs rather than being different distinct entities. CBT is based on certain fundamental principles.
- Cognition (thinking) is closely associated with emotion and behaviour.
- Changes in cognition (thinking) are likely to alter emotions and behaviour.
- Change in cognition is recognizable through close monitoring and observation.
- Cognition can be changed through voluntary efforts.
- Changes in cognition through voluntary effort can bring a change in emotions and behaviour.
- Similarly, changes in behaviour and emotion can also modify cognition.

Understanding the interconnectedness of cognition, emotion, and behaviour is the first step in cognitive behaviour therapy.

We can understand the concepts mentioned above by taking an example.

Say, a medical student went to the library with a plan to study for 2 hours; while going to the library, he felt motivated and was in a good mood. As he entered the library, he saw a friend standing at some distance. The student waived at his friend and said 'Hi'. The friend, however, didn't acknowledge him and walked away. Now, the medical student immediately had a thought 'the friend ignored me deliberately, he wanted to avoid me, everybody wants to avoid me, I will never make friends, what the point of studying if I have to live all alone my entire life'.

This thought is an example of an **'automatic negative thought'**. After he had this thought, the medical student started feeling sad (change in emotions) and went back to the hostel and slept (changes in behaviour). This example shows how automatic negative thoughts can change emotions as well as behaviour.

Often, individuals have certain faulty thinking patterns, called **cognitive distortions** or **cognitive errors** or maladaptive assumptions, that are responsible for the automatic negative thoughts.

Cognitive behavioural therapy targets and aims to correct the automatic negative thoughts and cognitive biases.

The therapy is carried out over multiple sessions. This therapy is useful in depression, anxiety disorders, obsessive-compulsive disorder, persistent auditory hallucination in schizophrenia, attention deficit hyperkinetic disorder and stress-related disorders.

COGNITIVE DISTORTIONS

Following is the list of common cognitive distortions (maladaptive assumptions):

- **All or nothing thinking:** Seeing things in black and white. For example, 'I failed to get a particular job, it means that I would never ever get any job'.
- **Approval seeking:** Belief that you should always be liked and loved by others; otherwise, life would be terrible.
- **Disqualifying positive:** A tendency to refuse to acknowledge the positive events in life and insist that they "don't count". For example, an engineer was praised by his manager for a particular work, however, the engineer thought, "he is praising me just to make me feel better; in reality, I don't deserve to be praised".
- **Emotional reasoning:** Belief that the emotions reflect reality. For example, if I have a bad feeling about a person, it means that the person, in reality, is a bad human being, even if I have no evidence to support the same.
- **Fallacy of fairness:** Tendency to judge a random negative event as an issue of justice. For example, after missing a flight due to heavy traffic, one thinks, "life is always unfair to me".
- **Jumping to conclusions:** Interpreting with minimal evidence. For example, a friend does not reply to the message, and the individual concludes that the friend hates him.
- **Labeling mislabeling:** Giving labels to self or others. For example, if the roommate did not clean the room once, the individual labels the roommate as a "lazy slob".
- **Magnification (catastrophising) and minimisation:** Focusing on the worst possible outcome is maximisation, and in its extreme form, it is called catastrophising. For example, if one loses a hundred rupee note and says that it is one of the biggest losses I ever had, it's maximisation. If the individual says that now there is nothing left in my life, it's catastrophisation.

  Minimisation is trying to minimise the importance of events. For example, an individual who was alcohol dependent, when criticised for his heavy drinking, said that "I don't really drink much, just a peg here and there".
- **Mental filtering/selective perception:** Picking a single negative detail while ignoring the rest. For example, at a party, everybody complimented the looks of an individual; however, a single person asked, "have you gained weight", and the individual gave all the importance to that one person's remark and ignored all the praise.
- **Overgeneralisation:** Considering a single adverse event and making a general rule out of it. For example, an individual made a mistake at work and then thought, "I always mess up everything". Labelling is an extreme form of overgeneralisation.
- **Personalisation:** Blaming oneself for events for which one is not responsible. For example, a wife blamed herself for her husband's extramarital affair.
- **Should statements:** Having many rules about how one and others should behave. For example, I should exercise daily; I should not be lazy.

Behaviour therapy: According to learning theory, maladaptive behaviours are learned by classical conditioning, operant conditioning and observational learning; and can be unlearnt. Many psychiatric disorders can be treated by behaviour therapy if the psychiatric symptoms are considered learned maladaptive behaviours. Behaviour therapy is a psychological treatment in which the maladaptive behaviours of patients are changed to improve their quality of life. It is particularly useful in children and in the treatment of phobias.

Some techniques used in behaviour therapy include:

A. **Systematic desensitisation:** This technique is based on the "**reciprocal inhibition**" principle. According to this principle, if an anxiety-provoking stimulus is given while a person is relaxed, the anxiety gets inhibited. For example, a person with a phobia of spiders, who is first made to relax; and then exposed to a spider, is likely to develop much lesser anxiety.

   The systematic desensitisation technique follows three steps: first, there is relaxation training, wherein the patient is taught to relax by using deep breathing or progressive muscle relaxation; second, there is a construction of a hierarchy in which the anxiety-provoking situations are listed from the least to the most anxiety-inducing situation. For example, for a person with a phobia of heights, the list may have "standing on the roof of a ten-storey building" at the top, "standing in the balcony on the second floor" in the middle and "standing on the third stair" at the bottom of the hierarchy; the third step is the desensitisation, wherein the person is exposed to the items in the hierarchy list and asked to relax simultaneously, starting with the least anxiety-provoking stimulus. As the patient masters the technique of relaxation in the presence of anxiety-provoking stimuli, he moves up to the next stimulus on the list. Systematic desensitisation is used to treat phobias, obsessive-compulsive disorders and certain sexual disorders.

B. **Therapeutic graded exposure or in vivo exposure (or exposure and response prevention):** It is similar to systematic desensitisation except that no relaxation techniques are used, and real-life situations are used. For example, if a patient is afraid of dogs, the exposure will start with looking at a picture of the dog, then looking at a video of the dog, then looking at a dog from a distance and finally holding a dog in arms. The patient learns to get habituated to anxiety (i.e., he learns that anxiety gradually decreases by itself). It is used in phobias and obsessive-compulsive disorder.

C. **Flooding (implosion):** Here, the patient is made to confront the feared situation directly, without any sequential exposure. No relaxation exercises are used either. The patient is exposed to the feared situation and experiences fear and anxiety, which gradually subsides as the patient is not allowed to escape.

D. **Modeling (participant modelling):** Here, the therapist himself makes contact with the phobic stimulus and demonstrates it to the patient. The patient learns by imitation and observation. For example, a therapist himself took a dog in his arms while a patient who had a phobia of dogs observed him. This technique is used in phobias as well as obsessive-compulsive disorders

E. **Assertiveness training:** Here, the person is taught to be assertive while asking for rights and while refusing unjust demands of others.

F. **Social skills training:** Usually used in patients with schizophrenia, it involves imparting skills required for dealing with others and living a social life.
G. **Aversive conditioning:** It is also called one-time conditioning. In this technique, a pleasurable stimulus is paired with a stimulus that causes an aversive reaction, leading to distaste for the pleasurable stimulus. For example, the use of antabuse (disulfiram) drug, which causes a bad reaction when mixed with alcohol, reduces the frequency of drinking in a person with alcohol dependence. Aversive conditioning has been used to treat unwanted behaviours (such as paraphilias). The patient is asked to imagine that he is indulging in the unwanted behaviour (such as a paraphilia), and immediately a painful stimulus (such as an electric shock) is given. An association gets created between the unwanted behaviour and painful stimulus, and the unwanted behaviour ceases. This technique is now rarely used due to ethical considerations.
H. **Token economy:** It is based on the principles of operant conditioning. The individual gets a token for every desirable behaviour, and these tokens can be redeemed for gifts or rewards. It is used primarily in the therapy of children.
I. **Biofeedback:** It is a treatment technique that uses the principles of operant conditioning. The biofeedback is based on the idea that the autonomic nervous system (which is usually involuntary) can be brought under voluntary control with the help of operant conditioning. It is used for the treatment of disorders that are caused by dysfunction in autonomic control, such as asthma, tension headaches, arrhythmias, etc. The technique uses a feedback instrument, the choice of which depends on the patient's problem. This instrument gives the patient feedback about the current status of a specific autonomic function. For example, an electromyogram (EMG) provides patient feedback on muscle tension in a particular muscle group. When the muscle tension is high, the EMG emits a higher tone, and when muscle tension is low (i.e., when the muscle is relaxed), the EMG emits a lower tone. Using feedback, the patient learns to control the muscle tone and hence can control symptoms caused by increased muscle tone (e.g., bruxism).

Family therapy: Family therapy is a form of psychotherapy that aims to alter the maladaptive family dynamics responsible for the causation or maintenance of the psychiatric disorder. Family therapy is influenced by various psychotherapy principles like: cognitive therapy, cognitive behaviour therapy, social learning theory, and operant conditioning. The therapy starts with setting specific goals. Family therapy helps facilitate communication among family members, correct distorted beliefs, improve interpersonal relationships, resolve conflicts, develop coping strategies to deal with day-to-day issues, and improve family functioning. It is more useful in dealing with complex relational issues and expressed emotions in patients with severe mental disorders (e.g., schizophrenia, bipolar disorder). It is also useful in psychosexual disorders, psychosomatic disorders, substance use disorders, parenting difficulties, and chronic medical illnesses.

Psychoanalysis: This technique has been covered in details in the Chapter 18 'Psychoanalysis'.

Substance use disorder – psychosocial treatment: Patients with substance use disorders (and other problematic behaviours) go through a series of changes before quitting substance use. Various models of these changes have been described; the most acceptable model is known as the **transtheoretical model of change**. According to this model, the following are the stages of change:
A. **Precontemplation:** In this stage, the substance user does not see any problem in his behaviour and does not think about quitting.
B. **Contemplation:** In this stage, the substance user starts realizing that he has a problem and is taking the substance excessively. He considers the pros and cons of stopping substance use. However, he is yet to take any decision.
C. **Preparation:** In this stage, the substance user decides to quit the substance and starts making a plan to quit.
D. **Action:** In this stage, the substance user stops taking the substance and makes changes in his behaviours (e.g., he stops meeting with friends who use drugs in an attempt to keep away himself from drugs) and starts taking treatment.
E. **Maintenance:** In this stage, the patient continues to stay away from substances (drugs) and continues with the treatment and other behaviours to prevent relapse. A patient may remain in the maintenance stage or may relapse and start taking substances again. Usually, a patient has few relapses before attaining complete abstinence (freedom) from the substance.

Various psychological treatment methods have been devised to help patients quit substance use and move from stages of precontemplation to maintenance. The commonly used techniques which focus on increasing the patient's motivation to quit the substance include motivation enhancement therapy or motivational interviewing.

Once the patient has reached the maintenance stage, relapse prevention techniques are used to prevent any relapses (return to the previous pattern of substance intake).

PSYCHOLOGICAL TESTING

Psychological tests help reach a psychiatric diagnosis and make deductions about the current and future functioning of the patients. There are separate tests to measure different domains of mental functions. Some of the commonly used tests include:

Intelligence tests: These are designed to measure the intelligence quotient (IQ). IQ is derived from the formula:

$$IQ = \text{Mental age (MA)}/\text{Chronological age (CA)} \times 100$$

In this formula, the maximum chronological age can be 15.

Now, much better and more precise tests have been devised to measure the intelligence, the commonly used tests include:
a. Wechsler adult intelligence scale
b. Malin's intelligence scale for Indian children (MISIC)

c. Bhatia's battery of performance tests of intelligence
d. Binet-Kamat test

Aptitude test: These psychometric tests measure aptitude or strength of skills in an individual. These are usually used in career counselling. For example, differential aptitude test (DAT).

Personality tests: These are of two types:
i. **Objective tests:** These are standardised tests that give numerical scores and can be analysed using standard result tables. For example, Minnesota Multiphasic Personality Inventory (MMPI).
ii. **Projective tests:** In these tests, patients are provided with ambiguous stimuli (unclear stimuli), and there are no right or wrong answers. It is believed that the patient's response to such an unclear stimulus reflects his internal thought processes and emotions. The patient "projects" his internal situation onto the test question and gives an answer, which an expert analyses to deduce the aspects of the patient's personality.

Some of the projective tests include:

Rorschach psychodiagnostik test: It was developed by Hermann Rorschach and contains 10 cards with ambiguous inkblot designs. Most of the cards are black, while cards 8, 9, 10 have various colours. The test is done in two phases: in the first one, the patient is shown the card and asked "what do you see in this card?" and the response is noted; in the second phase, they are asked queries about their response.

Thematic apperception test (TAT): It was developed by Henry Murray and Christina Morgan and adapted in the Hindi version by Dr Uma Mehrotra. Usually, 11 cards are used (10 cards with pictures plus one blank card). The individual has to develop a story regarding the characters shown in the picture. The stories are then interpreted to understand the individual's needs and presses (how they react to the environment).

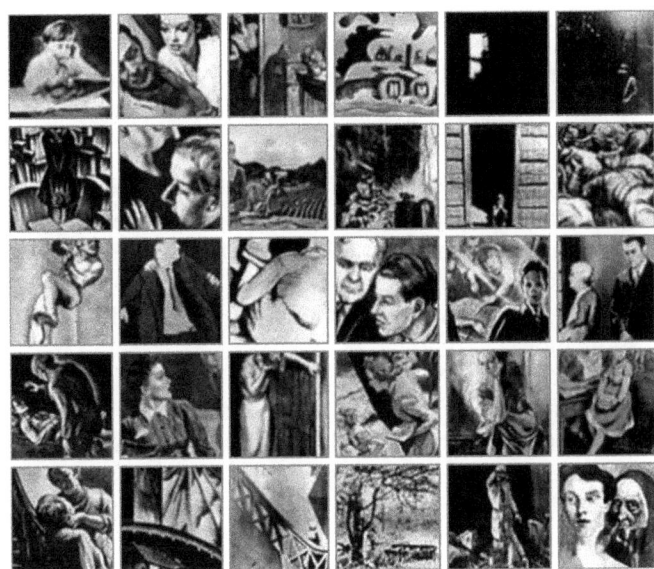

Fig. 20.2: Thematic apperception test cards.

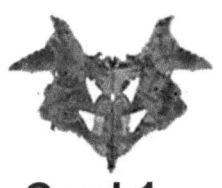

Card 1
Popular responses
bat, butterfly, moth

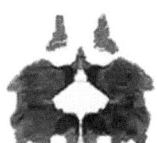

Card 2
Popular responses
two humans, four-legged animal, dog, elephant, bear

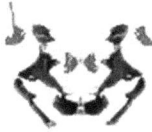

Card 3
Popular responses
two humans, human figures

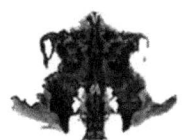

Card 4
Popular responses
animal hide, skin, rug

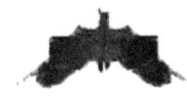

Card 5
Popular responses
bat, butterfly, moth

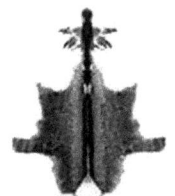

Card 6
Popular responses
animal hide, skin, rug

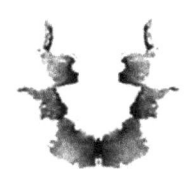

Card 7
Popular responses
human heads or faces

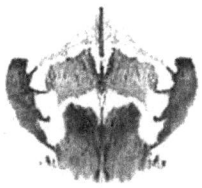

Card 8
Popular responses
animal: not cat or dog four-legged animal

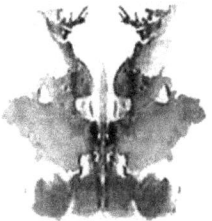

Card 9
Popular responses
human

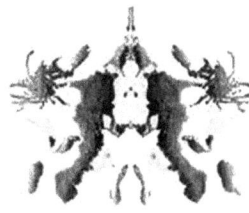

Card 10
Popular responses
crab, lobster, spider rabbit head, caterpillars, worms, snakes

Fig. 20.1: Rorschach test cards.

Draw-a-Person test (DAPT): Here, the individual has to draw a human figure that is then interpreted according to the guidelines.

Word association technique: It was first given by Carl Jung and is widely used to understand unconscious needs and processes. Here the examiner says a word and the individual answers with the first word that comes to their mind. For example, the clinician says sky, and the individual responds with 'blue'.

Sentence completion test: Here, individuals are given incomplete sentences and are asked to complete them. For example, a sentence may be like "I wish I.............."

Neuropsychological assessment for brain disorders or organic mental disorders: Several tests have been devised that extensively measure a wide range of cognitive functions like memory, motor functions, sensory functions, problem-solving, reading, writing, arithmetic, etc. Few such important tests include:
- Luria–Nebraska Neuropsychological battery
- Halstead–Reitan battery of neuropsychological tests
- **Bender–gestalt test (Bender visual motor gestalt test):** This test is used mainly as a screening tool for organic brain disorders.

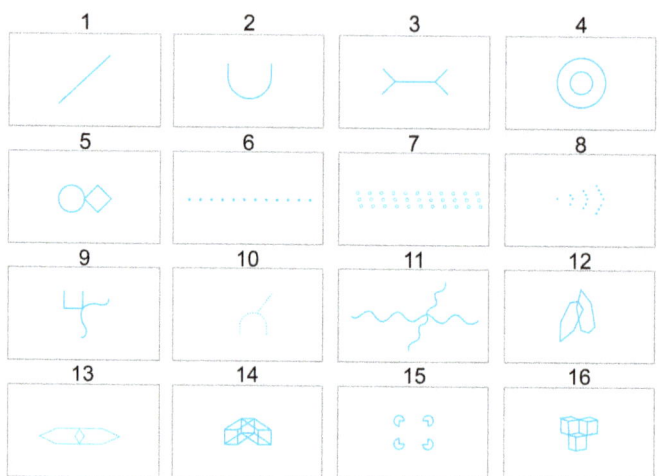

Fig. 20.3: bender gestalt test.

SUGGESTED READINGS

1. Simmons J, Griffiths R. CBT for Beginners. sage; 2017.
2. Wampold BE. The basics of psychotherapy: An introduction to theory and practice. American Psychological Association; 2019.
3. Geddes JR, Andreasen NC. New Oxford textbook of psychiatry. Oxford University Press, USA; 2020.
4. Boland R, Verduin M, Ruiz P, Shah A, Sadock B. Kaplan & Sadock's synopsis of psychiatry. 12th ed. Philadelphia: Wolters Kluwer; 2020.

21 Forensic Psychiatry

Vijay Niranjan, Praveen Tripathi

INTRODUCTION

Forensic psychiatry is a subspeciality of psychiatry that deals with issues arising in the interface between psychiatry and the law. While clinical psychiatry operates within the therapeutic context, forensic psychiatry operates within the legal context.

Forensic psychiatry covers a broad area; it deals with the matters related to criminal law, civil law, and the development and application of mental health legislation.

Reasons for Forensic Psychiatry Evaluations

A forensic psychiatric evaluation could be requested for various reasons. A criminal court may ask to assess a person's fitness to stand trial or determine the issue of criminal responsibility. A civil court may ask for a psychiatric assessment while assessing the need for guardianship, testamentary capacity, marital dispute or divorce on the grounds of mental illness, child custody and disability compensation, etc. Sometimes, the psychiatrist may receive a request from an employer asking for an opinion on an employee's mental condition and his/her fitness to continue in the job.

Forensic Psychiatric Assessment: Forensic Psychiatric Assessment Includes the Following

- A comprehensive psychiatric history including details of the events leading to the request, along with mental status examination.
- Marks of identification, photo-identity proof and a recent photograph of the person being examined are recorded.
- Hospitalisation may be required if there is a need for observation before giving a definite opinion on the diagnosis.
- If hospitalisation is not feasible, repeated assessments over a period should be conducted.
- Physical investigations should be ordered, depending on the case.
- Psychological testing for personality profile, intelligence, and cognitive functions may be needed.

Various aspects of forensic psychiatry are briefly discussed below.

CRIMINAL RESPONSIBILITY

Crime has two components: **Actus reus** and **mens rea**, i.e., guilty act against the law and evil intent, respectively. Thus for an act to be labelled as a crime, it should be against the law and be accompanied by evil intent.

To hold an individual criminally responsible, the intention needs to be proved. Whether a person with a mental illness can be held criminally responsible or not has been dealt with by multiple laws and has an interesting history with many high profile cases.

McNaughten Case and McNaughtens Rules

The case of Daniel McNaughten in 1843 got widespread public attention. McNaughten probably was suffering from schizophrenia and had a delusion that spies sent by catholic priests, with the help of Tories (the political party in power at that time), were following him and planning to harm him. He hence decided to kill the Tories Prime Minister, Sir Robert Peel. While attempting to kill the Prime Minister, he mistakenly shot and murdered the prime minister's private secretary, Edward Drummond.

During the trial, ten physicians found him insane and McNaughten was acquitted on the grounds of insanity. This led to a huge public outcry and resulted in the Lord chancellor putting five questions to a panel of judges to clarify the legal position. The answers came to be known as '**McNaughten's Rules**'.

McNaughten's rule states that "to establish a defense on the ground of insanity, it must be clearly proved that, at the time of committing the act, the party accused was laboring under such a defect of reason, from disease of mind, as not to know the nature and quality of the act he was doing or if he did know it, that he did not know he was doing what was wrong."

Insanity defense **(Section 84 IPC)** in the Indian context is adopted from McNaughten's rule. According to Section 84

IPC, "nothing is an offence which is done by a person who, at the time of doing it, by reason of unsoundness of mind, is incapable of knowing the nature of the act, or that he is doing what is either wrong or contrary to law."

The 'unsoundness of mind' should be established for the time when the crime was actually committed, and the burden of proving this lies on the accused.

Although not conclusive yet, there are a number of pointers that may indicate that the crime could have been a result of mental illness. These include an absence of motive in the crime, absence of secrecy while committing the crime, want of preparedness, use of needless force in the crime, and absence of accomplices in the act. Also, there is often indifference to the crime committed.

Other Judicial Rules/Acts for Criminal Responsibility: Some Other Rules that have Historical Significance Include

- **Durham's rule:** According to Durham's rule, "An accused person is not criminally responsible if the unlawful act is a product of mental disease or effect". It is also known as the 'Product rule'.
- **Curren's rule:** According to **Curren's** rule, "An accused person will not be held criminally responsible, if, at the time of committing act, he did not have the capacity to regulate his conduct to the requirement of law, as a result of mental disease or defect."
- **American law institute (ALI)/Brawner test** (modern penal code): In its model penal code, the ALI has recommended the following test, "A person is not responsible for criminal conduct if at the time of such conduct, as a result of mental disease or defect, he lacks substantial capacity either to appreciate the criminality (wrongfulness) of his conduct or to conform his conduct to the requirement of the law."
  This is the law in federal courts **today**.
- **Guilty but mentally ill (GBMI):** A new verdict GBMI, has been enacted by some states in the United States to reform the insanity defense. Defendants can be GBMI, if guilty of a crime and mentally ill at the time it was committed, but not legally insane at that time.
  For a GMBI verdict, the court still imposes a sentence, but the person receives psychiatric treatment.

Trial of a Person Suffering from Mental Illness

Mental illness may affect the capacity of a person to understand the legal proceedings being initiated against him and prepare a defence. In Indian law, Sections 328-339 of the Code of Criminal Procedure (CPC) 1973, provide guidelines for the trial of a person suspected to be suffering from a mental illness.

According to Section 328 IPC, if a magistrate has reasons to believe that the accused is of unsound mind and incapable of making his defense, the magistrate should inquire into the facts of unsoundness of mind and get the accused examined by a medical officer. If the magistrate is satisfied that the accused is of unsound mind, he shall postpone further proceedings in the case. The accused can then be detained in safe custody or be released pending investigation or trial if bail can be taken, and sufficient security is provided by a relative regarding treatment and care of the accused. The trial can resume only when the accused ceases to be of unsound mind.

CIVIL RESPONSIBILITY

Adoption

In adoption cases, a psychiatrist may be asked to give an opinion about the suitability of the prospective adopting parents. According to the Hindu Adoptions and Maintenance Act, 1956, any Hindu male "who is of sound mind and is not a minor" can adopt a child with the consent of his wife unless "she has been declared by a court... to be of unsound mind". Similarly, any Hindu female "who is of sound mind", is not a minor, and is not married, can adopt a child. If she is married, then her husband should also be of sound mind. The person giving the child for adoption should also be of sound mind.

Marriage and Divorce

According to the Hindu Marriage Act, if at the time of marriage, any party is incapable of giving a valid consent due to unsoundness of mind; or though capable of giving consent, has been suffering from a mental disorder of such a kind or to such an extent as to be unfit for marriage and the procreation of children; or has been subject to recurrent attacks of insanity or epilepsy, the marriage shall be voidable and can be annulled by a decree of nullity.

Insanity or unsoundness of mind is also grounds for divorce under the Muslim Marriage Act, 1939 and Parsi Marriage and Divorce Act, 1936.

Divorce can be granted under Section 13 of the Hindu Marriage Act on a petition filed by either spouse on the ground that the other party has been incurably of unsound mind or has been suffering continuously or intermittently from a mental disorder of such kind and to such extent that the petitioner cannot be reasonably expected to live with the respondent.

Contract

The law requires the individual to be of sound mind, to be considered competent for getting into a contract.

According to the Indian Contract Act 1872 (Section 11), "every person is competent to contract, who is of the age of majority... and who is of sound mind". A person is said to be of sound mind for the purpose of a contract if, at the time of making the contract, he can understand it and form a rational judgment as to its effect upon his interests.

Testamentary Capacity

Testamentary capacity refers to the ability of a person to make a will. Will is a legal document, and to be valid, the will needs to be signed by the testator in the presence of at least two witnesses. A will can be revoked or modified any time before the testator's death and comes into effect only after the testator's death.

According to Section 59 of the Indian Succession Act 1925, any person of sound mind can make a will. A person who has reached the age of majority can make a will. A person suffering from a mental disorder can make a will, provided he is capable of the required competency for making a will. Persons, who are ordinarily insane, may make a will during an interval while they are of sound mind.

No person can make a will while he is in such a state of mind, whether arising from intoxication or from illness or from any other cause, that he does not know what he is doing.

A psychiatrist may be asked to report whether a person is competent to make a will or not.

The following points are considered by psychiatrists during the evaluation:
1. Whether the will is being made voluntarily and in the absence of external pressure, coercion or compulsions
2. The person making a will should be aware of the act he is undertaking. The person should not be suffering from a mental disorder or be under the effect of some drugs to the extent that would interfere with his/her judgment.
3. The testator should have sufficient capacity to know the extent of his/her property and should also be aware of the potential beneficiaries.
4. The testator should be aware of the consequences of his/her decision and know the content of the will he/she is making.

MENTAL HEALTH LEGISLATION IN INDIA

Mental health legislation is essential for protecting the rights and dignity of persons with mental disorders and for developing accessible and effective mental health services.

During the British rule in India, few mental asylums were established, primarily with the aim of removing mentally ill patients from society. The British also brought about written laws, and the Indian Lunacy Act was promulgated in 1912.

The **Mental Health Act, 1987** replaced the Indian lunacy Act 1912. Mental Health Act, 1987 regulated the process of admission and discharge of the mentally ill in the country. It also provided mechanisms for monitoring and provisions for some basic rights of the mentally ill.

Mental Health Care Act 2017

The mental health legislation in force today is Mental Health Care Act.

This act received the assent of the President of India on the 7th April, 2017 after being passed by the parliament. This legislation is to protect, promote, and fulfil the rights of persons with mental illnesses. The act is progressive and rights-based in nature.

Salient features of this act:
1. **An elaborative definition of mental illness:** According to MHCA 2017, "mental illness" *means a substantial disorder of thinking, mood, perception, orientation or memory that grossly impairs judgment*, behaviour, capacity to recognise reality or ability to meet the ordinary demands of life, mental conditions associated with the abuse of alcohol and drugs, but does not include mental retardation.
2. The act provides for the establishment and functioning of various regulatory bodies like **Central and State Mental Health Authorities, Mental Health Review Commission and** Mental Health Review Boards.
3. **The act provides for various rights of the mentally ill:** Right to community living, right to dignity, right to equality and non-discrimination, right to information, right to confidentiality, right to personal communication, legal aid, and to make complaints, etc.
4. **Capacity to make mental healthcare and treatment decisions:** According to MHCA 2017, every person, including those with a mental illness, is assumed to have a capacity to decide about the kind of treatment (including admission) they want to have for their mental illness if they have the ability to:
   a. Understand the information given to them and based on which they have to decide (i.e., information about the illness, the symptoms, the treatment options available, etc.)
   b. Understand the consequences of their decisions (e.g., a patient who is having suicidal thoughts and not willing to take treatment should be able to understand that not taking treatment can be life-threatening for him)
   c. To communicate their decision by using speech or gestures.
5. **Advance directive:** Every person (who is not a minor) can make an advance directive that mentions:
   a. The way the person wishes to be treated for a mental illness.
   b. The way the person wishes not to be treated for a mental illness.

   The advance directive would be applicable only if the person loses the capacity to make mental healthcare or treatment decisions.

   It is the duty of the psychiatrist (or medical officer) in charge of treatment to ensure that treatment is being given according to the advance directive made by the patient. However, it is the patient's duty (or duty of caregiver or nominated representative) to provide access to the advance directive to the treating doctor. If there are unforeseen consequences due to following an advance directive, the doctor cannot be held liable for the same.
6. **Nominated representative:** Every person can appoint a nominated representative (who should not be minor and should be competent in discharging the duties as a nominated representative) and remove him if he wishes to. If a person loses the capacity to make mental healthcare or treatment decisions, the nominated representative will help (or will take) in making decisions about the treatment of the person.

7. **Admission:** The MHCA 2017 allows the following types of admissions:
   a. **Independent admissions:** Section 86 of MHCA is used for independent admissions, when the patient considers himself to have a mental illness and desires to be admitted to a mental health establishment. Independent admission (Section 86) has no limit on the duration of stay, and the patient can apply for discharge at any time. However, a mental health professional may prevent the discharge of a person admitted as an independent person under Section 86 for a period of 24 hours if his assessment is deemed necessary for admission under Section 89.
   b. **Supported admissions:** A person who needs admission, however, has lost the capacity to make mental healthcare or treatment decisions and hence needs a high level of support from the nominated representative, can be admitted as a 'supported admission' under Section 89 of MHCA. The nominated representative gives consent for admission in this case. The duration of admission under Section 89, is limited to 30 days; all such admissions need to be informed to the mental health board within 7 days of admission (for adults) and 3 days (for minors and females). During the admission or after 30 days, the patient can be reviewed for capacity and be discharged as an independent patient. If needed, the duration of admission can be extended for 90 days at first instance and later to 120 and 180 days after the board's approval (Section 90).
   c. **Emergency treatment:** Any registered medical practitioner can provide treatment to persons with mental illness, at a health establishment or in the community, in emergency situations, under section 94. The emergency treatment shall be limited to 72 hours or till the person with mental illness has been assessed at a mental health establishment, whichever is earlier. This section allows for emergency treatment at any centre, even those which are not licensed mental health establishments.
8. **Ban on direct electroconvulsive therapy** (ECT without the use of muscle relaxants and anaesthesia).
9. **Ban on ECT for minors:** In a rare case, if the psychiatrist in charge considers ECT is required for the treatment of a minor, he will have to take informed consent of the guardian and prior permission from the mental health review board.
10. **Ban on psychosurgery:** In a rare case, if the psychiatrist in charge considers psychosurgery, he will have to take informed consent of the patient and prior permission from the mental health review board.
11. **Decriminalisation of suicide:** Any person who attempts to commit suicide shall be presumed to be under severe stress and should not be tried or punished (MHCA 2017 repealed Section 309 of IPC, which provided for punishment in cases of attempted suicide).
12. **Restraints and seclusion:** A patient can be physically restrained only:
    a. If it is the only way to prevent harm to self or others.
    b. If it is authorised by the psychiatrist in charge.
13. The act specifies that every insurer should make provisions for medical insurance for the treatment of mental illnesses at par with physical illnesses.

Narcotic Drugs and Psychotropic Substances (NDPS) Act, 1985

The Narcotic Drugs and Psychotropic Act was enacted in 1985 and was amended in 1988, 2001, 2011, and 2014.

The act has strong provisions for controlling and regulating operations related to narcotic drugs and psychotropic substances.

According to Section 8 of the act, no person shall:
a. Cultivate any coca plant or opium poppy or cannabis plant or produce/possess/sell/transport any narcotic drug or psychotropic substances.

The NDPS Act makes a distinction between offences involving a small quantity of drugs (usually carried by addicts) and a commercial quantity of drugs. The law is much more stringent for people involved in drug commerce and who are caught with commercial quantities, with certain offences being punishable by the death penalty.

The act also allows the court to release rather than sentencing, an addict found guilty for offences relating to a small quantity of drugs for medical treatment at a government maintained or recognised hospital

Some of the quantities defined for common drugs and psychotropic substances in the NDPS Act are shown in **Table 21.1**.

Table 21.1: Quantities defined in NDPS act.

Drug/Psychotropic substance	Small quantity	Commercial quantity
Charas/Hashish	100 g	1 kg
Cocaine	2 g	100 g
Ganja	1 kg	20 kg
Heroin	5 g	250 g
Morphine	5 g	250 g
Opium	25 g	2.5 kg
Poppy Straw	1 kg	50 Kg

COTPA (Cigarettes and Other Tobacco Products Act) 2003

This act applies to all products containing tobacco in any form (smokeless and smoked tobacco). Some of the important sections include:
a. Prohibition of smoking in public places (Section 4)
b. Prohibition of advertisement of cigarettes and other tobacco products (Section 5)

c. Prohibition of sale of cigarettes or other tobacco products to minors and near educational institutes (Section 6)
d. Mandatory depiction of statutory warnings, including pictorial warnings on tobacco packs (Section 7)

Protection of Children from Sexual Offences Act (POCSO, 2012)

Protection of Children from Sexual Offences Act (2102) was passed to provide a legal framework for the protection of children from sexual offences. It is a gender-neutral act for both the children and the accused. It classifies various offences that can be punished, including:
a. Child pornography
b. Sexual harassment (e.g., use of sexually coloured language, making sexual gestures, etc.)
c. Sexual assault (involves inappropriate touch)
d. Penetrative sexual assault (involves vaginal/anal/oral/urethral penetration of child)
e. Aggravated penetrative sexual assault/aggravated sexual assault

The term '**aggravated**' is added with penetrative sexual assault/sexual assault in certain situations which are considered to be even more gruesome and include the following:
1. When perpetrated by persons in the position of authority such as police officers, armed forces, management or staff of jail/remand home/hospital, etc.
2. Where a gang is involved
3. Use of deadly weapons
4. Causing grievous hurt, attempts to murder, or that makes the female child pregnant
5. Done repeatedly or on a child below 12 years
6. In the course of communal or sectarian violence

The Protection of Women from Domestic Violence Act, 2005

Domestic Violence Act 2005 recognises domestic abuse as a punishable offence, and provides for emergency relief for the victims and legal recourse.

The act safeguards any woman who has been in a domestic relationship with the 'respondent' in the case. It thus also extends its provisions to those in live-in relationships. (Section 2).

The act mentions that any act/conduct/omission/commission that harms or injures or has the potential to harm or injure will be considered 'domestic violence' (Section 3). There are four categories of abuse namely: physical, sexual, verbal/emotional and economic.

Sections 18–23 provide options for legal redressal like: Protection orders, residence orders, monetary relief, custody for children, compensation orders, etc.

SUGGESTED READINGS

1. Gutheil T. Forensic Psychiatry as a Specialty. Psychiatric News. 2004;21:3-5.
2. Chadda RK. Forensic evaluations in psychiatry. Indian J Psychiatry. 2013;55:393-9.
3. Asokan TV. Forensic psychiatry in India: The road ahead. Indian J Psychiatry. 2014;56:121-7.
4. Indian Penal Code (1860) Bare Act, Eastern Book Company, Lucknow.
5. Criminal Procedure Code, 1973. Commercial Law Publishers (India): Delhi, 2007.
6. Hindu Adoption and Maintenance Act, 1956. Commercial Law Publishers (India): Delhi, 2007.
7. Hindu Marriage Act, 1955. Commercial Law Publishers (India): Delhi, 2007.
8. Nambi S. Marriage, mental health and the Indian legislation. Indian J Psychiatry. 2005;47:3-14.
9. Indian Contract Act (1872) Bare Act, Eastern Book Company, Lucknow.
10. Indian Succession Act, 1925. Commercial Law Publishers (India): Delhi, 2007.
11. Jiloha RC. Mental capacity/testamentary capacity. Clinical Practice Guidelines of the Indian Psychiatric Society. Forensic Psychiatry. 2009;20-34.
12. Nambi S, Ilango S, Prabha L. Forensic psychiatry in India: Past, present, and future. Indian J Psychiatry. 2016;58:175-80.
13. Dhanasekaran S, Kar SK, Tripathi A. The mental health care bill: changes and appraisal. Delhi Psychiatry J. 2014;17:160-6.
14. The Narcotic Drugs and Psychotropic Substances (Amendment) Act, 2014 (Act 16 of 2014).
15. The Protection of Children from Sexual Offences Act, 2012 (32 of 2012).
16. The protection of women from domestic violence act, 2005 Act no. 43 of 2005.

22. Community Psychiatry

Sujita Kumar Kar

PS19.1	Describe the relevance, role, and status of community psychiatry
PS19.2	Describe the objectives strategies and contents of the National Mental Health Programme
PS19.3	Describe and discuss the basic legal and ethical issues in psychiatry

INTRODUCTION

Community psychiatry is a subspeciality of psychiatry that deals with mental health issues in a community setting. Community psychiatry attempts to understand the needs of individuals who have a mental illness in the community settings and works to reintegrate them into the mainstream of society.

The scope of community psychiatry as a discipline includes providing basic mental health services at the doorsteps (in the community), strengthening psychosocial support, improving community mental health awareness, creating opportunities for the patients with mental illnesses at the community level, protecting the rights of mentally ill at the community level and creating self-help groups. Community psychiatry involves developing strategies for successfully delivering community mental health services and their monitoring, regulation, and protection.

Community mental healthcare aims to promote mental health and prevent mental illnesses in the community. It involves working on the deficits (disability) of individuals who have mental illnesses and attempts to restore the skills. Simultaneously, it also emphasises the strengths and capabilities of the individual for leading a dignified and productive life in society.

Studies reveal that many patients with mental illnesses (nearly one-third with chronic mental illnesses) remain untreated in the community. They are often subjected to abuse and neglect. Their mental health needs are not met adequately. The community mental health service model also targets the mental health needs of this population.

HISTORY OF COMMUNITY PSYCHIATRY

In the early days, patients with mental illnesses were segregated from the mainstream of society and were kept isolated in the asylums. As specific treatments (medications) were not available for mental illnesses, often these patients were subjected to unscientific and inhumane methods to correct or reform their behaviour. In the early part of the nineteenth century, movements against the inhumane treatment of the mentally ill emerged. In the 1950s, such movements gained momentum, and the focus of psychiatric disorders treatment started shifting towards community care through social reintegration. In western countries, the wave of community psychiatry was quite evident between 1950 to 1970. Funding for community mental health services and the generation of research evidence regarding the effectiveness of community mental health services were landmark events during this period.

The World Health Organisation (WHO) has taken several initiatives to develop the community mental health model. In a recent survey, WHO sought an opinion from 78 experts from 42 different countries to expand mental health services at the community level by deinstitutionalisation (deinstitutionalisation is the process of moving out the mentally ill from state institutions, such as mental asylums and providing treatment at the community level). On the basis of this survey, the principles for deinstitutionalisation were identified. These include:

1. Community based mental healthcare services must be in place
2. Commitment by the mental health workforce to bring a change
3. Extensive political support is crucial
4. Timing is the key
5. Additional financial resources are needed

An action plan has been laid down by WHO, known as **Mental Health Action Plan 2013–2030**. For community-level care, it focuses on reducing the stigma associated with mental illnesses, protecting the rights of the mentally ill, and facilitating the delivery of comprehensive and integrated mental health and social care service.

COMMUNITY PSYCHIATRY IN INDIA

The community psychiatry movement in India was influenced mainly by the western model of community psychiatry practice. In 1946, the "Bhore Committee" recommended the establishment of mental health units in general hospital medical settings, which subsequently moved in the direction of the development of community mental health units.

It took about 36 years after the **Bhore committee's** recommendation to initiate the community mental health programme. In 1982, a milestone was achieved in the history of Indian mental healthcare with the launch of **National Mental Health Programme (NMHP)**. NHMP emphasised community mental health and accelerated the decentralisation of mental healthcare, thereby decreasing the burden of mental healthcare on the mental hospitals and tertiary care hospitals by creating community mental health clinics.

In the 2001 Erwadi tragedy, 26 patients with psychiatric illness who were kept chained, in a religious place were killed in a fire. The gruesome event shocked mental health professionals, policymakers, media, politicians and the general public. It also made society aware of the exploitation of the rights of mentally ill persons in the community. In the subsequent years, this event influenced many processes like- the implementation of the law to its full extent, modifications in the laws related to mental health, and protection of rights of the mentally ill in the community.

Research in Community Psychiatry in India

Many epidemiological studies on the prevalence of psychiatric disorders in the community were conducted after 1960. But these studies were conducted in specific populations of specific regions of India, limiting their generalisability. The epidemiological studies attempted to see the prevalence of psychiatric disorders in various populations (hospital settings, community settings, geriatric populations, pediatric populations, women, victims of disaster, high-risk populations). Different sampling techniques and assessment tools were used for conducting these studies.

Some landmark studies like: the International Pilot Study of Schizophrenia (IPSS), the Determinants of the Outcome of Severe Mental Disorders (DOSMED) and the Study of Factors Affecting the Course and Outcome of Schizophrenia (SOFACOS) were conducted in community settings to study the outcome of schizophrenia. These studies enriched the understanding of the community perspective of severe mental disorders in India.

Other than these studies, studies to evaluate the disability, scope for rehabilitation, stigma and attitude towards mental illness, the burden of care of mental illnesses in the caregivers of the patients and pathways of care of mental illnesses were conducted to understand the ground reality of mental health services in the community.

NATIONAL MENTAL HEALTH PROGRAM

The National Mental Health Programme (NMHP) was launched in August 1982. The NMHP planned to implement mental health services in the community by developing district mental health units and school mental health programs. To achieve this goal, there was an intense need for trained manpower in mental health; hence the development of trained mental health personnel was one of the major agendas of NMHP.

NMHP stated three major objectives:
1. To make basic mental healthcare available, accessible, and affordable for every individual in the community who needs it.
2. To facilitate the utilisation of mental health knowledge in the community for the development of healthcare and social care.
3. To encourage community participation in mental health service development and delivery.

For the successful implementation of NMHP, various approaches have been suggested. These incude development of mental health resources (infrastructure and trained human resources), uniform distribution of resources in the community, integrating the mental healthcare with mainstream general healthcare, and proper planning and evaluation of the programme. In 1996, **District Mental Health Programme (DMHP)** was added to NMHP for effective utilisation of mental health services at the community level. In 2003, two schemes (modernisation of the mental hospitals and up-gradation of psychiatric departments of general hospitals and medical colleges) were introduced under NMHP. In the year 2009, the manpower development scheme was introduced under NMHP.

The district mental health program (DMHP) aims to:
- Provide basic mental health services in the community-based setting (both in the hospital setting as well as through outreach clinics).
- Training of mental health manpower (at district as well as subdistrict level).
- Conducting mental health sensitisation and awareness programs.
- Encouraging community participation in mental health service delivery.

The district mental health program initiated activities in the public-private partnership model. The non-government organisations were provided with financial support to carry out mental health-related activities in the community. To provide rehabilitation services to patients with mental illnesses, daycare centres, residential/long-stay homes, and community and primary health centres are being provided financial support or technical support by the government of India. By February 2017, DMHP had been implemented in 241 districts of the country.

To improve the mental healthcare as well as research, assistance has been provided to tertiary care centres. Many mental hospitals and psychiatric units of medical colleges have been converted to centres of excellence. These institutes are provided with the additional financial support of 33 crores to develop infrastructure, train manpower, carry out research activities, and provide mental healthcare in the hospital setting. Similarly, to meet the need for psychiatrists in the country, many medical college psychiatric units have been provided financial and technical assistance to start the post-graduate courses or increase the number of post-graduate seats in psychiatry. NMHP also provides support to carry out surveys, research, develop IEC (information, education and communication) materials, monitoring of mental health activities at different levels and conduct training programs/workshops.

CURRENT MENTAL HEALTH SCENE IN INDIA

As per the Mental Health Atlas – 2017 released by WHO, the Indian government spends 1.3% of the total health budget on mental health. India has 0.29 psychiatrists, 0.07 psychologists, 0.06 social workers, and 0.8 mental health nurses per lakh of the population.

India has a dedicated legislation for mental health (Mental Health Care Act, 2017) and a program for mental health (National Mental Health Programme).

National Mental Health Survey (2015–2016)

The National Mental Health Survey (NMHS) was a landmark and one of the largest epidemiological study on psychiatric disorders in the community, sponsored by the Ministry of Health and Family Welfare and led by the National Institute of Mental Health And Neuro-Sciences (NIMHANS), Bengaluru. This survey was conducted in 12 states (Tamil Nadu, Kerala, Rajasthan, Gujarat, Punjab, Uttar Pradesh, Madhya Pradesh, Chhattisgarh, Jharkhand, West Bengal, Manipur and Assam) of the country. In the survey, Mini International Neuropsychiatric Inventory (MINI 6.0) was used to screen for mental health morbidity in the community. In addition to recording the prevalence of various psychiatric disorders in the community, the survey also evaluated the existing mental health infrastructure, human resources in mental healthcare, healthcare utilisation, treatment gap, disability due to mental health and pattern of help-seeking behaviour for mental illnesses, in the country.

In the National Mental Health Survey, the sample size of the surveyed population was 34,802 (from 12 representative states of India). As the study participants were adults (above 18 years of age), the prevalence results were applicable to this population only.

In the surveyed population, the current and lifetime prevalence of psychiatric disorders (not including Tobacco use disorder) was found to be 10.6% and 13.7%, respectively.

Table 22.1 below mentions the current prevalence of various mental illnesses in India.

Table 22.1: Current prevalence of various psychiatric disorders in the adult population of India as per NMHS 2015–2016.

Psychiatric disorders	Current prevalence
Alcohol use disorder	4.6%
Tobacco use disorder	13.1%
Other substance use disorder	0.6%
Schizophrenia and other psychotic disorders	0.4%
Bipolar affective disorder	0.3%
Depressive disorder	2.7%
Neurotic and stress-related disorders	3.5%

Depressive disorder was found to be quite common in the urban metro population, with the highest prevalence among women in the 40–49 years of age group.

The treatment gap was also calculated for various psychiatric disorders in the national mental health survey. The treatment gap is the percentage of individuals who are in need of care but are not receiving the treatment. The treatment gap was found to be highest for alcohol use disorder (86.3%) and lowest for bipolar affective disorder (70.4%). For psychotic disorders, major depressive disorder and neurotic disorders, treatment gaps were 75.5%, 85.2% and 83.2%, respectively.

In this survey, it was also found that there is a scarcity of mental health manpower, scarcity of budget for mental health, lack of infrastructure to meet the needs of mental healthcare in the community, partial implementation of mental health law, poor supply of essential psychotropic medication, poor coordination and monitoring of mental health activities across the states which participated in the survey.

To Deliver Optimal

Mental health services at the community level, there is a need for inter-sectoral collaboration (coordination of different government sectors like: the Ministry of Health, Ministry of Social Welfare and so on), community participation and effective public-private partnership (a collaboration of public sectors with non-governmental organisations). An effective mental healthcare service in the community also needs huge trained mental health manpower (psychiatrists, clinical psychologists, psychiatric social workers and psychiatric nurses). Family (caregivers) and the community too play pivotal roles in facilitating mental health services in the community.

SUGGESTED READINGS

1. World Health Organization (WHO). Mental Health Atlas 2017.
2. https://www.who.int/mental_health/evidence/atlas/profiles-2017/IND.pdf
3. Innovation in deinstitutionalization: a WHO expert survey. WHO, 2014. http://www.lisboninstitutegmh.org/assets/docs/publications/9789241506816_eng.pdf
4. World Health Organization (WHO). Mental health action plan 2013–2020. http://www.who.int/mental_health/action_plan_2013/en/
5. Gururaj G, Varghese M, Benegal V, Rao GN, Pathak K, Singh LK, et al. National Mental Health Survey of India, 2015-16: Summary. Bengaluru, National Institute of Mental Health and Neuro Sciences, NIMHANS Publication No. 128, 2016.
6. Math SB, Srinivasaraju R. Indian psychiatric epidemiological studies: Learning from the past. Indian J Psychiatry. 2010;52,(Suppl S3):95-103.
7. Wig NN, Murthy SR. The birth of national mental health program for India. Indian J Psychiatry. 2015;57:315-9.
8. Directorate General Of Health Services. Ministry of Health & Family Welfare. Government of India http://dghs.gov.in/content/1350_3_NationalMentalHealthProgramme.aspx [Last accessed on 21-02-2017].

INDEX

Page numbers followed by *f* refer to figure; and *t* refer to table.

A

Abdominal pain 89
Abreaction 77, 150
Acamprosate 89
Accelerated detoxification 91
Acceptance 70
Acetylcholine levels 98
Acne 46
Acrophobia 54
Actigraphy 123
Acting out 153
Adaptive functioning 147
Addictive behaviours 95
Addictive disorders 83, 95
Adenylyl cyclase, activity of 157
Adequacy 2
Adjustment disorder 69
  and depression 70
  management 69
  symptoms 69
Adoption 168
  studies 16
Adrenal hyperplasia, congenital 131
Aducanumab 104
Advance directive 169
Advanced sleep phase type 127
Aggression, episodes of significant 64
Agitation 99
Agnosia 101
Agoraphobia 51, 53
  aetiology 53
  differential diagnoses 53
  epidemiology 53
  treatment 53
Agranulocytosis 24
Agreeableness 109
Ailurophobia 54
Aim inhibition 153
Akathisia
  acute 21
  management of 20
Alanine aminotransferase 88
Alcohol 85
  absorption 86
  acute effects of 86
  concentration, absolute 85*t*
  dependence 87
    questionnaire, severity of 88
  intoxication, symptoms of 86*t*
  mellanby effect 86
  metabolism 86
  rate of oxidation of 86
  reverse tolerance 86
  use disorder 53, 85, 87, 174
    identification test 88
    treatment of 88
  withdrawal 87
    delirium 87
    seizures 87, 89
Alcoholic
  anonymous 90
  blackout 86
Alcohol-induced
  anxiety disorders 87
  bipolar disorders 87
  dementia 87
  depressive disorders 87
  disorders 87
  persistent amnestic disorder 87
  psychotic disorders 87
  sexual dysfunction 87
  sleep disorder 87
Alertness 97
Alexithymia 5
Algophobia 54
Alogia 14
Alpha activity 123
Alpha-adrenergic agonist 140
Alpha-synuclein 106
Alprazolam 52
Alprostadil, method of use of 134
Altered sensorium 98
Altruism 154
Altruistic suicide 48
Alzheimer's disease 34, 102-106, 127
  brain atrophy in 102*f*
  early-onset 102
    autosomal dominant familial 103
  genetic factors 103
  hallmark of 102
  late-onset 102, 103
  management of 104
  risk factors 102
  treatment of 104
Ambient temperature 123
Ambitendency 15
Ambivalence 12
Amenorrhea 37, 117
American law institute 168
Amisulpride 23
Amitriptyline 68
Amnesia 100
Amnestic disorders 107
Amnestic syndromes 87
Amotivational syndrome 93
Amoxapine 37
Amphetamine 94
Amphetamine-like compounds 94
Amphetamines 94
Amygdala 32
Amygdalotomy 158
Amyloid cascade hypothesis 103
Amyloid deposits 102
Amyloid precursor protein 103
Amyloid β-peptide 102
Anaesthetic agents 156
Anal stage 154
Anankastic personality disorder 115
Anger 70
Anger outbursts 112
Angry mood 144
Anhedonia 5, 14
Anhedonia and loss of interest 29
Anniversary reaction 71
Anomic suicide 48
Anorexia nervosa 117
Anorgasmia 135
Anterior cingulate cortex 32
Anterior cingulate syndrome 107
Anterograde amnesia 86, 88
Antiandrogens 65
Anticholinergic agents 99
Anticholinergics 21
Anticipation 154
Anticipatory anxiety 51
Antidepressants 36
Antiepileptic medications 105
Antipsychotics 20, 21, 136
  atypical 22
  first-generation 21
  intramuscular injections of 24
  low dose 111
  medications 14
  newer drugs 23
  poor compliance with 24
  second-generation 20, 22
  typical 21

Antisocial personality disorder 64, 78, 85, 111
Antisuicidal agent 45
Anxiety 50, 95
 and fear 50
 symptoms of 50, 104
Anxiety disorders 73, 140
 classification of 51
Anxiolytics 111
Anxious personality disorder 114
Apathy 14
Aphasia 100
Appetite, increased 92
Apraxia 100
Aptitude test 165
Argumentative behaviour 144
Aripiprazole 22-24
Arousal disorder 128, 133
Arousal symptoms 67
Ascending reticular activating system 98
Asenapine 23
Asociality 14
Aspartate aminotransferase 88
Asperger's syndrome 143
Assertive community treatment 24
Assertiveness training 163
Association, loosening of 7
Asthenic 13
Ataxia 46, 87
Athletic 13
Attention 8
Attention deficit hyperactivity disorder 34, 94, 139
 aetiology 140
 clinical features 139
 management 140
Attenuated psychosis syndrome 26
Audible thoughts 13, 14
Auditory disturbances 26
Auditory hallucination 6
 third-person 13
Autism 12, 148
 development of 142
Autism spectrum disorder 140
 aetiology 141
 associated symptoms of 141
 core symptoms of 140
Autistic spectrum disorders 140
Autoimmune disorders 99
Automatic negative thought 162
Automatic obedience 15
Automatic pulling 62
Autoprosopagnosia 101
Aversive conditioning 164
Avoidance 51
Avoidant personality disorder 114
Avoidant restrictive food intake disorder 120
Avolition 14
Awakening, early morning 123
Azapirones 57

B

Ban on
 direct electroconvulsive therapy 170
 ECT for minors 170
 psychosurgery 170
Bargaining 70
Basal ganglia and cerebellum 17
Basic arousal 97
Beck depression inventory 35, 44
Beggar's disguise 26
Behavioural 72
 factors 85
 induced insufficient sleep syndrome 126
 model 67
 phenomena 128
 repetitive patterns of 141
 theory 55, 59, 73, 76
 therapy 55, 95, 144, 163
Bender gestalt test 166*f*
Bender visual motor gestalt test 166
Bender-gestalt test 166
Benzodiazepines 21, 25, 52, 53, 56, 61, 68, 69, 76, 89, 95, 124
 receptor agonists 124
 short-acting 89
Bereavement and depression 71
Beta activity 123
Beta-blockers 57, 112
Bhore Committee's 173
Bimodal distribution 13
Binge eating disorder 119, 120
Binswanger disease 105
Biofeedback 164
Biological antagonism 156
Biological theories 73
Biopsychosocial model 85
Bipolar affective disorder 174
Bipolar and related disorders 40
Bipolar depression 45
Bipolar disorder 40, 43, 44
 cases of 43
 developing 43
 prevalence of 43
 types of 25, 42
Bizarre delusions 8
Bleuler, four a's of 12*t*
Blood alcohol concentration 86, 88
Blotter acid 93
Bobo doll 162
Bodily distress disorder 72, 73
Body dysmorphic disorder 58, 61
Body integrity dysphoria 73
Bone mineral density 118
Borderline intellectual functioning 147
Borderline personality disorder 111, 112, 153
Bradycardia 95
Brain-derived neurotrophic factor 33
Brain disorders 166

Brain reward pathway 85
Brawner test 168
Bremelanotide 133
Brepiprazole 23
Brexanolone 46
Brexpiprazole 23
Briquet's syndrome 72
Bulimia nervosa 118, 119
 aetiology 120
 subtypes 119
 treatment 120
Buprenorphine 91
Bupropion 136
Butyrophenones 21

C

Caffeine 94, 95
Callouses 119
Calluses on knuckles 119*f*
Camphor, injections of 156
Cannabinoids 92
Cannabis 92, 93, 95
 and cannabis use disorders 92
 dependence 92
 flashbacks 93
 induced psychotic disorder 92
 plant and seeds 92*f*
 preparations 92, 92*t*
 related disorders 92
 use 17
Capgras syndrome 26
Capsulotomy 61
Carbamazepine 61, 68, 89, 112
 use in pregnancy 47
Carbidopa 106
Carbohydrate deficit transferrin 88
Cardiac arrhythmias 89
Cardiac side effects 22
Cardiovascular disorders 51
Cardiovascular system 77
Cariprazine 23
Carphologia 98
Castration anxiety 154
Cataplexy 126
Catastrophic
 misinterpretation of benign sensations 52
 reaction 101
Catatonia 14
 associated with schizophrenia 24
Catatonic
 schizophrenia 18
 symptoms 14
Catha edulis 94
Caudate tractotomy 61
Central and State Mental Health Authorities 169
Central nervous system depressant 86
Central nervous system disorders 99
Cerebral ventricles 17

Chief complaints 3
Child psychiatry 139
Childhood disintegrative disorder 143
Chlordiazepoxide 89
Chlorpromazine 20-22
Cholecystokinin 52
Cholinergic neurons, disorders of 103
Cholinesterase inhibitors 104
Chromosome
   1 103
   14 103
   18*q* and 22*q* 43
   21 103
   22 16
Chromosomes hormones 130
Chronic fatigue syndrome 74
Chronic obstructive pulmonary disease 77
Chronotherapy 128
Cigarettes and Other Tobacco Products Act 2003 170
Cingulotomy 61
Circadian rhythm disorders 128
Circadian rhythm sleep disorder 127
   types of 127
Circumstantiality 6
Civil responsibility 168
Clang associations 7
Claustrophobia 54
Clomipramine 61
Clonazepam 52
Clonidine 91, 140
Closed-ended questions 2
Clozapine 22, 23, 106
Clumsy child syndrome 144
Cluster 45
   A personality disorders 110
   B personality disorder 111
   C personality disorder 114
   seizures 87
Coarse tremors 46, 87
Cocaine 93
   bugs 94
   induced depressive disorders 34
Cognition 6
Cognitive
   accomplishments 160
   behaviour therapy 24, 36, 52-54, 56, 62, 64, 65, 68, 73, 74, 96, 120, 124, 162
   decline 11
   deficits, presence of 98
   development stages 160
   distortions 34, 162, 163
   disturbances 30, 41, 106
   errors 162
   functions 97
      progressive impairment of 100
   impairment 93, 100
   model 67
   remediation therapy 24
   restructuring 125

symptoms 15
theory 34, 52, 60
therapy 36
Coma 97
Communication disorders 148
Community psychiatry 172
   in India 172
   scope of 172
Complex motor tics 143
Complex vocal tics 143
Complicated bereavement 71
Compulsive sexual behaviour disorder 65
Conation, symptoms of 14
Concentration 8
Concrete operational stage 160
Condensation 151
Conduct disorder 140, 145
   aetiology 145
   clinical features and diagnosis 145
   course and prognosis 145
   treatment 145
Confabulations 88
Confusion assessment method 99
Confusional state 99
Congestive heart failure 89
Conjunctiva, reddening of 92
Conscientiousness 109
Consciousness
   and cognition 97
   clouding of 82
   content of 97
   disturbances of 100
   level of 97, 98
Conservation 160
Contamination 59
Contemplation 90, 164
Continuous positive airway pressure 127
Contract 168
Conversion disorder 72, 74, 78, 150
   aetiology of 76
   treatment of 76
Coping strategy 66
Coprophilia 137
Copy number variations, role of 142
Coronary artery disease 89
Coronary heart disease 115
Corpus callosum 88
Cortical and subcortical dementias 101
Cortical dementias 101
Cortical dysfunction, early appearance of 101
Cortico-striatal-thalamic-cortical 59
Cortico-striatothalamic circuit 143
Cortisol 131
   hypersecretion 33
   levels 33
Cotard's syndrome 7
Cowper's gland 130
Crack 94
Cranial electrical stimulation 158

Creutzfeldt-Jakob disease 101, 106
   treatment of 107
Criminal responsibility 167, 168
Crisis intervention 69
Criticism 111
   and hostility 20
Culture bound syndromes 78
Curren's rule 168
Cushing's syndrome 99
Cyclothymic disorder 45
Cynophobia 54
Cyproterone 65

D

Dantrolene 22
de Clerambault syndrome 7
Dealing with stressor 76
Death and dying 70
   stages of 70
Debriefing 69
Deceitfulness 111
Deep brain stimulation 68, 158
Deep tendon reflexes 46
Defense mechanism 66, 110, 152
   in psychiatric disorders 154
Defiant behaviour 144
Delayed ejaculation 135
   treatment 136
Delayed grief 71
Delayed sleep phase type 127
Deliberate fire setting 64
Delirium 37, 98, 99, 107, 157
   clinical diagnosis 99
   major causes of 99
   tremens 89
   versus dementia 99
   versus schizophrenia 99
Delusion 7 14, 16, 98, 99
   and hallucinations 153
   of enormity 7
   of grandeur or grandiosity 7
   of guilt 7
   of halitosis 26
   of infidelity 7
   of jealousy 7
   of love 7
   of negation 7
   of persecution 7, 26
   of reference 7
Delusional disorder 26, 74
   development of 26
Delusional parasitosis 26
Delusional perception 13
Dementia 99, 100, 106, 107
   due to Creutzfeldt-Jakob disease 106
   due to Huntington's disease 106
   epidemiology 100
   forms of 107
   of the Alzheimer type 102

praecox 11, 28
pugilistica 103
reversible causes of 101
symptoms 100
treatment of 106
types of 102
Denial 153
and shock 70
Dental enamel, loss of 119
Dependence 83
Dependent personality disorder 114
Depersonalisation 82
Depressed mood 5, 29,104
Depression 6, 70, 107
acute, treatment of 44
aetiology of 32
and anxiety disorders 85
final neurobiological model of 33
neuroanatomy of 32
psychosocial theories of 33
with suicide risk 157
Depressive disorder 28, 40, 42, 73, 174
major 28, 34, 157
clinical features and diagnosis 29
epidemiology 29
versus bipolar disorder 42
Depressive type 25
Derailment 7
Derealisation disorder 82
Dermatoglyphics, abnormal 141
Desensitisation 61
Desire phase, disorders of 133
Desmopressin 146
Detoxification 88, 91
Deutetrabenazine 22
Developmental coordination disorder 143, 144
Dexamethasone suppression test 33
in depression 33
Dhat syndrome 78
Diacetylmorphine 90
Dialectical behaviour therapy 113
Diarrhoea 91
Diathesis-stress model 82
Diazepam 89
DiGeorge syndrome 16
Digit repetition test 8
Digit span test 8
Digital gaming 96
Diphenhydramine 21
Discrepancy 78
Disinhibited social engagement disorder 70
Disobedience and hostility 144
Disorders specifically associated with stress 66
Disorganisation symptoms 14
Disorganised
behaviour 14
thought and speech 14

Displacement 151, 153
Disqualifying positive 163
Disruptive behaviour disorders 144
Dissociation 153
Dissociative 81
amnesia, types 81
continuous amnesia 81
generalised amnesia 81
localised amnesia 81
selective amnesia 81
systematised amnesia 81
anaesthetics 93
disorder 80, 82, 150, 154
aetiology of 82
development of 80
primary gain 80
secondary gain 80
tertiary gain 80
treatment of 82
fugue 81
identity disorder 80, 153
trance 81
Distortion 153
Distractibility 41
District Mental Health Programme 173
Disulfiram 89
Disulfiram acts 89
Diurnal bladder control, development of 145
Dizygotic concordance rate 13, 52, 85
Dizygotic twins 43, 110
Donepezil 104
Dopamine 17, 86, 131
4 receptor gene 140
norepinephrine reuptake inhibitor 140
receptor antagonists 21
receptor supersensitivity 22
transporter gene 140
Dopaminergic activity 89
Dorsolateral prefrontal cortex 32
Dorsolateral syndrome 107
Down's syndrome 103, 104
Downward drift hypothesis 13
Draw-a-person test 166
Dream
interpretation of 151
work 151
Droperidol 21
Drowsiness and paradoxical trouble sleeping 95
Drug abuse 17
Drug-induced parkinsonism 21
DSM-5 and ICD-11 classification 18
Dual-sex therapy 134
Durham's rule 168
Dysarthria 46
Dyspareunia 136
Dysphoric mania 40
Dystonia, acute 21

E

Eating disorders 117
aetiology 118
epidemiology 118
subtypes 118
treatment 118
Ebstein's anomaly 46, 47
Echo de pensee 13
Echolalia 15
Echopraxia 15
Ecstasy 40
Eddy currents 35
Educational history 4
EEG rhythms 123t
Ego 152
dystonic 8, 58
unconscious component of 152
Egocentric 160
Egoistic suicide 48
Ekbom syndrome 129
Elation 40
Electra complex 154
Electroconvulsive therapy 24, 35, 156, 157
Electroconvulsive therapy, types 156
Electrode placement 156
Electrolyte disturbances 99
Electrophysiology 18
Elevated mood 40
Elimination disorders 145
Embarrassment 53
Emergency treatment 170
Emil kraepelin 11, 28
Emile durkheim 48
Emotional
coldness 111
disturbances 5, 98
neuroanatomical substrate of 5
passivity of 12
reasoning 163
response 66
unstable 112
Empathy 2
Emptiness, chronic feeling of 112
Encopresis
aetiology 146
treatment 146
Endocrine 46
disorders 51, 77, 99, 107
side effects 22
Energy, loss of 30
Enuresis 146
treatment 146
Environmental measures 99
Ephedrine 94
Episodic illness 11, 25
Episodic memory deficits 100
Epstein–Barr virus 74
Erectile disorder 133, 134
aetiology 133

Erectile dysfunction 133
Ernst Kretschmer 13
Erotomania 7
Erotomanic type 26
Erythroxylum coca 93
Estrogen 131
Eszopiclone 124
Ethyl alcohol 85
Eugen bleuler 11
Euphoria 40
Euphoric mania 40, 45
Euphoric mood 5
Exaggerated emotions 113
Exaltation 40
Examination
   classification 9
   general physical examination 4
   higher mental functions 8
   mental status examination 4
   systemic examination 4
Excessive
   concern 119
   devotion 115
   rigidity 115
   self-importance 113
   sleepiness 125
   thoughts 72
   worries 56
Excitement 14
   disorders of 133
   phase 130
Excoriation disorder 62
Executive function disturbances 101
Executive organ 152
Exhibitionistic disorder 137
Expected panic attacks 51
Expressed emotions 19, 20
External genitalia 130
Extracellular deposits 103
Extrapyramidal side effects 21
Extrapyramidal symptoms 21
Extraversion 109
Eye movement desensitisation 68
Eyeballs, deviation of 21
Eye-opener 88

F

Facial abnormality 88
Facial flushing 89
Factitious disorder 77, 78
   treatment 78
Faecal continence 145
Fallacy of fairness 163
False belief 7
False pregnancy 74
Family
   and marital therapy 90
   interventions 24
   of origin 3

   of procreation 3
   therapy 164
   tree 3
Fantasy lover syndrome 7
Fear-related disorders 50
Feeling 72
   of gratification 64
   of impending doom 51
Female orgasm disorder 135
   treatment 135
Female sexual interest 133
   aetiology 133
   treatment 133
Fetal alcohol syndrome 88
Fetishistic disorder 137
Fingerprints 141
Flashbacks 67
Flexibility, lack of 115
Flibanserin 133
Floccillations 98
Flooding 55, 163
Flu-like syndrome 91
Flupenthixol 21, 24
Fluphenazine 21, 24
Focused pulling 62
Forensic psychiatric assessment 167
Forensic psychiatry 167
   evaluations, reasons for 167
Formal operational stage 161
Formal thought disorders 14
Fragile X syndrome 141
Freebasing 94
Free-floating anxiety 56
Fregoli syndrome 26
Frontotemporal dementia 101, 105
   treatment of 105
Frotteuristic disorder 137
Fun in life 115
Functional disorders 97
Functional hallucinations 6
Functional mental disorders 9
Functional neurological symptom
   disorder 74

G

Gaining weight, intense fear of 117
Galantamine 104
Gamblers anonymous 96
Gambling disorder 96
Gamma-glutamyl transferase 88
Ganser's syndrome 82
Gastric acid, loss of 119
Gastrointestinal symptoms 46
Gastrointestinal system 77
Gedankenlautwerden 13
Gegenhalten 15
Gender dysphoria 131, 132
   aetiology of 132
   cases of 132
Gender identity 130

Gender incongruence 131, 132
Genderqueers 132
General adaptation syndrome 77
Generalised anxiety disorder 51, 56
   aetiology 56
   comorbidity 56
   differential diagnosis 56
   psychological factors 56
   treatment 56
Genetic 16, 52
   abnormalities 137
   factors 67
Genetic syndrome 16
Genital sensate focus 134
Genito-pelvic pain 136
Granulovacuolar degeneration 103
Gridiron abdomen 78
Grief disorder, prolonged 70
Grief reactions
   abnormal 71
   complicated 71
Grimacing 15
Guilty mentally ill 168
Gynaecomastia 37

H

Habit reversal 144
   technique 62
Hair loss 46
Hair-pulling disorder 62
Hallmark symptom 53
Hallucinations 5, 14, 16, 99
Hallucinogens 93
   intoxication 93
   persisting perception disorder 93
   treatment 93
Haloperidol 21, 24, 61
Hamilton rating scale for depression 35, 44
Harmful pattern, use of alcohol 87
Head injury 137
Headache 45
Hebephrenic schizophrenia 18
Heller's syndrome 143
Hemizygous 22q11.2 deletions 16
Hemp insanity 92
Hepatic encephalopathy 99
Heroin 90
High potency 21
Hippocampus 32
Histrionic personality disorder 111, 113
Hoarding disorder 58, 61
   treatment 62
Homicide 15, 44
Homosexuality 131
   prevalence of 131
Hoover's sign 75
   positive 75
Hopelessness 47

Hormonal
  contraceptives 136
  disorders 137
    dysregulation 33, 43
    treatment 132
Hospital addiction 77
Human leukocyte antigens class II 126
Humiliation 53
Humour 154
Huntington's disease, treatment of 106
Hyperactive delirium 98
Hyperactivity and impulsivity 139
Hypercalcaemia 99
Hyperdopaminergic state 17, 43
Hyper-excited state 88
Hypermagnesaemia 99
Hypernatraemia 99
Hyperphagia 125
Hyperprolactinaemia 22
Hyperreflexia 37
Hypersexuality 125
Hypersomnia 125
  due to drugs 127
  due to medical condition 127
  in context of sleep-related breathing disorder 127
  types of 125
Hypersomnolence disorder 125
Hyperthyroidism 99
Hypertrophic grief 71
Hypervigilance 67
Hypnagogic hallucinations 6, 126
Hypnopompic hallucinations 6, 126
Hypoactive delirium 98
Hypocalcaemia 99
Hypochondriasis 58, 63
Hypocretin, deficiency of 126
Hypodopaminergic state 17
Hypofrontality in schizophrenia 17
Hypokalaemia 119
Hypomagnesaemia 99
Hypomania, treatment of 44
Hypomanic episode 41
Hyponatraemia 99
Hypotension 91
Hypothalamic pituitary adrenal 33
Hypothalamus 126, 127
Hypothetico-deductive reasoning 161
Hypothyroidism 34, 46

I

Ibogaine 93
Id 152
Ideas, flight of 6, 41
Identifying data 2
Identity, disturbances of 112
Idiopathic hypersomnia 125
Idiosyncratic alcohol intoxication 86
Illness anxiety disorder 72-74
Illness, course of 3
Illusions 5
Iloperidone 22
Imaginal exposure 55
Imagined abandonment 112
Imipramine 68, 146
Immature defenses 153
Immigration 17
Immune-mediated disorder 126
Immunological mechanisms 33
Implosion 55, 163
Impressionistic speech 113
Impulse control disorders 64, 153
Impulsivity 112
In vivo exposure 55, 163
Inappropriate affect 14
Incoherence 7
Increased goal-directed activities 41
Indecisiveness 115
Indifference towards praise 111
Induced delusional disorder 26
Induced movement 15
Infection, maternal exposure to 16
Inflated self-esteem 41
Informants 2
  chronological information 2
  closeness with the patient 2
  coherence 2
  concern with the patient 2
  consistency 2
Information processing speed 15
Inhalants solvents 95
Insight oriented psychotherapy 56
Insomnias 91, 99, 104, 123
  pharmacological management of 124
  treatment 124
  types 124
    adjustment 124
    due to drug use 124
    due to medical disorders 124
    idiopathic 124
    inadequate sleep hygiene 124
    psychophysiological 124
    sleep state misperception 124
    subjective 124
Instability of self-image 112
Instinctual drives 151
Intellectual development, disorders of 147
Intellectual disability 141, 147
  aetiology 148
  degrees of severity of 147
  diagnosis 147
  management of 148
    primary prevention 148
    secondary prevention 148
    tertiary prevention 148
  mild 147
  moderate 147
  profound 147
  severe 147
Intellectual functioning 147
  general level of 146
Intellectualisation 153
Intelligence 8
  quotient 147
  tests 164
Intermetamorphosis, syndrome of 26
Intermittent explosive disorder 64
Internal genitalia 130
International classification of diseases 9, 116
International Pilot Study of Schizophrenia 19, 173
Interpersonal relationships, unstable 112
Intoxication 83, 91, 92
  acute 86
Intracellular inclusions 103
Intravaginal ejaculatory latency time 135
Intrusive thought 59, 160
Irregular sleep-wake type 127
Irresistible sleep episodes 126
Irritability 92, 141
  and aggressiveness 112
Irritable mood 40, 144
Isocarboxazid 35
Isolation of affect 153

J

Jealous type 26
Jet lag type 127
Judgment 9
Judicial rules 168
Jumping to conclusions 163

K

Key informant technique 84
Kindling 34
  effect 44
Kleine-Levin syndrome 125
Kleptomania 64, 137
Kluver-Bucy syndrome 105
Koro 78
Korsakoff syndrome 88, 107

L

La belle indifference 75
Labeling mislabeling 163
Lacrimation 91
Lamotrigine 44
Language
  comprehension 15
  disturbances 98, 141
Latah 78
Learned helplessness, theory of 34
Learning disorders 140
  developmental 146
  diagnosis of specific 147
  types of 146
Learning theory 76, 161
Lethargy 97
Leukocytosis 22
Levodopa 106

Lewy body dementia 106
   treatment of 106
Life events and environmental stress 33
Lifelong erectile disorder 134
Light therapy 128
Limbic system 5, 17
Lithium 44, 45
Lithium responsiveness, correlates of 45
Lithium toxicity 46
Lithium use in pregnancy 47
Logoclonia 15
Lorazepam 89
Low birth weight 88
Lurasidone 23
Lysergic acid diethylamide 93, 94

M

Magical thinking 111
Magnan phenomenon 94
Magnetic seizure therapy 158
Magnification and minimisation 163
Malafide intention 2
Male hypoactive sexual desire disorder 133
   aetiology 133
   treatment 133
Malingering 78
Mammillary bodies 88
Mania 6
   acute, treatment of 44
Mania a potu 86
Manic episode 40, 157
Manic-depressive psychosis 11
Mannerisms 15
Marchiafava–Bignami disease 88
Marital status 48
Marriage and divorce 168
Masked depression 29
Masturbation 131
Mature defenses 154
McNaughten's case and rules 167
Mean corpuscular volume 88
Medical disorders 20, 51
Medically unexplained symptoms 72
Medication-induced
   bipolar disorder 43
   sexual dysfunction 136
Medicolegal history 4
Medroxyprogesterone 65
Melatonin 128
   influences circadian rhythm 128
   receptor agonist 124
Memory 8
   deficits 98
      different kinds of 100
   disturbances 157
   immediate 8
   recent 8
   remote 8
   working 8, 15

Menstrual
   history 4
   related hypersomnia 125
Mental and behavioural disorders 83
Mental compulsions 59
Mental disorders
   diagnostic and statistical manual of 9
   severe 19, 137
Mental distress gets 73
Mental filtering 163
Mental health 48, 84
   Act, 1987 169
   action plan 2013–2030 172
   care act 2017 169
   care and treatment decisions 169
   legislation in India 169
   review commission 169
   scene in India 174
   services 174
Mental illness 169
Mental retardation 19, 147
Mentalisation-based therapy 113
Mentally ill 172
Mesocortical tract 17
Mesolimbic tract 17
Metabolic
   acidosis 36, 119
   alkalosis 119
Methadone 91
Methylenedioxymethamphetamine 94
Methylphenidate 94, 140
Metoidioplasty 132
Metonyms 7
Micropsychotic episodes 112
Migraine 45
Mind
   components of 152f
      ego 152f
      id 152f
      superego 152f
   disorders of 97
   theory of 141
Minimal brain dysfunction 139
Mini-mental status examination 99, 100, 104
Minnesota multiphasic personality inventory 165
Mirtazapine 136
Misnomer 117
Mixed anxiety and depressive disorder 57
Modafinil 126, 140
Modelling, participant modelling 55, 163
Monoamine
   hypothesis of depression 33
   oxidase A 110
   oxidase inhibitors 35, 52, 68
Monozygotic concordance 43
   rate 13, 85
Montgomery Asberg Depression Rating Scale 35, 44

Mood
   and affect 4
      affective flattening 5
      appropriateness and congruency 5
      fluctuations 5
      labile mood 5
      quality 5
   congruent psychotic features 30
   disorders 28, 40, 140
      classification 28
   disturbances 29, 40
   elevation of 5
   incongruent psychotic features 30
   stabilisers 47
      use of 47
   symptoms 101
Morbid jealousy 7
Motivational enhancement therapy 90
Motor activity 4
   decreased psychomotor activity 4
   increased psychomotor activity 4
Motor disorders 143
Motor symptoms 14, 74
   early presentation of 101
Motor tics 143
Movement disorders 21, 23
Movement, loss of 106
Multi-infarct dementia 105
Multiple personality disorder 80
Multiple sleep latency test 125
Münchhausen syndrome 77, 78
Muscarinic anticholinergics 156
Muscle dysmorphia 61
Muscle relaxants 157
Muscle tone, loss of 123
Musculoskeletal system 77
Mutism 14
Myalgic encephalomyelitis 74
Myoclonus 37
Myoglobinuria 22
Mysophobia 54

N

Naloxone 91
Naltrexone 89, 91
Narcissistic defenses 153
Narcissistic personality disorder 111, 113
Narcolepsy 126
   with cataplexy 126
   without cataplexy 126
Narcotic Drugs and Psychotropic Substances Act, 1985 170
Narrow therapeutic index 46
Nasal spray of naloxone 92
National Mental Health Program 173
National Mental Health Survey 29, 43, 84, 174
Nature versus nurture 16
Necrophilia 137
Negativism 15

Neologism 7
Neural tube defects 47
Neuritic plaques 102
Neuroanatomical and neuropathological factors 17
Neurobiological
  factors 56, 67
  theories 82
Neurobiology 17, 32, 85, 118
Neurochemical factors 54
Neurochemistry 33, 103
Neurocognitive disorders 97
  major 100
Neurodevelopmental disorders 148
Neurofibrillary tangles 102, 103
Neuroimaging 43
Neuroimmunology 59
Neuroleptic malignant syndrome 22, 99, 157
Neurological
  disorders 20, 51, 60, 137
  signs 101
  symptoms 101, 102
Neuropathology 102
Neurosis 10, 154
  development of 153
Neurotic
  and stress-related disorders 174
  defenses 153
  illness develops 154
  symptoms 19
Neuroticism 109
Neurotransmitter 52, 59, 110
  disturbances 145
Neutropenia 45
  mild 24
  moderate 24
  severe 24
Nicotine
  craving for 94
  replacement therapy 95
Night eating syndrome 120
Nightmare disorder 129
Nigrostriatal
  pathway 21
  tract 21
Nihilistic delusion 7
Nocturnal
  and morning erections 134
  bladder control, development of 145
  enuresis 129
  panic attacks 51
Nominated representative 169
Nonarteritic ischemic optic neuropathy 134
Nongenital sensate focus 134
Nonrapid eye movement sleep 122
  arousal disorders 128
  parasomnias 128
Norepinephrine
  dopamine disinhibitor 133
  reuptake inhibitor 140
Normal functions, loss of 14

Normal human sexuality 130
Nucleus accumbens 21
Nymphomania 65

O

Objective tests 165
Observational learning 162
Obsessions 8, 58
Obsessive-compulsive disorder 45, 52, 58, 60, 115, 153, 154, 157
  aetiology 59
  comorbidity 60
  course and prognosis 60
  differential diagnosis 60
  epidemiology 59
  treatment 60, 61
Obstetric complications 16
Obstructive sleep apnoea 127
Obtundation 97
Occupational delirium 98
Oculogyric crisis 21f
Oedipus complex 55, 154
Olanzapine 22, 24, 61
Olfactory bulb 33
Olfactory reference disorder 58, 63
Olfactory reference syndrome 26
Omega sign 30, 30f
Oneroid state 97
Open-ended questions 2
Openness to experience 109
Operant conditioning, types of 161t
Ophthalmoplegia 87
  starts 88
Opioid antagonist treatment 91
Opioid substitution therapy 91
Opioids 86, 90
Oppositional defiant disorder 144
  aetiology 144
  clinical features and diagnosis 144
  course and prognosis 145
  treatment 145
Oral phentolamine 134
Orbital prefrontal cortex 32
Orbitofrontal syndrome 107
Orchiectomy 132
Organic erectile disorder 133, 134
Organic mental disorders 9, 97, 166
Organic versus functional mental disorders 9
Orgasm phase, disorders of 135
Othello syndrome 7
Overactive amygdala 67
Overdose treatment 91
Overgeneralisation 163
Oxytocin 131

P

P300 wave 18
Painful coitus 136
Painful consequences, high potential for 41

Palilalia 15
Paliperidone 22, 24
Pananxiety 19
Panic attack 51
Panic disorder 51, 53
  aetiology 52
  differential diagnosis 51
  epidemiology 51
Panneurosis 19
Pansexuality 19
Paradoxical
  intention 125
  sleep 123
  suicide 30
Paranoia 93
Paranoid
  personality disorder 110
  schizophrenia 18, 94
Paraphilic disorders 137
  features of 137t
Parasomnias 128
  associated with REM sleep disorders 128
Parkinson's disease 34, 106, 157
Parkinsonian symptoms 106
Parotid gland enlargement 119
Partial dissociative identity disorder 81
Partialism 137
Passive death wishes 30
Passive-aggressive behaviour 153
Pathological doubt 59
Patient-doctor relationship 1, 2
Pavor nocturnus 128
Peculiar and odd interpersonal relationships 111
Pedophilic disorder 136, 137
Penfluridol 21
Penile erection 123
Penile prosthetic implants 134
Penis envy 154
Pentagastrin 52
Perceptual abnormalities 98
Perfectionism 115
Periodic limb movement disorder 129
Perphenazine 21
Perseveration 6, 15
Persistent
  anxiety symptoms 19
  complex bereavement disorder 70
  motor 144
Person suffering from mental illness 168
Personal judgment 9
Personalisation 163
Personality changes 101
Personality disorder 109, 110
  aetiology 110
  anankastia in 116
  borderline pattern 116
  classification of 110
  detachment in 116
  disinhibition in 116
  dissociality in 116

epidemiology 110
mild 116
moderate 116
negative affectivity in 116
severe 116
Personality tests 165
Pfropf schizophrenia 19
Phallic stage 154
Phalloplasty 132
Pharmacotherapy and psychotherapy, combination of 36
Phencyclidine intoxication 93
Phenelzine 35
Phenothiazines 21
Phenylketonuria 104
Phenylpropanolamine 94
Phobia 19, 54, 154
development of 153
types of 54t
Phosphodiesterase-5 inhibitors 134
Phototherapy 35, 128
Physical disorders 87
Physical health 48, 84
Pica 120
Pick's disease 101, 105
Piloerection 91
Pimavanserin 23
Pipotiazine 24
Pleasurable activities, exclusion of 115
Pleasure principle 152
Polysomnography 123, 125
Polysurgical addiction 77
Ponto-geniculo-occipital spikes 123
Poor
concentration 95
tolerance to criticism 113
Possession trance disorder 81
Postcoital
dysphoria 136
headache 136
Post-operative delirium 99
Postpartum
blues 46
depression 46
psychosis 46
Post-traumatic stress disorder 66
aetiology 67
clinical features and diagnosis 67
comorbidity 68
epidemiology 67
management 68
Posturing 14, 14f
Prazosin 68
Precocious skills 141
Precontemplation 90
Prefrontal cortex 17, 32, 33
Pregnancy
and use of mood stabilisers 47
psychiatric aspects of 46
Premature ejaculation 135
acquired 135

aetiology 135
lifetime 135
treatment 135
Premorbid personality 4, 111
Preoccupation with rules 115
Preoperational stage 160
Present illness, history of 3
Pressured speech 41
Privacy and confidentiality 1
Prochlorperazine 21
Procognitive agents 104
Progesterone 131
Progressive nonfluent aphasia 105
Projective identification 153
Prolactin 131
Property, destruction of 145
Prophylaxis in bipolar I disorder 45
Propositional thought 161
Propranolol 46
Prosopagnosia 101
Protection of Children from Sexual Offences Act, 2012 171
Protection of Women from Domestic Violence Act, 2005 171
Protein kinase B 141
Protracted withdrawal 87
Proverb testing 9
Provocative behaviour 113
Pseudocholinesterase deficiency 157
Pseudocyesis 74
Pseudodementia 30, 107
Pseudoephedrine 94
Pseudohallucinations 6
Pseudoneurotic schizophrenia 19
Pseudoseizure 75
Psoriasis 46
Psychiatric disorders 20, 51, 60, 66, 87, 97
prevalence of 174t
treatment of 156, 158
Psychiatric interview 1, 1f
Psychiatry, history taking in 2
Psychoactive substance abuse history 4
Psychoanalysis 55, 150, 164
father of 150
Psychoanalytic
oriented therapy 36
theories 52, 55
view 76
Psychodynamic
psychotherapy 68
theory 34, 60, 73, 82
Psychoeducation 45
Psychogenic
nonepileptic seizures 75
origin 72
Psychological
erectile disorder 134
factors affecting 77
first aid 69
interventions 69, 169
processes 1

symptoms 50
testing 164
theories 52, 59, 67, 150, 160
Psychomotor
activity, disturbances of 98
agitation 29, 41
disturbance 41, 29
retardation 29
Psychoses 10
versus neuroses 10
Psychosexual, stages of development 154
Psychosocial
interventions 105, 140
treatment 24, 91
Psychosurgery 158
Psychotherapy 52, 53, 68, 69, 114, 144, 162
approaches of 162
types of 162t
Psychotic disorders 10, 25, 60
primary 11
Psychotic symptoms 14, 101
Puberty-blocking endocrine treatment 132
Puerperal psychosis 46
Pulmonary disorders 99
Pupillary dilatation 93
Purging disorder 120
Purging type 118
Pyknic 13
Pyromania 64

Q

Quetiapine 22, 44, 61, 106

R

Rapamycin 141
Rapid eye movement 112
sleep 122, 123
Rapidly changing magnetic fields 158
Rapport 2
Rationalisation 153
Reaction formation 153
Reactive attachment disorder 70
Reality principle 152
Reciprocal inhibition 163
Recovery, complete cure 19
Recurrent deliberate self-harm 112
Reflex hallucinations 6
Regression 153
Reinforcement
negative 85
positive 85
Relapse prevention 90
Relaxation therapy and feedback 125
Remorse and guilt, lack of 112
Renal failure 22
Repression 151, 153
Research domain criterion 10
Research in community psychiatry in India 173

Index

Residual
    ataxia 87
    schizophrenia 18
Resistant schizophrenia, treatment 23
Respiratory depression 91
Respiratory disorders 51
Respiratory system 77
Responsible behaviour, lack of 112
Restless legs syndrome 129
Restlessness 21
Restraints and seclusion 170
Restricting type 118
Retrograde amnesia 88, 157
Rett's disorder 143
Rett's syndrome 143
Reversed biological symptoms 31
Reversibility 160
Reversible and irreversible dementia 101
Reward deficiency syndrome 85
Rhinorrhea 91
Right thing 152
Risperidone 22-24, 61
Rivastigmine 104
Rorschach
    psychodiagnostik test 165
    test cards 165*f*
Rumination-regurgitation disorder 120

S

Safety and comfort 2
Salivary cortisol levels 33
Salvia divinorum 93
Satyriasis 65
Scars on knuckles 119
Scatologia 137
Schizoaffective disorder 21, 25
Schizoid personality disorder 110, 111
Schizophrenia 10, 11, 13, 16, 19, 60, 97, 111, 157, 174
    and 22*q*11. 2 deletion syndrome 16
    and bipolar disorder 10
    continuous 18
    course and outcome of 19
    episode of 20
    experience 14
    first episode 18
    late-onset 13
    mania 137
    multiple episodes 18
    onset of 66
    prognosis in 24
    simple 18
    tracts in 17*f*
    types of 18, 19
Schizophreniform disorder 25
    diagnosis of 25
Schizotypal personality disorder 110, 111
Schneiderian first-rank symptoms 12*t*
Screening test 88
Scrotoplasty 132
Sedation 22

Sedative-hypnotics 95
Seizures 157
    prolonged 157
    symptoms 75
    versus pseudoseizure, clinical manifestations in 75*f*
Selective mutism 57
Selective perception 163
Selective serotonin reuptake inhibitors 37, 52, 68, 105, 144
    use of 74
Selegiline 106
Semans technique 135
Semantic dementia 105
Semantic memory deficits 100
Semicoma 97
Senile plaques 103
Sense of
    control 56
    entitlement 113
Sensorimotor stage 160
Sensory
    impairment 26
    symptoms 74
Sentence completion test 166
Separation anxiety disorder 51, 57
Serial seven subtraction test 8
Serious mental disorders 11
Serotonin 17, 131
    dopamine antagonists 22
    levels, increased 142
    norepinephrine reuptake inhibitors 35, 52, 68
    syndrome 37, 99
    transporter gene 32
Sertindole 22
Sex addiction 65
Sexual
    and marital history 4
    behaviour 130
    disorders 130
    dysfunctions 133, 136
    identity 130
    impulses 65
    masochism disorder 137
    orientation 130
    response cycle 130
        phases 130
    sadism disorder 137
    violation 69
Sexually seductive 113
Shared psychotic disorders 26
Sick role 78
Sigmund Freud proposed 52
Significant
    improvement 19
    symptoms 19
Similarities testing 9
Simple motor tics 143
Single-gene disorders 141
Situational panic attacks 51

Skills training 24
Skin popping 90*f*
Sleep
    and EEG rhythms 123
    attacks 126
    decreased need for 40
    deprivation 35
    disorders 122
        assessment of 123
    disturbances 29
    latency 123
    maintenance insomnia 123
    onset insomnia 123
    paralysis 126
    physiology of 122
    related bruxism 129
    related movement disorders 129
    restriction therapy 125
    spindles 122
    talking 128
    terror 128
    wake disorders 123
    walking 128
Slow-wave sleep 122
Small caudate nucleus, bilaterally 59
Small stature 88
Snowball technique 84
Social and geographical risk factors 17
Social anxiety disorder 51, 53
    aetiology 54
    comorbidity 53
    differential diagnosis 54
    epidemiology 53
    treatment 54
Social
    inhibition 114
    judgment 9
    phobia 53
    skills training 142, 164
    smile 141
Sociocultural factors 118
Sodium diet 46
Sodium oxybate 127
Soft neurological signs 43, 140
Soft signs in schizophrenia 18
Somatic passivity 13
Somatic symptom disorder 72, 63
    aetiology 73
    diagnosis of 73
    versus illness anxiety disorder 74
Somatic therapies 156
Somatic type 26
Somnambulism 128
Somniloquy 128
Somnolence 97
Specific learning disorders 146
Specific phobia 51, 54
    aetiology 54
    comorbidity 54
    differential diagnosis 55
    epidemiology 54
    treatment 55

Specifiers
   for bipolar and related disorders 42
   severity 31
   with anxious distress 31
   with atypical features 31
   with catatonia 31
   with melancholic features 31
   with mixed features 31
   with peripartum onset 31
   with psychotic features 31
   with seasonal pattern 31
Speech 4
   speed of 4
   spontaneity 4
   tone 4
   volume 4
Sphygmomanometer cuff 157
Spina bifida 47
Spiteful 144
Squeeze technique 135
Stabilisation phase 20
Stable phase 20
Stealing, episodes of 64
Stereotactic
   limbic leucotomy 158
   subcaudate tractotomy 158
   movement disorder 143, 144
Stereotypy 15
Stimulants 93
   induced psychotic disorders 94
   intoxication 94
   withdrawal 94
Stimulus control therapy 124
Stinginess 115
Stomach cancer, evidence of 63
Stop-start technique 135
Streptococcus 143
Stress (acute) disorder, treatment of 25, 68, 69
Stressor 67
   diagnostic and statistical manual of 69
Structural theory of mind 151
Stupor 14, 97
Subclinical hypothyroidism 33
Subcortical dementia 101, 106
Subcortical types 101
Subcutaneous injection 133
Subjective doubles, syndrome of 26
Sublimation 154
Substance use disorder 83, 84, 153
   aetiology 85
   comorbidity 85
   epidemiology 84
   prevalence of 84
   psychosocial treatment 164
Succinylcholine 157
Sudden contraction 21
Suggestibility, high degree of 113
Suicidal behaviour 112
Suicidal intent 30
   signs of 47

Suicidal thoughts 30, 71
Suicide 15, 47
   decriminalisation of 170
   risk of 44
Sundowner syndrome 101
Sundowning 98
Superego 152
Supportive psychotherapy 56
Suppression 154
Suprachiasmatic nucleus 127
Symbolic representation 151
Sympathy 2
Synesthesia 6, 92
Synthetic cannabinoids 95
Systematic desensitisation 55, 163
Systemic lupus erythematosus 77

T

Tachycardia 93
Talkativeness, increased 41
Tangentiality 7
Tardive dyskinesia 22
Tau protein, intraneuronal aggregates of 102
Teeth, loss of 119*f*
Temperament 109
Tension and arousal, increasing 64
Test judgment 9
Testamentary capacity 168
Testosterone 131
Tetrabenazine 22, 106
Tetrahydrocannabinol 92
Thalidomide 142
Thanatophobia 54
Thiamine deficiency 88, 107
Thinking
   and speech, oddities of 111
   disorders of continuity of 6
   negative 30
   primary process 151
Thioridazine 21, 22
Thiothixene 21
Thioxanthenes 21
Thought 6
   alienation 8
   block 6
   broadcast 5, 8, 12
   disorders of 6
      content of 7
      form of 6
      possession of 8
      stream of 6
   flow of 6
   insertion 8, 12
   withdrawal 8, 12
Tic disorder 60, 143
Tobacco use disorder 29, 174
Token economy 164
Tolerance 83
Tombstone 103
Tongue, movements of 22

Topographical theory of mind, part of 151
   conscious 151
   preconscious 151
   unconscious 151
Torpor 97
Torticollis 21
Tourette's disorder 143
   course and prognosis 143
   diagnosis of 143
   management 143
Tourette's syndrome 140
Trance disorder 81
Transcranial direct current stimulation 158
Transcranial magnetic stimulation 35, 158
Transference 150
Transgender 132
Transient hallucinations 71
Transient psychotic disorders 25
Transsexuals 132
Transtheoretical model of change 89, 164
Transvestic disorder 137
Tranylcypromine 35
Traumatic bereavement 71
Traumatic brain injury 107
Trazodone 68
Tremor entrainment test 75
Tremulousness 87
Trichobezoar in trichotillomania 62*f*
Trichotillomania 62
   and excoriation disorder 58
Tricyclic antidepressant 36, 52, 61, 68, 146
Trifluoperazine 21
Trigger points 77
Tryptophan hydroxylase 48
Tuberoinfundibular tract 22
Tuberous sclerosis complex 2 141
Twilight state 97

U

Unconscious conflicts 152
Undoing 153
Universal sleep hygiene 124
Unshakeable belief 7
Urban areas 17
Uremic encephalopathy 99
Urophilia 137
Use disorder 84

V

Vacuum pump 134
Vagal nerve stimulation 35
Vaginismus 136
Vaginoplasty 132
Vagus nerve stimulation 158
Valbenazine 22
Valence systems
   negative 10
   positive 10

Valproate 47, 68, 112
    use in pregnancy 47
Valproic acid 142
Van Gogh syndrome 19
Varenicline 95, 95
Vascular dementia 105
    diagnosis of 105
    treatment of 105
Vasovagal response 54
Velocardiofacial syndrome 16
Venlafaxine 57
Ventral tegmental 21
Ventromedial prefrontal cortex 32
Veraguth fold 30, 30f
Verbal declarative memory 15
Video-gaming 96
Vilazodone 37
Vindictive 144
Vineland
    adaptive behaviour scale 148
    social maturity scale 148
Violence 15
Vision loss 98
Visual disturbances 26

Visual hallucinations 82
Visuospatial
    ability disturbances 98
    skills deficits 100
Vitamin B12 107
Vocal tic disorder 144
Vocal tics 143
    simple 143
Voices
    giving running commentary 13
    heard arguing 13
Volatile solvents 95
Volition, passivity of 12
Vorbeigehen 82
Voyeuristic disorders 137

W

Wakefulness test, maintenance of 125
Waxy flexibility 14
Weak leg 75
Weight
    and appetite changes 29
    gain, stopping 119
Wernicke's encephalopathy 87, 99

Wernicke–Korsakoff syndrome 87, 89
Widmark formula 88
Wish fulfilment 151
Withdrawal symptoms 83, 91, 92
Word approximations 7
Word association technique 166

X

Xenophobia 54

Y

Yawning 91
Young mania rating scale 44

Z

Z track technique 24
Zaleplon 124
Ziprasidone 22
Zolpidem 104, 124
Zoophilia 137
Zotepine 23
Zuclopenthixol 24

EU GSPR Authorised Reprsentative
Logos Europe, 9 rue Nicolas Poussin
1700, La Rochelle, France
Phone: +33 (0) 6 67 93 73 78
E-mail: contact@logoseurope.eu

www.ingramcontent.com/pod-product-compliance
Ingram Content Group UK Ltd.
Pitfield, Milton Keynes, MK11 3LW, UK
UKHW050431150426
5217IPUK00019B/1334